# Principles of Basic Trauma Nursing

## First Edition

By
**Brita M. O'Carroll, RN, BS, MEd, CPUR**

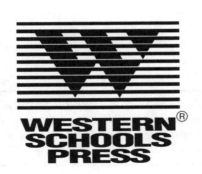

WESTERN®
SCHOOLS
PRESS

21 Bristol Drive
South Easton, MA 02375
1-800-618-1670

## ABOUT THE AUTHOR

**Brita M. O'Carroll, RN, BS, MEd, CPUR,** was educated at Duke University, Columbia University, New York University and the University of North Florida. She has experience in clinical nursing, health information management, as an educator, a regional director for emergency medical services, international research and is a published freelance writer. Ms. O'Carroll has made presentations at national and international conferences and is a Fellow in the Royal Society for the Promotion of Health and the International Council on Alcohol and Addictions.

## ABOUT THE SUBJECT MATTER EXPERT

**Ann L. West, MSN, RN, CNS, CEN,** is a cardiothoracic surgery policy, procedure, and education special-ist for a hospital in northwest Ohio. She is a past president of the Emergency Nurses Association-Ohio State Council. Ms. West has been the staff educator at the Medical College of Ohio and was the trauma nurse coordi-nator and then the pulmonary/critical care clinical nurse specialist. She has been an emergency nurse and edu-cator for 20 years. Ms. West served on the Ohio State Trauma Coalition for two years and is a state, local, and national writer and speaker on trauma and pulmonary topics.

**Copy Editor:** Michelle Gyure

**Typesetter:** Kathy Johnson

**Indexer:** Sylvia Coates

Western Schools' courses are designed to provide nursing professionals with the educational information they need to enhance their career development. The information provided within these course materials is the result of research and consultation with prominent nursing and medical authorities and is, to the best of our knowledge, current and accurate. However, the courses and course materials are provided with the understanding that Western Schools is not engaged in offering legal, nursing, medical, or other professional advice.

Western Schools' courses and course materials are not meant to act as a substitute for seeking out professional advice or conducting individual research. When the information provided in the courses and course materials is applied to individual circumstances, all recommendations must be considered in light of the uniqueness pertaining to each situation.

Western Schools' course materials are intended solely for *your* use and *not* for the benefit of providing advice or recommenda-tions to third parties. Western Schools devoids itself of any responsibility for adverse consequences resulting from the failure to seek nursing, medical, or other professional advice. Western Schools further devoids itself of any responsibility for updating or revising any programs or publications presented, published, distributed, or sponsored by Western Schools unless otherwise agreed to as part of an individual purchase contract.

**ISBN:** 1-57801-044-6

# IMPORTANT: Read these instructions *BEFORE* proceeding!

Enclosed with your course book you will find the FasTrax® answer sheet. Use this form to answer all the final exam questions that appear in this course book. If you are completing more than one course, be sure to write your answers on the appropriate answer sheet. Full instructions and complete grading details are printed on the FasTrax instruction sheet, also enclosed with your order. Please review them before starting. *If you are mailing your answer sheet(s) to Western Schools, we recommend you make a copy as a backup.*

## ABOUT THIS COURSE

A "Pretest" is provided with each course to test your current knowledge base regarding the subject matter contained within this course. Your "Final Exam" is a multiple choice examination. **You will find the exam questions at the end of each chapter.** Some smaller hour courses include the exam at the end of the book.

In the event the course has less than 100 questions, mark your answers to the questions in the course book and leave the remaining answer boxes on the FasTrax answer sheet blank. **Use a <u>black pen</u> to fill in your answer sheet.**

## A PASSING SCORE

You must score 70% or better in order to pass this course and receive your Certificate of Completion. Should you fail to achieve the required score, we will send you an additional FasTrax answer sheet so that you may make a second attempt to pass the course. Western Schools will allow you three chances to pass the same course...*at no extra charge!* After three failed attempts to pass the same course, your file will be closed.

## RECORDING YOUR HOURS

Please monitor the time it takes to complete this course using the handy log sheet on the other side of this page. See below for transferring study hours to the course evaluation.

## COURSE EVALUATIONS

In this course book you will find a short evaluation about the course you are soon to complete. This information is vital to providing the school with feedback on this course. The course evaluation answer section is in the lower right hand corner of the FasTrax answer sheet marked "Evaluation" with answers marked 1–25. Your answers are important to us, please take five minutes to complete the evaluation.

On the back of the FasTrax instruction sheet there is additional space to make any comments about the course, the school, and suggested new curriculum. Please mail the FasTrax instruction sheet, with your comments, back to Western Schools in the envelope provided with your course order.

## TRANSFERRING STUDY TIME

Upon completion of the course, transfer the total study time from your log sheet to question #25 in the Course Evaluation. The answers will be in ranges, please choose the proper hour range that best represents your study time. You MUST log your study time under question #25 on the course evaluation.

## EXTENSIONS

You have 2 years from the date of enrollment to complete this course. A six (6) month extension may be purchased. If after 30 months from the original enrollment date you do not complete the course, *your file will be closed and no certificate can be issued.*

## CHANGE OF ADDRESS?

In the event you have moved during the completion of this course please call our student services department at 1-800-618-1670 and we will update your file.

## A GUARANTEE YOU'LL GIVE HIGH HONORS TO

If any continuing education course fails to meet your expectations or if you are not satisfied in any manner, for any reason, you may return it for an exchange or a refund (less shipping and handling) within 30 days. Software, video and audio courses must be returned unopened.

*Thank you for enrolling at Western Schools!*

WESTERN SCHOOLS
P.O. Box 1930
Brockton, MA 02303
(800) 618-1670

# Principles of Basic Trauma Nursing

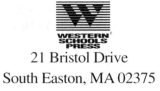

WESTERN®
SCHOOLS
PRESS

21 Bristol Drive
South Easton, MA 02375

Please use this log to total the number of hours you spend reading the text and taking the final examination (use 50-min hours).

| Date | Hours Spent |
|------|-------------|
| _____ | _____ |
| _____ | _____ |
| _____ | _____ |
| _____ | _____ |
| _____ | _____ |
| _____ | _____ |
| _____ | _____ |
| _____ | _____ |
| _____ | _____ |
| _____ | _____ |
| _____ | _____ |
| _____ | _____ |
| _____ | _____ |

**TOTAL** [          ]

**Please log your study hours with submission of your final exam. To log your study time, fill in the appropriate circle under question 25 of the FasTrax® answer sheet under the "Evaluation" section.**

Please choose the answer that represents the total study hours it took you to complete this 30 hour course.

    A. less than 25 hours          C. 29–32 hours

    B. 25–28 hours               D. greater than 32 hours

# Principles of Basic Trauma Nursing

## WESTERN SCHOOLS' NURSING
## CONTINUING EDUCATION EVALUATION

Instructions: Mark your answers to the following questions with a black pen on the "Evaluation" section of your FasTrax® answer sheet provided with this course. You should not return this sheet. Please use the scale below to rate the following statements:

A   Agree Strongly                    C   Disagree Somewhat
B   Agree Somewhat                     D   Disagree Strongly

The course content met the following education objectives:

1. Describes the basic concepts of trauma nursing and the emergency medical system.
2. Identifies the basics of trauma nursing including assessment and triage.
3. Identifies appropriate airway management techniques in the trauma patient.
4. Describes the principles of managing shock and cardiac arrest.
5. Describes the principles of the proper management of head injuries.
6. Recognizes the causes and management of maxillofacial and neck trauma.
7. Identifies appropriate strategies for the recognition and management of eye trauma.
8. Describes the proper procedures for managing spinal injuries.
9. Indicates the major nursing strategies for managing thoracic trauma.
10. Describes the key components of managing abdominal trauma.
11. Recognizes the various types of genitourinary trauma and appropriate treatment strategies.
12. Describes the principles of treating gynecologic and obstetric trauma.
13. Identifies the proper procedures for managing orthopedic and neuromuscular trauma.
14. Describes the concepts important in the management of burn injuries.
15. Identifies the important strategies in the management of pediatric patients suffering traumatic injuries.
16. Recognizes the signs and symptoms of elder trauma, abuse and neglect.
17. Identifies the psychosocial issues affecting patients who have experienced a traumatic injury.
18. Describes the process of organ donation and tissue transplantation.
19. The content of this course was relevant to the objectives.
20. This offering met my professional education needs.
21. The objectives met the overall purpose/goal of the course.
22. The content of this course was appropriate for home study.
23. The course was generally well written and the subject matter explained thoroughly. (If no, please explain on the back of the FasTrax instruction sheet.)

24. The final examination was well written and at an appropriate level for the content of the course.

25. **PLEASE LOG YOUR STUDY HOURS WITH SUBMISSION OF YOUR FINAL EXAM.** Please choose which best represents the total study hours it took to complete this 30 hour course.

   A. less than 25 hours

   B. 25–28 hours

   C. 29–32 hours

   D. greater than 32 hours

# CONTENTS

**Evaluation** ......................................................................v

**Pretest** .......................................................................xix

**Introduction** ...............................................................xxiii

***Chapter 1* About Trauma** ...................................................1

    Introduction .................................................................1

    Trauma Defined ...............................................................1

    Epidemiology .................................................................2

    Injuries Associated with Trauma ..............................................2

        Motor Vehicle Crashes ..................................................2

        Falls ...................................................................3

        Intentional Trauma .....................................................3

        Rape ...................................................................4

        Firearms ...............................................................4

        Burns ..................................................................4

        Recreational Activities ..................................................4

        Drowning and Near Drowning .............................................4

    Means of Impact Trauma ......................................................5

        Types of Injuries .......................................................5

        Means of Impact ........................................................5

    Levels of Trauma Care ........................................................5

        Prehospital Care .......................................................6

        Acute Hospital Care ....................................................6

        Long-Term Care and Rehabilitation .......................................7

        Classification of Trauma Centers .........................................7

    Summary .....................................................................8

    Exam Questions ..............................................................9

***Chapter 2* Basics of Trauma Nursing** ......................................11

    Introduction ................................................................11

    The Trauma Nursing Process .................................................12

    Patient Assessment ..........................................................12

        Primary Assessment ....................................................13

        Secondary (General or Routine) Assessment ..............................14

    Major Body Areas ...........................................................15

        Head ..................................................................15

        Neck ..................................................................16

Chest . . . . . . . . . . . . . . . . . . . . . . . . . . . . . . . . . . . . . . . . . . . . . . . . . . . . . . . . . . .16

Abdomen . . . . . . . . . . . . . . . . . . . . . . . . . . . . . . . . . . . . . . . . . . . . . . . . . . . . . . .16

Extremities . . . . . . . . . . . . . . . . . . . . . . . . . . . . . . . . . . . . . . . . . . . . . . . . . . . . . .16

Triage . . . . . . . . . . . . . . . . . . . . . . . . . . . . . . . . . . . . . . . . . . . . . . . . . . . . . . . . . . . . . . .16

Urgency . . . . . . . . . . . . . . . . . . . . . . . . . . . . . . . . . . . . . . . . . . . . . . . . . . . . . . . .19

Triage Nursing . . . . . . . . . . . . . . . . . . . . . . . . . . . . . . . . . . . . . . . . . . . . . . . . . . .19

Summary . . . . . . . . . . . . . . . . . . . . . . . . . . . . . . . . . . . . . . . . . . . . . . . . . . . . . . . . . . . . .19

Exam Questions . . . . . . . . . . . . . . . . . . . . . . . . . . . . . . . . . . . . . . . . . . . . . . . . . . . . . . .21

*Chapter 3* **Airway Management** . . . . . . . . . . . . . . . . . . . . . . . . . . . . . . . . . . . . . . . . .**23**

Introduction . . . . . . . . . . . . . . . . . . . . . . . . . . . . . . . . . . . . . . . . . . . . . . . . . . . . . . . . . .23

Basic Anatomy and Physiology of the Airway . . . . . . . . . . . . . . . . . . . . . . . . . . . . . . . .24

Upper Airways . . . . . . . . . . . . . . . . . . . . . . . . . . . . . . . . . . . . . . . . . . . . . . . . . . . .24

Lower Airways . . . . . . . . . . . . . . . . . . . . . . . . . . . . . . . . . . . . . . . . . . . . . . . . . . . .25

Pediatrics . . . . . . . . . . . . . . . . . . . . . . . . . . . . . . . . . . . . . . . . . . . . . . . . . . . . . . . .25

Injury and Obstruction . . . . . . . . . . . . . . . . . . . . . . . . . . . . . . . . . . . . . . . . . . . . . . . . . .26

Assessment . . . . . . . . . . . . . . . . . . . . . . . . . . . . . . . . . . . . . . . . . . . . . . . . . . . . . . . . . . .26

Look . . . . . . . . . . . . . . . . . . . . . . . . . . . . . . . . . . . . . . . . . . . . . . . . . . . . . . . . . . . .26

Listen . . . . . . . . . . . . . . . . . . . . . . . . . . . . . . . . . . . . . . . . . . . . . . . . . . . . . . . . . . .26

Feel . . . . . . . . . . . . . . . . . . . . . . . . . . . . . . . . . . . . . . . . . . . . . . . . . . . . . . . . . . . .27

Airway Management and Stabilization . . . . . . . . . . . . . . . . . . . . . . . . . . . . . . . . . . . . . .27

Basic Management Techniques . . . . . . . . . . . . . . . . . . . . . . . . . . . . . . . . . . . . . . . .27

Mechanical Methods for Airway Control (Airway Adjuncts) . . . . . . . . . . . . . . . . . . .29

Nursing Strategies . . . . . . . . . . . . . . . . . . . . . . . . . . . . . . . . . . . . . . . . . . . . . . . . . . . . .30

Summary . . . . . . . . . . . . . . . . . . . . . . . . . . . . . . . . . . . . . . . . . . . . . . . . . . . . . . . . . . . . .30

Exam Questions . . . . . . . . . . . . . . . . . . . . . . . . . . . . . . . . . . . . . . . . . . . . . . . . . . . . . . .31

*Chapter 4* **Shock and Cardiac Arrest** . . . . . . . . . . . . . . . . . . . . . . . . . . . . . . . . . . . . . .**33**

Introduction . . . . . . . . . . . . . . . . . . . . . . . . . . . . . . . . . . . . . . . . . . . . . . . . . . . . . . . . . .33

Shock . . . . . . . . . . . . . . . . . . . . . . . . . . . . . . . . . . . . . . . . . . . . . . . . . . . . . . . . . . . . . . . .33

Physiology . . . . . . . . . . . . . . . . . . . . . . . . . . . . . . . . . . . . . . . . . . . . . . . . . . . . . . . .34

Recognizing Shock . . . . . . . . . . . . . . . . . . . . . . . . . . . . . . . . . . . . . . . . . . . . . . . . .34

Types, Assessment, and Management of Shock . . . . . . . . . . . . . . . . . . . . . . . . . . . . . . .36

Hypovolemic (Low Volume) Shock . . . . . . . . . . . . . . . . . . . . . . . . . . . . . . . . . . . . .36

Cardiogenic (Low Output) Shock . . . . . . . . . . . . . . . . . . . . . . . . . . . . . . . . . . . . . .38

Distributive or Vasogenic Shock . . . . . . . . . . . . . . . . . . . . . . . . . . . . . . . . . . . . . . .39

(Flow) Obstruction Shock . . . . . . . . . . . . . . . . . . . . . . . . . . . . . . . . . . . . . . . . . . . .41

Other Types of Shock . . . . . . . . . . . . . . . . . . . . . . . . . . . . . . . . . . . . . . . . . . . . . . .41

Nursing Strategies for the Patient in Shock . . . . . . . . . . . . . . . . . . . . . . . . . . . . . . . . . .42

Examples of Nursing Diagnoses Related to Shock . . . . . . . . . . . . . . . . . . . . . . . . . . . . .43

Basic Cardiovascular Anatomy and Physiology . . . . . . . . . . . . . . . . . . . . . . . . . . . . . . .43

Heart . . . . . . . . . . . . . . . . . . . . . . . . . . . . . . . . . . . . . . . . . . . . . . . . . . . . . . . . . . . .43

Vessels . . . . . . . . . . . . . . . . . . . . . . . . . . . . . . . . . . . . . . . . . . . . . . .44

Lungs . . . . . . . . . . . . . . . . . . . . . . . . . . . . . . . . . . . . . . . . . . . . . . . .45

Blood . . . . . . . . . . . . . . . . . . . . . . . . . . . . . . . . . . . . . . . . . . . . . . . .45

Injury, the Heart and Cardiac Arrest . . . . . . . . . . . . . . . . . . . . . . . . . . . . .46

Considerations Regarding Resuscitation . . . . . . . . . . . . . . . . . . . . . . . . . .46

Summary . . . . . . . . . . . . . . . . . . . . . . . . . . . . . . . . . . . . . . . . . . . . . . . .47

Exam Questions . . . . . . . . . . . . . . . . . . . . . . . . . . . . . . . . . . . . . . . . . . .49

*Chapter 5* **Head Injury** . . . . . . . . . . . . . . . . . . . . . . . . . . . . . . . . . . . . . **.51**

Introduction . . . . . . . . . . . . . . . . . . . . . . . . . . . . . . . . . . . . . . . . . . . . . .51

Anatomy and Physiology . . . . . . . . . . . . . . . . . . . . . . . . . . . . . . . . . . . . .52

Scalp . . . . . . . . . . . . . . . . . . . . . . . . . . . . . . . . . . . . . . . . . . . . . . . .52

Skull . . . . . . . . . . . . . . . . . . . . . . . . . . . . . . . . . . . . . . . . . . . . . . . .52

Meninges . . . . . . . . . . . . . . . . . . . . . . . . . . . . . . . . . . . . . . . . . . . . .52

Brain . . . . . . . . . . . . . . . . . . . . . . . . . . . . . . . . . . . . . . . . . . . . . . . .53

Cranial Nerves . . . . . . . . . . . . . . . . . . . . . . . . . . . . . . . . . . . . . . . . .53

Pediatric Differences . . . . . . . . . . . . . . . . . . . . . . . . . . . . . . . . . . . . .53

Conditions of Head Injuries . . . . . . . . . . . . . . . . . . . . . . . . . . . . . . . . . . .54

Pathophysiology . . . . . . . . . . . . . . . . . . . . . . . . . . . . . . . . . . . . . . . .54

Specific Head Injuries . . . . . . . . . . . . . . . . . . . . . . . . . . . . . . . . . . . .54

Focal Injuries . . . . . . . . . . . . . . . . . . . . . . . . . . . . . . . . . . . . . . . . . . . . .55

Scalp Laceration . . . . . . . . . . . . . . . . . . . . . . . . . . . . . . . . . . . . . . . .55

Skull Fracture . . . . . . . . . . . . . . . . . . . . . . . . . . . . . . . . . . . . . . . . . .55

Contusion . . . . . . . . . . . . . . . . . . . . . . . . . . . . . . . . . . . . . . . . . . . . .55

Epidural Hematoma . . . . . . . . . . . . . . . . . . . . . . . . . . . . . . . . . . . . . .55

Subdural Hematoma . . . . . . . . . . . . . . . . . . . . . . . . . . . . . . . . . . . . . .56

Other Focal Injuries . . . . . . . . . . . . . . . . . . . . . . . . . . . . . . . . . . . . . .56

Diffuse Injuries . . . . . . . . . . . . . . . . . . . . . . . . . . . . . . . . . . . . . . . . . . . .56

Concussion . . . . . . . . . . . . . . . . . . . . . . . . . . . . . . . . . . . . . . . . . . . .57

Diffuse Axonal Injury (DAI) . . . . . . . . . . . . . . . . . . . . . . . . . . . . . . . .57

Patient Assessment . . . . . . . . . . . . . . . . . . . . . . . . . . . . . . . . . . . . . . . . .57

Nursing Strategies for the Head Injury Patient . . . . . . . . . . . . . . . . . . . . . .58

Examples of Nursing Diagnoses Related to Head Injury . . . . . . . . . . . . . . . .59

Summary . . . . . . . . . . . . . . . . . . . . . . . . . . . . . . . . . . . . . . . . . . . . . . . .59

Exam Questions . . . . . . . . . . . . . . . . . . . . . . . . . . . . . . . . . . . . . . . . . . .61

*Chapter 6* **Maxillofacial and Neck Trauma** . . . . . . . . . . . . . . . . . . . . . . . . **.63**

Introduction . . . . . . . . . . . . . . . . . . . . . . . . . . . . . . . . . . . . . . . . . . . . . .63

Anatomy and Physiology . . . . . . . . . . . . . . . . . . . . . . . . . . . . . . . . . . . . .63

Facial Structures . . . . . . . . . . . . . . . . . . . . . . . . . . . . . . . . . . . . . . . .63

Cranial Nerves . . . . . . . . . . . . . . . . . . . . . . . . . . . . . . . . . . . . . . . . . .64

Upper Airway . . . . . . . . . . . . . . . . . . . . . . . . . . . . . . . . . . . . . . . . . .64

Major Vessels . . . . . . . . . . . . . . . . . . . . . . . . . . . . . . . . . . . . . . . . . . . . . . . . . .65

Mechanism of Injury . . . . . . . . . . . . . . . . . . . . . . . . . . . . . . . . . . . . . . . . . . . . . . . .65

Maxillofacial and Neck Injuries . . . . . . . . . . . . . . . . . . . . . . . . . . . . . . . . . . . . . . . . .66

Soft-Tissue Trauma . . . . . . . . . . . . . . . . . . . . . . . . . . . . . . . . . . . . . . . . . . . . .66

Major Vessel Injury . . . . . . . . . . . . . . . . . . . . . . . . . . . . . . . . . . . . . . . . . . . . .67

Fracture . . . . . . . . . . . . . . . . . . . . . . . . . . . . . . . . . . . . . . . . . . . . . . . . . . . . . .67

Assessment . . . . . . . . . . . . . . . . . . . . . . . . . . . . . . . . . . . . . . . . . . . . . . . . . . . . . . . .69

Primary Assessment . . . . . . . . . . . . . . . . . . . . . . . . . . . . . . . . . . . . . . . . . . . . .69

Secondary Assessment . . . . . . . . . . . . . . . . . . . . . . . . . . . . . . . . . . . . . . . . . . .69

Nursing Strategies for the Maxillofacial and Neck Trauma Patient . . . . . . . . . . . . . . .70

Examples of Nursing Diagnoses Related to Maxillofacial and Neck Injuries . . . . . . . . .72

Summary . . . . . . . . . . . . . . . . . . . . . . . . . . . . . . . . . . . . . . . . . . . . . . . . . . . . . . . . . .72

Exam Questions . . . . . . . . . . . . . . . . . . . . . . . . . . . . . . . . . . . . . . . . . . . . . . . . . . . . .73

**Chapter 7  Ocular Trauma** . . . . . . . . . . . . . . . . . . . . . . . . . . . . . . . . . . . . . . . . . . . . .**75**

Introduction . . . . . . . . . . . . . . . . . . . . . . . . . . . . . . . . . . . . . . . . . . . . . . . . . . . . . . . .75

Anatomy and Physiology . . . . . . . . . . . . . . . . . . . . . . . . . . . . . . . . . . . . . . . . . . . . . . .75

Mechanism of Injury . . . . . . . . . . . . . . . . . . . . . . . . . . . . . . . . . . . . . . . . . . . . . . . . . .77

Ocular Injuries and Interventions . . . . . . . . . . . . . . . . . . . . . . . . . . . . . . . . . . . . . . . .77

Periorbital Injury . . . . . . . . . . . . . . . . . . . . . . . . . . . . . . . . . . . . . . . . . . . . . . . .77

Foreign Body . . . . . . . . . . . . . . . . . . . . . . . . . . . . . . . . . . . . . . . . . . . . . . . . . . .77

Contusion . . . . . . . . . . . . . . . . . . . . . . . . . . . . . . . . . . . . . . . . . . . . . . . . . . . . .78

Corneal Abrasion . . . . . . . . . . . . . . . . . . . . . . . . . . . . . . . . . . . . . . . . . . . . . . . .78

Corneal Laceration . . . . . . . . . . . . . . . . . . . . . . . . . . . . . . . . . . . . . . . . . . . . . . .78

Conjunctival Laceration . . . . . . . . . . . . . . . . . . . . . . . . . . . . . . . . . . . . . . . . . . .79

Subconjunctival Hemorrhage . . . . . . . . . . . . . . . . . . . . . . . . . . . . . . . . . . . . . . .79

Avulsion . . . . . . . . . . . . . . . . . . . . . . . . . . . . . . . . . . . . . . . . . . . . . . . . . . . . . .79

Hyphema . . . . . . . . . . . . . . . . . . . . . . . . . . . . . . . . . . . . . . . . . . . . . . . . . . . . . .79

Iris Injury . . . . . . . . . . . . . . . . . . . . . . . . . . . . . . . . . . . . . . . . . . . . . . . . . . . . .80

Lens Injury . . . . . . . . . . . . . . . . . . . . . . . . . . . . . . . . . . . . . . . . . . . . . . . . . . . .80

Retinal Detachment . . . . . . . . . . . . . . . . . . . . . . . . . . . . . . . . . . . . . . . . . . . . . .80

Burn Injury . . . . . . . . . . . . . . . . . . . . . . . . . . . . . . . . . . . . . . . . . . . . . . . . . . . .80

Perforation or Rupture of the Globe . . . . . . . . . . . . . . . . . . . . . . . . . . . . . . . . . .81

Orbital Fracture . . . . . . . . . . . . . . . . . . . . . . . . . . . . . . . . . . . . . . . . . . . . . . . . .82

Contact Lenses And Prostheses . . . . . . . . . . . . . . . . . . . . . . . . . . . . . . . . . . . . .82

Assessment . . . . . . . . . . . . . . . . . . . . . . . . . . . . . . . . . . . . . . . . . . . . . . . . . . . . . . . . .83

Nursing Strategies for the Patient with Ocular Trauma . . . . . . . . . . . . . . . . . . . . . . . .84

Examples of Nursing Diagnoses Related to Ocular Trauma . . . . . . . . . . . . . . . . . . . . .85

Summary . . . . . . . . . . . . . . . . . . . . . . . . . . . . . . . . . . . . . . . . . . . . . . . . . . . . . . . . . .85

Exam Questions . . . . . . . . . . . . . . . . . . . . . . . . . . . . . . . . . . . . . . . . . . . . . . . . . . . . .87

*Chapter 8* **Trauma to the Spine** . . . . . . . . . . . . . . . . . . . . . . . . . . . . . . . . . . . . . . . . . . . . . . . . . . . **.89**

Introduction . . . . . . . . . . . . . . . . . . . . . . . . . . . . . . . . . . . . . . . . . . . . . . . . .89

Anatomy and Physiology . . . . . . . . . . . . . . . . . . . . . . . . . . . . . . . . . . . . . . .90

    Overview . . . . . . . . . . . . . . . . . . . . . . . . . . . . . . . . . . . . . . . . . . . . . . .90

The Spinal Cord . . . . . . . . . . . . . . . . . . . . . . . . . . . . . . . . . . . . . . . . . . . . . .92

Mechanism of Injury . . . . . . . . . . . . . . . . . . . . . . . . . . . . . . . . . . . . . . . . . .92

Spinal Cord and Spinal Column Injuries . . . . . . . . . . . . . . . . . . . . . . . . . . . .95

    Spinal Shock . . . . . . . . . . . . . . . . . . . . . . . . . . . . . . . . . . . . . . . . . . . .95

    Autonomic Dysreflexia . . . . . . . . . . . . . . . . . . . . . . . . . . . . . . . . . . . . .95

    Cervical Injury . . . . . . . . . . . . . . . . . . . . . . . . . . . . . . . . . . . . . . . . . .96

    Thoracic Injury . . . . . . . . . . . . . . . . . . . . . . . . . . . . . . . . . . . . . . . . .96

    Lumbar Injury . . . . . . . . . . . . . . . . . . . . . . . . . . . . . . . . . . . . . . . . . .96

    Incomplete Spinal Cord Injury . . . . . . . . . . . . . . . . . . . . . . . . . . . . . . .96

    Penetrating Injury . . . . . . . . . . . . . . . . . . . . . . . . . . . . . . . . . . . . . . .96

    Impalement . . . . . . . . . . . . . . . . . . . . . . . . . . . . . . . . . . . . . . . . . . . .96

    Injury Without Radiographic Abnormality . . . . . . . . . . . . . . . . . . . . . . .97

Assessment . . . . . . . . . . . . . . . . . . . . . . . . . . . . . . . . . . . . . . . . . . . . . . . . .97

    Signs (Observable Physical Findings) . . . . . . . . . . . . . . . . . . . . . . . . . .97

    Inspection . . . . . . . . . . . . . . . . . . . . . . . . . . . . . . . . . . . . . . . . . . . . .98

    Palpation . . . . . . . . . . . . . . . . . . . . . . . . . . . . . . . . . . . . . . . . . . . . . .98

    Symptoms (Patient Complaints) . . . . . . . . . . . . . . . . . . . . . . . . . . . . . .98

    History . . . . . . . . . . . . . . . . . . . . . . . . . . . . . . . . . . . . . . . . . . . . . . .99

Nursing Strategies for the Patient with Spinal Cord and Column Injuries . . . . . . . . . . . . . . . . . . . . . . . . . .99

    Stabilization . . . . . . . . . . . . . . . . . . . . . . . . . . . . . . . . . . . . . . . . . . .99

    Immobilization . . . . . . . . . . . . . . . . . . . . . . . . . . . . . . . . . . . . . . . .100

    Circulation . . . . . . . . . . . . . . . . . . . . . . . . . . . . . . . . . . . . . . . . . . .100

    Full Evaluation/Other Measures . . . . . . . . . . . . . . . . . . . . . . . . . . . .100

    Pharmacological Management . . . . . . . . . . . . . . . . . . . . . . . . . . . . . .101

Examples of Nursing Diagnoses Related to Spinal Cord and Spinal Column Trauma . . . . . . . . . . . . . .101

Summary . . . . . . . . . . . . . . . . . . . . . . . . . . . . . . . . . . . . . . . . . . . . . . . . .101

Exam Questions . . . . . . . . . . . . . . . . . . . . . . . . . . . . . . . . . . . . . . . . . . . . .103

*Chapter 9* **Thoracic Trauma** . . . . . . . . . . . . . . . . . . . . . . . . . . . . . . . . . . . . . . . . . . . . . . . . . . . . . **.105**

Introduction . . . . . . . . . . . . . . . . . . . . . . . . . . . . . . . . . . . . . . . . . . . . . . .105

Anatomy and Physiology . . . . . . . . . . . . . . . . . . . . . . . . . . . . . . . . . . . . . .106

    Pulmonary System . . . . . . . . . . . . . . . . . . . . . . . . . . . . . . . . . . . . . .106

    Cardiovascular System . . . . . . . . . . . . . . . . . . . . . . . . . . . . . . . . . . .108

Mechanism of Injury . . . . . . . . . . . . . . . . . . . . . . . . . . . . . . . . . . . . . . . . .108

    Blunt Trauma . . . . . . . . . . . . . . . . . . . . . . . . . . . . . . . . . . . . . . . . .108

    Penetrating Object . . . . . . . . . . . . . . . . . . . . . . . . . . . . . . . . . . . . . .109

    Compression . . . . . . . . . . . . . . . . . . . . . . . . . . . . . . . . . . . . . . . . . .109

Injury to the Back of the Chest . . . . . . . . . . . . . . . . . . . . . . . . . . . . . . . . . . . . . . . . .109

Categories of Chest Trauma . . . . . . . . . . . . . . . . . . . . . . . . . . . . . . . . . . . . . . . . . . .109

Thoracic Injuries and Interventions . . . . . . . . . . . . . . . . . . . . . . . . . . . . . . . . . . . . . . . . .109

Chest Wall Injury . . . . . . . . . . . . . . . . . . . . . . . . . . . . . . . . . . . . . . . . . . . . . . . . . . . .109

Pulmonary Injury . . . . . . . . . . . . . . . . . . . . . . . . . . . . . . . . . . . . . . . . . . . . . . . . . . . .111

Cardiac and Great Vessel Injuries . . . . . . . . . . . . . . . . . . . . . . . . . . . . . . . . . . . . . .113

Complications of Chest Injury . . . . . . . . . . . . . . . . . . . . . . . . . . . . . . . . . . . . . . . . . . . . . .114

Subcutaneous Emphysema . . . . . . . . . . . . . . . . . . . . . . . . . . . . . . . . . . . . . . . . . . . .114

Pneumothorax . . . . . . . . . . . . . . . . . . . . . . . . . . . . . . . . . . . . . . . . . . . . . . . . . . . . . .114

Tension Pneumothorax . . . . . . . . . . . . . . . . . . . . . . . . . . . . . . . . . . . . . . . . . . . . . . .114

Open Pneumothorax/Sucking Chest Wound . . . . . . . . . . . . . . . . . . . . . . . . . . . . . .115

Hemothorax . . . . . . . . . . . . . . . . . . . . . . . . . . . . . . . . . . . . . . . . . . . . . . . . . . . . . . . .115

Traumatic Asphyxia . . . . . . . . . . . . . . . . . . . . . . . . . . . . . . . . . . . . . . . . . . . . . . . . . .116

Cardiac Tamponade . . . . . . . . . . . . . . . . . . . . . . . . . . . . . . . . . . . . . . . . . . . . . . . . . .116

Assessment . . . . . . . . . . . . . . . . . . . . . . . . . . . . . . . . . . . . . . . . . . . . . . . . . . . . . . . . . . . .117

Signs and Symptoms . . . . . . . . . . . . . . . . . . . . . . . . . . . . . . . . . . . . . . . . . . . . . . . . .117

Nursing Strategies for the Patient with Thoracic Injury . . . . . . . . . . . . . . . . . . . . . . . . .118

Examples of Nursing Diagnoses Related to Patients with Thoracic Trauma . . . . . . . . . . .120

Summary . . . . . . . . . . . . . . . . . . . . . . . . . . . . . . . . . . . . . . . . . . . . . . . . . . . . . . . . . . . . .120

Exam Questions . . . . . . . . . . . . . . . . . . . . . . . . . . . . . . . . . . . . . . . . . . . . . . . . . . . . . . . .121

*Chapter 10* **Abdominal Trauma** . . . . . . . . . . . . . . . . . . . . . . . . . . . . . . . . . . . . . . . . . . . .**123**

Introduction . . . . . . . . . . . . . . . . . . . . . . . . . . . . . . . . . . . . . . . . . . . . . . . . . . . . . . . . . . .123

Anatomy and Physiology . . . . . . . . . . . . . . . . . . . . . . . . . . . . . . . . . . . . . . . . . . . . . . . . .123

Organs . . . . . . . . . . . . . . . . . . . . . . . . . . . . . . . . . . . . . . . . . . . . . . . . . . . . . . . . . . . . . . .124

Peritoneal Space . . . . . . . . . . . . . . . . . . . . . . . . . . . . . . . . . . . . . . . . . . . . . . . . . . . .124

Retroperitoneal Space . . . . . . . . . . . . . . . . . . . . . . . . . . . . . . . . . . . . . . . . . . . . . . . .127

Mechanism of Injury . . . . . . . . . . . . . . . . . . . . . . . . . . . . . . . . . . . . . . . . . . . . . . . . . . . . .127

Closed/Blunt Injury . . . . . . . . . . . . . . . . . . . . . . . . . . . . . . . . . . . . . . . . . . . . . . . . . .127

Open/Penetrating Injury . . . . . . . . . . . . . . . . . . . . . . . . . . . . . . . . . . . . . . . . . . . . . .127

Abdominal Injuries and Interventions . . . . . . . . . . . . . . . . . . . . . . . . . . . . . . . . . . . . . . .128

Diaphragm . . . . . . . . . . . . . . . . . . . . . . . . . . . . . . . . . . . . . . . . . . . . . . . . . . . . . . . . .128

Stomach . . . . . . . . . . . . . . . . . . . . . . . . . . . . . . . . . . . . . . . . . . . . . . . . . . . . . . . . . . .128

Bowel . . . . . . . . . . . . . . . . . . . . . . . . . . . . . . . . . . . . . . . . . . . . . . . . . . . . . . . . . . . . .130

Liver . . . . . . . . . . . . . . . . . . . . . . . . . . . . . . . . . . . . . . . . . . . . . . . . . . . . . . . . . . . . . .130

Spleen . . . . . . . . . . . . . . . . . . . . . . . . . . . . . . . . . . . . . . . . . . . . . . . . . . . . . . . . . . . . .130

Pancreas . . . . . . . . . . . . . . . . . . . . . . . . . . . . . . . . . . . . . . . . . . . . . . . . . . . . . . . . . . .131

Pelvic Fracture . . . . . . . . . . . . . . . . . . . . . . . . . . . . . . . . . . . . . . . . . . . . . . . . . . . . . .131

Vascular Structures . . . . . . . . . . . . . . . . . . . . . . . . . . . . . . . . . . . . . . . . . . . . . . . . . .131

Foreign Body . . . . . . . . . . . . . . . . . . . . . . . . . . . . . . . . . . . . . . . . . . . . . . . . . . . . . . .132

Assessment . . . . . . . . . . . . . . . . . . . . . . . . . . . . . . . . . . . . . . . . . . . . . . . . . . . . . . . . . . . .132

Diagnostic Tests . . . . . . . . . . . . . . . . . . . . . . . . . . . . . . . . . . . . . . . . . . . . . . . . . . . . . . .132

Assessment Principles . . . . . . . . . . . . . . . . . . . . . . . . . . . . . . . . . . . . . . . . . . . . . . . . . .132

Signs and Symptoms . . . . . . . . . . . . . . . . . . . . . . . . . . . . . . . . . . . . . . . . . . . . . . . . . . .133

Nursing Strategies for the Patient with Abdominal Trauma . . . . . . . . . . . . . . . . . . . . . . . . . . . . .134

Examples of Nursing Diagnoses Related to Abdominal Injury . . . . . . . . . . . . . . . . . . . . . . . . . . .135

Summary . . . . . . . . . . . . . . . . . . . . . . . . . . . . . . . . . . . . . . . . . . . . . . . . . . . . . . . . . . . . . . . . . .135

Exam Questions . . . . . . . . . . . . . . . . . . . . . . . . . . . . . . . . . . . . . . . . . . . . . . . . . . . . . . . . . . . .137

*Chapter 11* **Genitourinary Trauma** . . . . . . . . . . . . . . . . . . . . . . . . . . . . . . . . . . . . . . .**139**

Introduction . . . . . . . . . . . . . . . . . . . . . . . . . . . . . . . . . . . . . . . . . . . . . . . . . . . . . . . . . . . . . .139

Anatomy and Physiology . . . . . . . . . . . . . . . . . . . . . . . . . . . . . . . . . . . . . . . . . . . . . . . . . . .140

Urinary System . . . . . . . . . . . . . . . . . . . . . . . . . . . . . . . . . . . . . . . . . . . . . . . . . . . . . .140

Genital/Reproductive System . . . . . . . . . . . . . . . . . . . . . . . . . . . . . . . . . . . . . . . . . .141

Mechanism of Injury . . . . . . . . . . . . . . . . . . . . . . . . . . . . . . . . . . . . . . . . . . . . . . . . . . . . . . .144

Genitourinary Injuries and Interventions . . . . . . . . . . . . . . . . . . . . . . . . . . . . . . . . . . . . . . .144

Urinary Injury . . . . . . . . . . . . . . . . . . . . . . . . . . . . . . . . . . . . . . . . . . . . . . . . . . . . . . .144

Genital Injury . . . . . . . . . . . . . . . . . . . . . . . . . . . . . . . . . . . . . . . . . . . . . . . . . . . . . . .148

Assessment . . . . . . . . . . . . . . . . . . . . . . . . . . . . . . . . . . . . . . . . . . . . . . . . . . . . . . . . . . . . . .150

Nursing Strategies for the Patient with Genitourinary Trauma . . . . . . . . . . . . . . . . . . . . . . . .151

Examples of Nursing Diagnoses Related to Genitourinary Trauma . . . . . . . . . . . . . . . . . . . . .151

Summary . . . . . . . . . . . . . . . . . . . . . . . . . . . . . . . . . . . . . . . . . . . . . . . . . . . . . . . . . . . . . . . . . .151

Exam Questions . . . . . . . . . . . . . . . . . . . . . . . . . . . . . . . . . . . . . . . . . . . . . . . . . . . . . . . . . . . .153

*Chapter 12* **Obstetric and Gynecologic Trauma** . . . . . . . . . . . . . . . . . . . . . . . . . . . . . . .**155**

Introduction . . . . . . . . . . . . . . . . . . . . . . . . . . . . . . . . . . . . . . . . . . . . . . . . . . . . . . . . . . . . . .155

Changes in Anatomy and Physiology During Pregnancy . . . . . . . . . . . . . . . . . . . . . . . . . . . .155

Terminology . . . . . . . . . . . . . . . . . . . . . . . . . . . . . . . . . . . . . . . . . . . . . . . . . . . . . . . .155

Structures, Organs, and Systems . . . . . . . . . . . . . . . . . . . . . . . . . . . . . . . . . . . . . . . . .156

Mechanism of Injury . . . . . . . . . . . . . . . . . . . . . . . . . . . . . . . . . . . . . . . . . . . . . . . . . . . . . . .160

Obstetric Injury, Complications, and Interventions . . . . . . . . . . . . . . . . . . . . . . . . . . . . . . . .161

Blunt Trauma . . . . . . . . . . . . . . . . . . . . . . . . . . . . . . . . . . . . . . . . . . . . . . . . . . . . . . . .161

Penetrating Injury . . . . . . . . . . . . . . . . . . . . . . . . . . . . . . . . . . . . . . . . . . . . . . . . . . . .162

Assessment . . . . . . . . . . . . . . . . . . . . . . . . . . . . . . . . . . . . . . . . . . . . . . . . . . . . . . . . . . . . . .162

Diagnostic Tests . . . . . . . . . . . . . . . . . . . . . . . . . . . . . . . . . . . . . . . . . . . . . . . . . . . . .162

Assessment Principles . . . . . . . . . . . . . . . . . . . . . . . . . . . . . . . . . . . . . . . . . . . . . . . . .162

Nursing Strategies for the Patient with Obstetric Trauma . . . . . . . . . . . . . . . . . . . . . . . . . . . .164

Examples of Nursing Diagnoses Related to Obstetric Trauma . . . . . . . . . . . . . . . . . . . . . . . . .165

Gynecologic Trauma . . . . . . . . . . . . . . . . . . . . . . . . . . . . . . . . . . . . . . . . . . . . . . . . . . . . . . .165

Nursing Strategies for the Patient with Gynecologic Trauma . . . . . . . . . . . . . . . . . . . . . . . . . .166

Examples of Nursing Diagnoses Related to Gynecologic Trauma . . . . . . . . . . . . . . . . . . . . . .166

Summary . . . . . . . . . . . . . . . . . . . . . . . . . . . . . . . . . . . . . . . . . . . . . . . . . . . . . . . . . . . . . . . . . .167

Exam Questions . . . . . . . . . . . . . . . . . . . . . . . . . . . . . . . . . . . . . . . . . . . . . . . . . . . . . . . . . . . .169

*Chapter 13* **Orthopedic and Neurovascular Trauma** . . . . . . . . . . . . . . . . . . . . . . . . . . . . . . . . . . . . . . . . .**171**

Introduction . . . . . . . . . . . . . . . . . . . . . . . . . . . . . . . . . . . . . . . . . . . . . . . . . . . . . . . . . . . . . . . . . . . . . . .171

Anatomy and Physiology . . . . . . . . . . . . . . . . . . . . . . . . . . . . . . . . . . . . . . . . . . . . . . . . . . . . . . . . . . .171

    Bones . . . . . . . . . . . . . . . . . . . . . . . . . . . . . . . . . . . . . . . . . . . . . . . . . . . . . . . . . . . . . . . . . . . . .171

    Joints . . . . . . . . . . . . . . . . . . . . . . . . . . . . . . . . . . . . . . . . . . . . . . . . . . . . . . . . . . . . . . . . . . . . .172

    Muscle . . . . . . . . . . . . . . . . . . . . . . . . . . . . . . . . . . . . . . . . . . . . . . . . . . . . . . . . . . . . . . . . . . . .172

    Ligaments . . . . . . . . . . . . . . . . . . . . . . . . . . . . . . . . . . . . . . . . . . . . . . . . . . . . . . . . . . . . . . . . .173

    Tendons . . . . . . . . . . . . . . . . . . . . . . . . . . . . . . . . . . . . . . . . . . . . . . . . . . . . . . . . . . . . . . . . . . .173

    Cartilage . . . . . . . . . . . . . . . . . . . . . . . . . . . . . . . . . . . . . . . . . . . . . . . . . . . . . . . . . . . . . . . . . . .173

Mechanism of Injury . . . . . . . . . . . . . . . . . . . . . . . . . . . . . . . . . . . . . . . . . . . . . . . . . . . . . . . . . . . . . .173

Orthopedic Trauma and Associated Neurovascular Problems . . . . . . . . . . . . . . . . . . . . . . . . . . . . .174

    Types of Orthopedic Injuries . . . . . . . . . . . . . . . . . . . . . . . . . . . . . . . . . . . . . . . . . . . . . . . . . .174

Assessment . . . . . . . . . . . . . . . . . . . . . . . . . . . . . . . . . . . . . . . . . . . . . . . . . . . . . . . . . . . . . . . . . . . . . .185

Nursing Strategies for the Patient with Orthopedic Trauma and Associated Neurovascular Problems . .186

Examples of Nursing Diagnoses Related to Orthopedic Trauma and Associated Neurovascular

    Problems . . . . . . . . . . . . . . . . . . . . . . . . . . . . . . . . . . . . . . . . . . . . . . . . . . . . . . . . . . . . . . . . . .187

Summary . . . . . . . . . . . . . . . . . . . . . . . . . . . . . . . . . . . . . . . . . . . . . . . . . . . . . . . . . . . . . . . . . . . . . . . .187

Exam Questions . . . . . . . . . . . . . . . . . . . . . . . . . . . . . . . . . . . . . . . . . . . . . . . . . . . . . . . . . . . . . . . . . .189

*Chapter 14* **Burn Injuries** . . . . . . . . . . . . . . . . . . . . . . . . . . . . . . . . . . . . . . . . . . . . . . . . . . . . . . . . . . . . . . . .**191**

Introduction . . . . . . . . . . . . . . . . . . . . . . . . . . . . . . . . . . . . . . . . . . . . . . . . . . . . . . . . . . . . . . . . . . . . . . .191

Epidemiology . . . . . . . . . . . . . . . . . . . . . . . . . . . . . . . . . . . . . . . . . . . . . . . . . . . . . . . . . . . . . . . . . . . . .191

Anatomy and Functions of the Skin . . . . . . . . . . . . . . . . . . . . . . . . . . . . . . . . . . . . . . . . . . . . . . . . . .192

    Anatomy . . . . . . . . . . . . . . . . . . . . . . . . . . . . . . . . . . . . . . . . . . . . . . . . . . . . . . . . . . . . . . . . . . .192

    Functions . . . . . . . . . . . . . . . . . . . . . . . . . . . . . . . . . . . . . . . . . . . . . . . . . . . . . . . . . . . . . . . . . .192

Pathopsysiology . . . . . . . . . . . . . . . . . . . . . . . . . . . . . . . . . . . . . . . . . . . . . . . . . . . . . . . . . . . . . . . . . .193

    Zones of Damage . . . . . . . . . . . . . . . . . . . . . . . . . . . . . . . . . . . . . . . . . . . . . . . . . . . . . . . . . . .193

    Pulmonary Response to Smoke Inhalation . . . . . . . . . . . . . . . . . . . . . . . . . . . . . . . . . . . . . . . .194

Mechanism of Injury . . . . . . . . . . . . . . . . . . . . . . . . . . . . . . . . . . . . . . . . . . . . . . . . . . . . . . . . . . . . . .195

Burn Injuries . . . . . . . . . . . . . . . . . . . . . . . . . . . . . . . . . . . . . . . . . . . . . . . . . . . . . . . . . . . . . . . . . . . . .195

    Thermal Burns . . . . . . . . . . . . . . . . . . . . . . . . . . . . . . . . . . . . . . . . . . . . . . . . . . . . . . . . . . . . . .195

    Light Burns . . . . . . . . . . . . . . . . . . . . . . . . . . . . . . . . . . . . . . . . . . . . . . . . . . . . . . . . . . . . . . . .198

    Chemical Burns . . . . . . . . . . . . . . . . . . . . . . . . . . . . . . . . . . . . . . . . . . . . . . . . . . . . . . . . . . . . .198

    Electrical Burns . . . . . . . . . . . . . . . . . . . . . . . . . . . . . . . . . . . . . . . . . . . . . . . . . . . . . . . . . . . . .199

    Nuclear Radiation Burns . . . . . . . . . . . . . . . . . . . . . . . . . . . . . . . . . . . . . . . . . . . . . . . . . . . . . .200

Assessment . . . . . . . . . . . . . . . . . . . . . . . . . . . . . . . . . . . . . . . . . . . . . . . . . . . . . . . . . . . . . . . . . . . . . .200

    Assessment Principles . . . . . . . . . . . . . . . . . . . . . . . . . . . . . . . . . . . . . . . . . . . . . . . . . . . . . . . .200

    Assessing a Burn Injury . . . . . . . . . . . . . . . . . . . . . . . . . . . . . . . . . . . . . . . . . . . . . . . . . . . . . . .201

Nursing Strategies for the Patient with Burn Injuries . . . . . . . . . . . . . . . . . . . . . . . . . . . . . . . . . . .202

    Airway . . . . . . . . . . . . . . . . . . . . . . . . . . . . . . . . . . . . . . . . . . . . . . . . . . . . . . . . . . . . . . . . . . . .202

    Breathing . . . . . . . . . . . . . . . . . . . . . . . . . . . . . . . . . . . . . . . . . . . . . . . . . . . . . . . . . . . . . . . . . .202

                Circulation . . . . . . . . . . . . . . . . . . . . . . . . . . . . . . . . . . . . . . . . . . . . . . . . . . . . .202

                Temperature Regulation . . . . . . . . . . . . . . . . . . . . . . . . . . . . . . . . . . . . . . . . . . . .203

                Wound Care . . . . . . . . . . . . . . . . . . . . . . . . . . . . . . . . . . . . . . . . . . . . . . . . . . . . .203

        Examples of Nursing Diagnoses Related to Burn Injury . . . . . . . . . . . . . . . . . . . . . . . . . . .204

        Summary . . . . . . . . . . . . . . . . . . . . . . . . . . . . . . . . . . . . . . . . . . . . . . . . . . . . . . . . . . . .204

        Exam Questions . . . . . . . . . . . . . . . . . . . . . . . . . . . . . . . . . . . . . . . . . . . . . . . . . . . . . . .205

*Chapter 15* **Pediatric Trauma and Child Maltreatment** . . . . . . . . . . . . . . . . . . . . . . . . . . . . . . .**207**

        Introduction . . . . . . . . . . . . . . . . . . . . . . . . . . . . . . . . . . . . . . . . . . . . . . . . . . . . . . . . . .207

        Epidemiology and Mechanisms of Injury . . . . . . . . . . . . . . . . . . . . . . . . . . . . . . . . . . . . . .208

        Anatomy and Physical Characteristics of Children and Adolescents . . . . . . . . . . . . . . . . . . .210

                Physical Growth . . . . . . . . . . . . . . . . . . . . . . . . . . . . . . . . . . . . . . . . . . . . . . . . . .210

                Metabolism, Fluid, and Electrolyte Balance . . . . . . . . . . . . . . . . . . . . . . . . . . . . . .210

                Thermoregulation . . . . . . . . . . . . . . . . . . . . . . . . . . . . . . . . . . . . . . . . . . . . . . . . .211

                Respiratory System . . . . . . . . . . . . . . . . . . . . . . . . . . . . . . . . . . . . . . . . . . . . . . .211

                Cardiovascular System . . . . . . . . . . . . . . . . . . . . . . . . . . . . . . . . . . . . . . . . . . . . .212

                Neurologic System . . . . . . . . . . . . . . . . . . . . . . . . . . . . . . . . . . . . . . . . . . . . . . . .212

                Musculoskeletal System . . . . . . . . . . . . . . . . . . . . . . . . . . . . . . . . . . . . . . . . . . . .213

                Gastrointestinal and Genitourinary Systems . . . . . . . . . . . . . . . . . . . . . . . . . . . . . .213

        Predominant Pediatric Trauma . . . . . . . . . . . . . . . . . . . . . . . . . . . . . . . . . . . . . . . . . . . . . .213

                Head Injury . . . . . . . . . . . . . . . . . . . . . . . . . . . . . . . . . . . . . . . . . . . . . . . . . . . . . .213

                Spinal Cord Injury . . . . . . . . . . . . . . . . . . . . . . . . . . . . . . . . . . . . . . . . . . . . . . . .214

                Thoracic Injury . . . . . . . . . . . . . . . . . . . . . . . . . . . . . . . . . . . . . . . . . . . . . . . . . .215

                Abdominal Injury . . . . . . . . . . . . . . . . . . . . . . . . . . . . . . . . . . . . . . . . . . . . . . . . .215

                Genitourinary Injury . . . . . . . . . . . . . . . . . . . . . . . . . . . . . . . . . . . . . . . . . . . . . . .216

                Musculoskeletal Injury . . . . . . . . . . . . . . . . . . . . . . . . . . . . . . . . . . . . . . . . . . . . .217

                Burn Injury . . . . . . . . . . . . . . . . . . . . . . . . . . . . . . . . . . . . . . . . . . . . . . . . . . . . . .218

        Maltreatment of Children . . . . . . . . . . . . . . . . . . . . . . . . . . . . . . . . . . . . . . . . . . . . . . . . . .218

                Neglect . . . . . . . . . . . . . . . . . . . . . . . . . . . . . . . . . . . . . . . . . . . . . . . . . . . . . . . . .218

                Physical Abuse . . . . . . . . . . . . . . . . . . . . . . . . . . . . . . . . . . . . . . . . . . . . . . . . . . .218

                Sexual Abuse . . . . . . . . . . . . . . . . . . . . . . . . . . . . . . . . . . . . . . . . . . . . . . . . . . . .219

                Emotional Abuse . . . . . . . . . . . . . . . . . . . . . . . . . . . . . . . . . . . . . . . . . . . . . . . . .220

                Significant Clinical Findings . . . . . . . . . . . . . . . . . . . . . . . . . . . . . . . . . . . . . . . . .220

        Assessment . . . . . . . . . . . . . . . . . . . . . . . . . . . . . . . . . . . . . . . . . . . . . . . . . . . . . . . . . . . .222

                Initial Assessment . . . . . . . . . . . . . . . . . . . . . . . . . . . . . . . . . . . . . . . . . . . . . . . . .222

                History . . . . . . . . . . . . . . . . . . . . . . . . . . . . . . . . . . . . . . . . . . . . . . . . . . . . . . . . .224

        Nursing Strategies for the Pediatric Trauma/Child Maltreatment Patient . . . . . . . . . . . . . . . . .224

        Examples of Nursing Diagnoses for the Pediatric Trauma/Child Maltreatment Patients . . . . . . . . . . . .225

        Summary . . . . . . . . . . . . . . . . . . . . . . . . . . . . . . . . . . . . . . . . . . . . . . . . . . . . . . . . . . . . . .226

        Exam Questions . . . . . . . . . . . . . . . . . . . . . . . . . . . . . . . . . . . . . . . . . . . . . . . . . . . . . . . . .227

*Chapter 16* **Elder Trauma, Abuse, and Neglect** .............................................229

   Introduction .............................................................229

   Epidemiology and Mechanisms of Injury .......................................230

      Falls ...............................................................230

      Motor Vehicle Crashes ...............................................230

      Pedestrian vs Motor Vehicle Accidents ..................................231

      Burns ..............................................................231

      Injury Related to Violence ............................................231

      Abuse and Neglect ..................................................231

   Changes in Aging .......................................................232

      Cardiovascular System ...............................................232

      Respiratory System ..................................................232

      Nervous System .....................................................233

      Musculoskeletal System ..............................................233

      Renal ..............................................................234

      Metabolic and Hepatic Changes .......................................234

      Thermoregulation ...................................................234

      Comorbid Conditions ................................................234

   Elder Abuse and Neglect .................................................234

      Primary Categories of Elder Mistreatment ...............................234

      Risk Factors Associated with Elder Abuse ...............................235

      Signs and Symptoms .................................................235

   Assessment .............................................................236

      Assessment Principles ................................................236

      Resuscitation and Initial Assessment ...................................236

      Secondary Survey ...................................................236

   Nursing Strategies for the Elder Trauma or Maltreatment Patient ................237

      Trauma ............................................................237

      Abuse and Neglect ..................................................238

   Examples of Nursing Diagnoses Related to the Elder Trauma or Maltreatment Patient .............238

   Summary ...............................................................239

   Exam Questions .........................................................241

*Chapter 17* **Psychosocial Considerations** .........................................**243**

   Introduction .............................................................243

   A General Perspective of Psychosocial Aspects of Trauma .......................243

   Trauma and Stress .......................................................244

   Responses to Trauma .....................................................245

      Denial .............................................................245

      Anger .............................................................245

      Bargaining .........................................................246

Depression . . . . . . . . . . . . . . . . . . . . . . . . . . . . . . . . . . . . . . . . . . . . . . . . . . . . . . . . . . . . . . . . . .246

Acceptance . . . . . . . . . . . . . . . . . . . . . . . . . . . . . . . . . . . . . . . . . . . . . . . . . . . . . . . . . . . . . . . . . .246

Crisis Intervention . . . . . . . . . . . . . . . . . . . . . . . . . . . . . . . . . . . . . . . . . . . . . . . . . . . . . . . . . . . . . . .246

Suicide and Suicide Attempts . . . . . . . . . . . . . . . . . . . . . . . . . . . . . . . . . . . . . . . . . . . . . . . . . . . . . . . .247

Special Patients . . . . . . . . . . . . . . . . . . . . . . . . . . . . . . . . . . . . . . . . . . . . . . . . . . . . . . . . . . . . . . . . . .247

Hearing Impaired . . . . . . . . . . . . . . . . . . . . . . . . . . . . . . . . . . . . . . . . . . . . . . . . . . . . . . . . . . .248

Vision Impaired . . . . . . . . . . . . . . . . . . . . . . . . . . . . . . . . . . . . . . . . . . . . . . . . . . . . . . . . . . . .248

Other Disabilities . . . . . . . . . . . . . . . . . . . . . . . . . . . . . . . . . . . . . . . . . . . . . . . . . . . . . . . . . . .248

Non-English Speaking . . . . . . . . . . . . . . . . . . . . . . . . . . . . . . . . . . . . . . . . . . . . . . . . . . . . . . .248

Nursing Strategies for Meeting Psychosocial Needs of the Trauma Patient . . . . . . . . . . . . . . . . . . . . . .248

Examples of Nursing Diagnoses Related to the Psychosocial Considerations of Trauma . . . . . . . . . . .250

Summary . . . . . . . . . . . . . . . . . . . . . . . . . . . . . . . . . . . . . . . . . . . . . . . . . . . . . . . . . . . . . . . . . . . . . . .250

Exam Questions . . . . . . . . . . . . . . . . . . . . . . . . . . . . . . . . . . . . . . . . . . . . . . . . . . . . . . . . . . . . . . . . . .253

*Chapter 18* **Organ Donation** . . . . . . . . . . . . . . . . . . . . . . . . . . . . . . . . . . . . . . . . . . . . . . . . . . . .**255**

Introduction . . . . . . . . . . . . . . . . . . . . . . . . . . . . . . . . . . . . . . . . . . . . . . . . . . . . . . . . . . . . . . . . . . . . . .255

Historical Background . . . . . . . . . . . . . . . . . . . . . . . . . . . . . . . . . . . . . . . . . . . . . . . . . . . . . . . . . . . . . .256

Legislative Background . . . . . . . . . . . . . . . . . . . . . . . . . . . . . . . . . . . . . . . . . . . . . . . . . . . . . . . . . . . . .257

The Donation Process . . . . . . . . . . . . . . . . . . . . . . . . . . . . . . . . . . . . . . . . . . . . . . . . . . . . . . . . . . . . . .258

Recognition of Donors . . . . . . . . . . . . . . . . . . . . . . . . . . . . . . . . . . . . . . . . . . . . . . . . . . . . . . .259

Criteria for Donors . . . . . . . . . . . . . . . . . . . . . . . . . . . . . . . . . . . . . . . . . . . . . . . . . . . . . . . . . .260

Determination of Death . . . . . . . . . . . . . . . . . . . . . . . . . . . . . . . . . . . . . . . . . . . . . . . . . . . . . . .260

Donor Evaluation . . . . . . . . . . . . . . . . . . . . . . . . . . . . . . . . . . . . . . . . . . . . . . . . . . . . . . . . . . .262

Medical Examiner Evaluation . . . . . . . . . . . . . . . . . . . . . . . . . . . . . . . . . . . . . . . . . . . . . . . . . .263

Hospital Requirements . . . . . . . . . . . . . . . . . . . . . . . . . . . . . . . . . . . . . . . . . . . . . . . . . . . . . . .263

Obtaining Consent . . . . . . . . . . . . . . . . . . . . . . . . . . . . . . . . . . . . . . . . . . . . . . . . . . . . . . . . . . .263

The Procurement Process . . . . . . . . . . . . . . . . . . . . . . . . . . . . . . . . . . . . . . . . . . . . . . . . . . . . . . . . . . .265

Tissue Procurement: Eyes, Corneas, Heart Valves, Bone, and Skin . . . . . . . . . . . . . . . . . . . .265

Solid-Organ Procurement: Heart, Lungs, Liver, Kidneys, and Pancreas . . . . . . . . . . . . . . . . . .267

Ethical Considerations . . . . . . . . . . . . . . . . . . . . . . . . . . . . . . . . . . . . . . . . . . . . . . . . . . . . . . . . . . . . .267

Financial Considerations . . . . . . . . . . . . . . . . . . . . . . . . . . . . . . . . . . . . . . . . . . . . . . . . . . . . . . . . . . .268

The Future of Transplantation . . . . . . . . . . . . . . . . . . . . . . . . . . . . . . . . . . . . . . . . . . . . . . . . . . . . . . .268

Nursing Strategies for Organ Donation . . . . . . . . . . . . . . . . . . . . . . . . . . . . . . . . . . . . . . . . . . . . . . . .269

Summary . . . . . . . . . . . . . . . . . . . . . . . . . . . . . . . . . . . . . . . . . . . . . . . . . . . . . . . . . . . . . . . . . . . . . . .269

Exam Questions . . . . . . . . . . . . . . . . . . . . . . . . . . . . . . . . . . . . . . . . . . . . . . . . . . . . . . . . . . . . . . . . . .271

**Glossary** . . . . . . . . . . . . . . . . . . . . . . . . . . . . . . . . . . . . . . . . . . . . . . . . . . . . . . . . . . . . . . . . . . . . . .**273**

**Bibliography** . . . . . . . . . . . . . . . . . . . . . . . . . . . . . . . . . . . . . . . . . . . . . . . . . . . . . . . . . . . . . . . . . .**277**

**Index** . . . . . . . . . . . . . . . . . . . . . . . . . . . . . . . . . . . . . . . . . . . . . . . . . . . . . . . . . . . . . . . . . . . . . . . .**283**

**Pretest Key** . . . . . . . . . . . . . . . . . . . . . . . . . . . . . . . . . . . . . . . . . . . . . . . . . . . . . . . . . . . . . . . . . .**296**

# PRETEST

Begin by taking the pretest. Compare your answers on the pretest to the answer key (located in the back of the book). Circle those test items that you missed. The pretest answer key indicates the course chapters where the content of that question is discussed.

Next, read each chapter. Focus special attention on the chapters where you made incorrect answer choices. Exam questions are provided at the end of each chapter so that you can assess your progress and understanding of the material.

1. Trauma has become such a national problem

    a. that it is the primary cause of death in the first 45 years of life.

    b. that all trauma is now treated in a trauma center.

    c. that trauma refers to any type of injury.

    d. that the patient must be treated within the first 3 hours.

2. Trauma is injury caused by a physical force causing harm to the body

    a. but not necessarily severe enough to cause a threat to life and limb.

    b. and is severe enough to be a potential threat to limb or life.

    c. and does not usually require immediate intervention.

    d. occurring most often to the elderly.

3. Epidemiology is the collection of data that form frequency and distribution patterns and

    a. it is only relative to medical illnesses, not trauma.

    b. only has to with infectious diseases.

    c. helps to determine causal factors and acts as a basis for prevention and control planning to reduce morbidity and mortality.

    d. is only used at the National Center for Health Statistics.

4. Six elements of nursing that form an organized structure for providing patient care are

    a. assessment, diagnosis, decision making, implementation and evaluation.

    b. assessment, nursing strategies, nursing diagnosis, education, intervention and evaluation.

    c. assessment, strategies, nursing diagnosis, planning, education and intervention.

    d. assessment, nursing diagnosis, planning, decision making, implementation and evaluation.

5. Nursing diagnosis

    a. was one of the first concepts in clinical nursing practice.

    b. gives the nurse latitude in acting independently and without a physician's order.

    c. has nothing to do with clinical diagnosis but is based upon implementation of the physician's orders.

    d. is based upon clinical nursing philosophy.

6. Life is dependent upon continuous and adequate breathing, and

    a. the body has a large oxygen reserve.

    b. when respiration ceases, the heart pumps faster to circulate existing oxygen.

    c. when respiration ceases, the only oxygen available to the body is that which remains in the lungs and bloodstream.

    d. respiration ceases only after the heart stops.

7. Management of the trauma patient

    a. requires training in advanced cardiac life support.

    b. begins with the ABCs.

    c. should only be conducted in a trauma center.

    d. should always begin with a history of the incident causing the injury.

8. Homeostasis refers to

    a. the body's performance of complicated functions.

    b. inadequate response to disturbances in the body's balance.

    c. swelling of the extremities after traumatic injury.

    d. the body's means for balancing its internal environment.

9. "Shock," a clinical syndrome, is

    a. a series of reactions to a mental or physical upset of the body's internal balance.

    b. a group of signs and symptoms that keeps the body's functions constant.

    c. caused only by trauma.

    d. it is represented by the cardiovascular triad.

10. As pressure increases in the head

    a. it causes the cerebral blood flow and oxygen to increase, resulting in the level of consciousness to diminish.

    b. it causes the brain to swell.

    c. it diminishes the cerebral blood flow and oxygen supply.

    d. the sympathetic response causes the blood pressure to drop.

11. With any head or neck injury the

    a. pupils should be checked immediately.

    b. primary assessment assumes there is a cerivcal fracture.

    c. skull should be checked first for a fracture.

    d. airway is usually obstructed.

12. Retinal detachment occurs

    a. when there is a corneal laceration.

    b. primarily to the elderly.

    c. when the patient has a cerebrovascular accident.

    d. from various medical causes or trauma.

13. The autonomic nervous system

    a. controls involuntary movements and has sympathetic and parasympathetic branches.

    b. lies outside the central nervous system.

    c. is functionally part of the somatic component of the nervous system.

    d. controls the cranial nerves.

14. The cardiovascular system is complex, and

   a.  it has a cranial and pulmonary intrasystem.

   b.  it is made up of systemic circulation and pulmonary circulation.

   c.  it has a high- and low-pressure subsystem to handle afterload.

   d.  becomes afterload once the blood leaves the heart.

15. Flail chest is

   a.  a serious contusion caused by trauma.

   b.  a complication of pneumonia.

   c.  when three or more ribs are broken, each in two places, and the part of the chest wall between the fractures becomes loose.

   d.  occurs from harsh coughing.

16. Abdominal trauma

   a.  is easily identified.

   b.  can be overlooked because outward signs may not be present.

   c.  occurs most often in children.

   d.  does not reflect a relationship between incidence and mechanism of injury.

17. Genitourinary injuries are not usually isolated to a particular organ but are associated with multiple injuries. Other characteristics of genitourinary injuries are

   a.  the anatomical location of the GU structures make life-threatening injuries likely.

   b.  it does not take much force to fracture a kidney.

   c.  penetrating mechanisms account for 80% of GU trauma injuries.

   d.  at least half of the patients with renal injuries also have skeletal or multiple trauma.

18. The most frequent obstetric trauma complication is

   a.  the onset of premature uterine contractions.

   b.  fracture of the pelvis penetrating the uterus.

   c.  that in the first trimester, it is unlikely that the fetus will be affected by the consequences of the mother's injuries, such as hypoxia and decreased perfusion.

   d.  torcolysis.

19. Posterior hip dislocation is a serious injury because

   a.  it is an injury of the elderly.

   b.  the patient may develop pneumonia.

   c.  of the likelihood of impaired blood supply to the femoral head and damage to the sciatic nerve.

   d.  it is difficult to treat without surgery.

20. The "rule of nines" is

   a.  a method of determining the correct amount of lactated Ringer's solution and the rate of administration for burn patients.

   b.  a method for rapid, accurate assessment of the amount of body surface area affected by burns.

   c.  a method for determining the depth of a burn.

   d.  the means to determine the depth of burns in each of nine body areas.

21. A child's ribs are flexible so that blunt trauma to the chest

   a.  will splinter the ribs when they fracture.

   b.  usually results in no injury.

   c.  usually results in contusion to the ribs instead of fractures.

   d.  is an indicator of child abuse.

22. Older people are living longer and are in better health than ever. Trauma in this age group

    a.  is not likely to be any more serious than the same trauma in a younger person.

    b.  is likely to be more serious than the same injury in a younger person.

    c.  accounts for the elderly comprising more than 50% of all trauma patients.

    d.  is not related to elder abuse.

23. Elder abuse is a concept that is being investigated to determine

    a.  if it is an actual problem for older people.

    b.  reasons for abuse and neglect, along with associated risk factors.

    c.  if criminal acts are involved in elder abuse.

    d.  why abuse only occurs in extended care facilities.

24. Why is it important to consider the psychosocial aspects of trauma in the patient's early management?

    a.  Because all trauma causes stress.

    b.  It isn't; this facet of care is not the responsibility of the trauma nurse.

    c.  It is the same as the psychiatric aspects of patient care.

    d.  This question is irrelevant.

25. Why does the gap between the need for organ and tissue transplants and the supply widen every day?

    a.  Not enough people are educated enough to make arrangements to donate their organs and tissues.

    b.  More people need tissues and organs than are dying.

    c.  Medical care for transplantation is too expensive.

    d.  Most people do not approve of transplantation.

# INTRODUCTION

Trauma is a national problem to such an extent that it is identified as the primary cause of death in the first 45 years of life. Injury can occur anywhere. Bodily harm caused by many kinds of external factors such as forceful action or thermal or chemical agents, can disfigure, cripple or kill.

Most trauma care is provided in the prehospital and emergency department environment. Ideally, serious trauma is treated in a trauma center. Because these centers are not within close proximity for many people requiring their expertise, patients may be assessed, stabilized, admitted or transferred by emergency departments in non-trauma center hospitals. Therefore, trauma patients are seen along with many other acute and nonacute problems. Management of the trauma patient must be conducted under specific guidelines, often in the midst of confusion.

Nursing in the trauma setting is never dull. It is exciting in the anticipation of the unknown case, precise in the known case and stressful. Probably no other aspect of nursing requires the assessment and care of the patient to function in such close coordination with the entire medical team. An organized and standardized approach is essential. Strong fundamental skills are requisite. These abilities critically affect the treatment and outcomes of injured patients, particularly in the first hour after the incident.

The purpose of this book is to provide a review of the fundamentals of the mechanisms of injury, problems associated with trauma and the related nursing diagnoses and interventions. The level of information is basic and targeted to those nurses wanting an introduction to trauma care, as well as a review for nurses working in emergency departments and prehospital trauma care situations.

Course content includes basic concepts of pediatric and adult trauma nursing, triage, airway management, shock/cardiac arrest, trauma to specific anatomic and physiologic systems, burns, elder trauma, psychosocial aspects, and organ donation.

It should be noted that in this book, the patient is referred to in the masculine gender only as a means of generally accepted grammar. The pretest will provide a guideline to determine special areas for you to concentrate on during your study. Exam questions are at the end of each chapter.

# CHAPTER 1

## ABOUT TRAUMA

### CHAPTER OBJECTIVE

Upon completion of this chapter, the reader will be able to describe the basic concepts of trauma nursing and the emergency medical system.

### LEARNING OBJECTIVES

Upon completion of this chapter, the reader should be able to:

1. Define trauma, its basic mechanisms and potential effects upon the body.
2. Identify at least five of the major causes of traumatic injury.
3. Describe the three major components of the emergency medical services system.
4. Identify the levels of care for the trauma patient.
5. Relate the relevance of the "golden hour" to the survival of the trauma patient.
6. Describe the scope of basic trauma nursing.

### INTRODUCTION

Trauma often occurs without warning and may cause life-altering damage to the patient and the patient's family, along with billions of dollars in lost annual productivity. It demands systematic and knowledgeable assessment and care with maximum efficiency.

The effective practitioner understands the needs of the injured patient, from the site of injury through the treatment environment.

Patient care should be planned and conducted so that the patient is assured of the best potential for recovery with the least amount of disability and that there is the best utilization of resources without unnecessary duplication of services.

### TRAUMA DEFINED

Trauma is physical injury and referred to as harm to the body caused by an external action such as an assaulting force, thermal or chemical agents. It is generally accepted that traumatic injury is defined as being severe enough to be a potential threat to life or limb, usually requiring immediate intervention.

The term "injury" has a Greek derivation meaning "wound." Many think of trauma or injury as being synonymous with "accident." However, accident has a random and unexpected, unable-to-be averted connotation, while trauma actually is a more broad concept, not necessarily unable to be prevented. In this book, the terms "injury" and "trauma" are used interchangeably, while "accident" is used to mean a reportable incident.

# EPIDEMIOLOGY

Epidemiology generally refers to the distribution and determinants of disease frequency in man. It is relative to trauma in the collection of data such as age, gender, race/ethnicity and geographic characteristics that form frequency and distribution patterns. The information helps to determine causal factors and act as a basis for prevention and control planning to reduce morbidity and mortality.

The National Center for Health Statistics gathers data about morbidity and mortality. The most recent published data are at least two years old and eight years of data are used to determine trends. For instance, in 1986, 2,105,361 deaths occurred in the United States, and increased to 2,286,000 in 1994. However, during the same period of time, the total deaths from all injuries, including accidents and adverse effects, homicides, suicides, legal intervention and all other causes, fell from 151,032 to 149,520. Nevertheless, by 1994, combined injury death data revealed trauma to be the fourth leading cause of death for all groups and ages combined.

Additional information about trauma in the United States includes:

- Death rates for injuries are comparable to those from cerebrovascular diseases.

- The most significant increase in the trauma death rate is in the 25- to 43-year-old group.

- Accidents and their adverse effects, excluding suicides and homicides, are the leading cause of death for people 45 and under, with more male deaths than female (National Trauma Data Bank, 1994).

- In 1993, more than 12,000 children under the age of 19 died as a result of trauma-related injuries, making trauma the leading cause of death during the childhood and adolescent years (Soud, 1998).

- Gender and age variances in injury deaths are related to the type of injury.

- Injury deaths and death rates also vary by race. For instance, Whites have a higher death rate from suicide than Blacks; Blacks have a higher death rate from accidents and their adverse effects than Whites.

- Violence is a major public health problem in the United States, with juveniles causing a large portion of this problem. Every year more than a million teenagers are robbed, assaulted or raped by their peers.

- Two-thirds of deaths from injuries are accidental; one-third are caused by suicide or homicide.

- Death rates regarding suicide, homicide and motor vehicle crashes show geographic differences.

The incidence and rate of injury occurring, but not causing death, is more difficult to determine. Some statistics reflect the magnitude of the problem. Yearly, one out of four Americans sustain an injury. 10% of visits to physician offices are injury related. For each death caused by injury, 19 people are hospitalized for nonfatal injuries (Sheehy & Jimmerson, 1994).

Injury occurs anywhere. However, some types of trauma tend to be associated with certain activities or populations.

Trauma is a serious public health problem in this country. Regardless of the circumstances, intentional or unintentional, most injuries are preventable.

# INJURIES ASSOCIATED WITH TRAUMA

## Motor Vehicle Crashes

The National Highway Traffic Safety Administration (NHTSA) publishes an annual report, *Traffic Safety Facts,* utilizing data from the Fatal Accident Reporting System (FARS) and the General Estimates System (GES).

Motor vehicle crashes are the leading cause of unintentional and work-related death in this country for the ages of 1–34 years. However, between 1966 and 1994, the number of traffic-related fatalities dropped from 50,894 to 40,676, with about 500,000 being hospitalized (Newberry, 1998).

Over half of the fatalities occur on Fridays, Saturdays, and Sundays. These statistics include occupants of the motor vehicles and pedestrians.

Pedestrian versus motor vehicle injuries have a high incidence in the pediatric population. Because children are smaller than adults, a unique pattern of injuries occurs with the vehicular trauma ranging from head to toe, rather than being confined to a particular site.

The decrease in motor vehicle-related deaths is due to many factors such as the development of emergency medical services systems, comprehensive safety and prevention programs, active campaigns against drunk driving, and wider use of seat belts and motorcycle and bicycle helmets. It is an excellent example of how the use of data provide information used in planning for prevention to lower the morbidity and mortality resulting from trauma.

## Falls

Falls are second to motor vehicle crashes in causing unintentional fatalities. At least 10,000 elderly people die each year. Falls by children are the major cause of nonfatal injury and a significant cause of unintentional death, particularly from head injuries.

## Intentional Trauma

Included are all aspects of violence: nonfatal assaults; homicides; suicides; and occasionally, burns, falls and motor vehicle crashes. Assault occurs when there is an intentional threat to injure

*and* the apparent ability to carry it out at that moment. Battery is the touching of another person without his consent, resulting in harmful contact. The definitions become clouded when the terms are used in legal and nonlegal contexts. Most intentional injury in this country is caused by interpersonal violence.

Much of the violence against children is directly related to the home environment. Along with societal violence such as gangs, the morbidity and mortality in children has changed the nature of their emergency department visits. In 1994, the National Clearinghouse on Child Abuse and Neglect reported more than 3 million incidents of child abuse and/or neglect; nearly half of them being less than a year old.

Victims of partner abuse in heterosexual relationships almost always are women (Sheehy, 1998). This may stem from the male's perception that the woman is his property, thus under his control. Abuse of pregnant women is not infrequent; and most of them are in the poverty-level sector. Because our society has had a high tolerance for this type of violence and a reluctance to report it until recently, it has been generally accepted. In recent years, domestic violence, both of partners and children, has become a social issue and recognized as serious public health problem.

The problem of intentional injury to the elderly has become a serious one as the number of older adults and those needing care has increased. Part of the problem is the lack of training and supervision of the caregiver in adequate facilities, or the elder person crammed into the home of a relative who is already stretched to the limit. A clear picture of the magnitude of this problem is difficult because of the lack of reporting. The case of an 80-year-old sustaining a head injury from "falling out of a wheelchair" is seen frequently in the emergency department. Further, quick, easy, and accurate assessment cannot be done from a cluster of sometimes-vague symptoms along with a nonspecific history.

Most of the murder-suicides are related to "amorous jealousy," typically of those involved in a relationship, recently estranged, or married, according to research conducted by Cornell University. If the murder-suicide extends outside the family, it may be due to external stresses in addition to familial problems, and the violence, usually with the use of a firearm, may include those known and unknown by the assailant.

## Rape

*The 1994 Uniform Crime Reports* of the Federal Bureau of Investigation maintains statistics only on the sexual assaults on women. Feared and misunderstood, where choice is taken away, it is not considered a crime of passion. One in four women will be sexually assaulted during her lifetime.

## Firearms

Firearm-related injuries and deaths have dramatically increased in the past decade, both in unintentional and intentional cases. Of the nearly 40,000 firearm deaths in 1994, about 30% were unintentional, frequently occurring in children. Of all firearm injuries to children under 18 years old, 50% to 60% involve the head. Firearm homicides have increased to the point that it is anticipated they will exceed motor vehicle-related deaths by 2003. Especially in teenagers, and primarily males, the intentional injuries and murders, have risen to almost epidemic proportions. Street gangs were responsible for over one-third of *all* homicides in Los Angeles in 1994.

## Burns

Severe burns are frightening and the survivor of a major burn is almost sure to end up with a permanent disfigurement and disability. An estimated 2 million people are burned each year, with 75,000 being hospitalized. Types of burns are thermal, being caused by fire or intense heat such as scalds;

electrical, such as current or lightning; chemical, either acid or alkaline; flash burns and radiation. The most common burn is sunburn. Fortunately, burn and fire-related injuries sustained in the home are on the decline, thanks to an increased use of fire safety devices and awareness programs.

## Recreational Activities

The degree of physical maturation, size and endurance is directly related to the degree of injury sustained by children and adults in sports, whether for recreation or competition (Wong, 1997). Proper matching regarding age, strength, agility, size and skill levels impact the prevention of recreational injuries, particularly when the sport involves physical contact. Large numbers of severe, crippling or fatal injuries occur to those ill matched or ill prepared for a particular activity. Overextension of physical abilities, poor equipment, or conditions contribute additional risks. The leading cause of serious sports injuries for boys is football and for girls is gymnastics. Bicycle accidents contribute over 600,000 visits to the emergency department each year. In-line skating, otherwise known as "wreckreation," contributes close to 100,000 visits to emergency departments in this country (Wreckreation, 1994).

## Drowning and Near Drowning

Drowning is the third leading cause of accidental death. It is the result of aspiration of fresh or salt water, each of which has different physiological effects. About 10% of the victims do not drown from aspiration of water but from asphyxiation due to closure of the glottis and laryngospasm. Pulmonary injury is worsened by contaminants such as chlorine, sand, algae and mud, thus making emergency management even more difficult and can cause death from related problems for the near-drowning victim. Associated injuries such as those to the head or spinal cord further complicate the recovery process.

# MEANS OF IMPACT TRAUMA

T rauma is now recognized as a disease process with the means of injury being a part of the etiology (Newberry, 1998). Physical injury results from energy that can originate from kinetic (motion or mechanical), chemical, electrical, thermal, or radiation sources.

## Types of Injuries

Blunt trauma does not cause an opening in the skin. Energy from blunt trauma is transmitted in all directions, which can cause organs and tissues to burst or break if the pressure becomes great enough. Determination of the extent of injury is difficult because blunt trauma is not as obvious as penetrating wounds, but may be more life threatening. This type of injury may be seen in vehicular injuries to the head, chest, abdomen, or extremities.

Foreign objects that are set in motion and enter the body cause penetrating injuries. The energy created by the force is dispersed into the surrounding tissues. Evaluation and assessment depends upon the wounding agent, how the energy is dispersed, proximity to the victim and the characteristics of the tissues involved.

## Means of Impact

An assaulting force of injury is either absorbed and redistributed in the body, or it is powerful enough to cause forcible disruption to the tissues. There are three basic mechanisms of kinetic energy: rapid forward deceleration, rapid vertical deceleration and penetration by a projectile (Campbell, 1988).

The sudden resistance to an object swiftly moving forward is rapid forward deceleration. A person moving forward who has an abrupt stop due to impacting an object will experience blunt trauma.

Rapid downward motion meeting sudden resistance is rapid vertical deceleration. For instance, when an individual falls and slams against the surface, the impact will force the energy upward and cause blunt trauma.

Blast injuries are often seen in conjunction with hazardous explosions where volatile materials are involved. When gas expands, an equal volume of air is displaced and follows the blast wave. Massive injuries such as burns, evisceration and traumatic amputation can result from the force of motion along with the force and contact of toxic substances. Three phases or impact points occur with blasts. The first is the concussive effect from an expanding mass of heated gas. These injuries may be severe but not obvious and easily overlooked. Examples are central nervous system damage, rupture of gas-containing organs and torn membranes and blood vessels. Secondary injuries come from high-velocity projectiles, such as glass and other debris. The third point of impact occurs if the victim is thrown through the air, becoming a missile and receiving rapid vertical deceleration trauma.

# LEVELS OF TRAUMA CARE

B y the mid-1960s, it was evident that there was an urgent nationwide need for emergency treatment for the ill and injured. Funeral homes were using hearses as ambulances and transporting patients, *after* they transported the dead, who were "guaranteed payment." Emergency "rooms" were more like clinics, rather than the departments we know today.

Designated trauma centers did not exist, nor did designated perinatal, poison control, cardiac, and other specialized emergency facilities. There were a few burn and spinal cord injury centers. Emergency medical services legislation had not been enacted, and there were no standards for ambulances, communications, or medical control.

Emergency medical technicians and paramedics did not exist and a specialty for emergency department nursing had not been developed. Basic and advanced life support had not been thought of or defined.

Emergency nursing is one of the few specialties for which the nurse is expected to have a wide range of in-depth knowledge and skills. No longer can one just become an emergency department nurse without additional didactic and clinical training.

In 1966, the first two trauma centers opened in Chicago and San Francisco. Within three short years, the concept of emergency medical services *systems* (EMSS) was developed as the means for a coordinated, systematic mechanism for providing emergent care from the scene through treatment and rehabilitation.

The emergency medical services systems that are now developed on a nationwide basis have been shown to (Peitzman, Rhodes, Schwab & Yearly, 1998):

- "Equalize access of persons in both rural and urban locations to similar levels of care.

- Reduce death and disability.

- Create a formalized continuum of care from the scene of the accident or injury through rehabilitation.

- Provide a mechanism for continuous quality improvement of the system."

There are three major components of the emergency medical services system: prehospital care, acute hospital care, and long-term care/rehabilitation.

## Prehospital Care

The prehospital care includes the following:

1. Discovery of injury: An injured person may be discovered by anyone anywhere. The period of delay from the traumatic incident to discovery usually varies with the population density.

2. Access to the EMS system: through 911 or some alternative dispatch system.

3. Lifesaving prehospital care includes:

    **Basic life support** measures include the administration of oxygen, control of bleeding by direct pressure, and the performance of cardiopulmonary resuscitation (CPR). Other skills include safe extrication and patient movement, splinting and fracture immobilization.

    **Advanced life support** measures require additional specialized advanced training in the assessment and treatment of the patient, including airway intubation and chest decompression; establishing intravenous lines; administration of medications and other advanced measures according to established protocols and/or under orders from a medical command.

    **Medical command** is usually directed by a physician responsible for the care provided by designated rescue units in a given area and under approved protocols or standing orders.

4. Triage or injury assessment determines the severity of the injury; where the injury is located; circumstances of the injury and other special circumstances, such as age extremes, existing medical conditions, and significant medical history. Prehospital triage directs the patient to the most suitable treatment facility.

5. Transport is by the fastest, most efficient and suitable means to a facility either under the direction of triage or protocols based on time, distance, patient stability and available skills of the prehospital providers.

## Acute Hospital Care

Trauma centers receive designation after meeting established criteria regarding the numbers and qualifications of the surgeons, who staff on a 24-hour-a-day basis. Other facilities and services include operating rooms, blood bank, radiology and so forth. Trauma centers have a team activation system that responds to a predetermined triage criteria identifying a severely injured patient. Team members have defined roles and responsibilities to provide systematic and coordinated care.

## Long-Term Care and Rehabilitation

The EMS system has established a dedicated link between inpatient treatment and rehabilitation to ensure the transition to long-term recovery.

The concept of the "golden hour," following injury was developed by Dr. R. Adams Cowley, director of the first statewide EMS system, which is in Maryland. It refers to the occurrence of death following injury as a function of time.

The three peaks of occurrence are immediate, early and late. Immediate deaths are caused by massive head injury, brain stem injury and major cardiovascular injury. Half of all trauma deaths are immediate, with most of these victims being unsalvageable (Peitzman et al., 1998). Early deaths occur within the first few hours, mostly from major torso trauma. Modern trauma centers often are able to save many of these patients; the term "golden hour," refers to this group of injuries. Dr. Cowley and the American College of Surgeons found that the survival of seriously injured patients was highest when intervention took place during the first hour after the incident, along with skilled prehospital and emergency department staff and a trauma surgeon being immediately available. Late deaths reflect 20% of all in-hospital deaths due to trauma. Prolonged critical periods cause organ failure and sepsis, which account for most of these deaths. Regardless of how soon resuscitation takes place, if it is inadequate and the care insufficient, organ failure will likely develop and the patient will ultimately succumb.

## Classification of Trauma Centers

In order to provide the best utilization and avoid duplication of services, the early emergency med-

ical services systems, in conjunction with the American College of Surgeons, devised a system for categorization of emergency departments. Included was the designation of specialized care centers for such acute problems as trauma, spinal cord injuries, burns, perinatal, poison control centers and other specialties. Additionally, standards were devised to designate skill and capability levels for the degree of care able to be provided by each hospital. These criteria provide the classification for Level I, II, and III facilities (Peitzman et al., 1998).

### Level I

Provides a trauma team 24 hours a day, 7 days a week, with complete resuscitative, operative, critical care and rehabilitative capabilities. The trauma team is usually headed by an attending trauma surgeon, emergency physician, trauma fellow or senior surgical resident. Level I centers demonstrate a commitment to education by providing physician training, research, community outreach and prevention programs. Because of the complexity of care that must be provided and the attending enormous expense to provide these services, Level I trauma centers are usually regional and based on documented need and population base. Even so, many of these trauma centers have closed down due to the lack of available funding.

### Level II

Emergency department capabilities are similar to those of Level I centers, but the trauma team is not necessarily in-house 24 hours a day; but must be able to meet the severely injured patient when he arrives. Clinical resources such as cardiac surgery, neurosurgery, replantation, microvascular surgery and so forth usually vary in availability. Research, education, and resident teaching programs are not required.

### Level III

These facilities are specifically set up for rural areas that are immediately inaccessible to Level I and II trauma centers. In-house surgical coverage on a 24-hour basis not only is not required, it is often impossible in rural areas. Often staff functions on an on-call basis. Accessibility to higher level facilities should be timely, usually by helicopter, and requires official transfer agreements.

Many seriously injured patients arrive at nontrauma centers needing rapid assessment, intervention and resuscitation, sometimes followed by transfer to a trauma center. It is the highly organized capabilities of the entire emergency medical services system, with multidisciplinary teams that enable the accessibility to necessary treatment.

# SUMMARY

Trauma can place the patient in danger of disability or the loss of limb or life. Injuries are a major public health issue. The best treatment requires rapid intervention with a skilled team working in a systematic and efficient manner. From the site of the injury through treatment and rehabilitation, planned protocols and medical direction ensure the patient will receive the level of treatment appropriate for the injury.

# EXAM QUESTIONS

## CHAPTER 1
### Questions 1–5

1. Trauma is a physical injury that

    a. is an external action causing harm to the body.

    b. is synonymous with "accident."

    c. is always preventable.

    d. must be treated in a Level I trauma center.

2. The most significant increase in the trauma death rate is in the age range of

    a. under one year old.

    b. those over 60 years.

    c. 25–43 years old.

    d. no particular age group.

3. The leading cause of death from trauma is

    a. firearms.

    b. intentional injury.

    c. motor vehicle crashes.

    d. child abuse.

4. Level of trauma care refers to the

    a. peaks of occurrence of death after trauma.

    b. degrees of patient assessment.

    c. level of hospital and emergency department capabilities.

    d. degree of trauma that has occurred.

5. The "golden hour" is

    a. the first hour the patient is in the emergency department.

    b. a concept developed by trauma nurses.

    c. time related to the optimal survival of the trauma patient.

    d. time spent during the assessment of the patient.

# CHAPTER 2

# BASICS OF TRAUMA NURSING

## CHAPTER OBJECTIVE

Upon completion of this chapter, the reader will be able to identify the basics of trauma nursing including assessment and triage.

## LEARNING OBJECTIVES

Upon completion of this chapter, the reader should be able to:

1. Identify two functions unique to trauma nursing.

2. Relate the means of kinetic energy to the type of injuries likely to occur.

3. Recognize the importance of trauma patient assessment and identify the four components of the principles of trauma assessment described by the American College of Surgeons.

4. Identify the purpose and process of primary and secondary assessment.

5. Define the trauma nursing triage process.

## INTRODUCTION

Traumatic injury can be severe enough to be a threat to life and limb. It requires immediate attention, otherwise known as emergency treatment and care. Trauma nurses are required to have more extensive skills and knowledge than any other specialty, including knowledge of medical illness and care along with the identification and treatment of the injury. This course deals with the aspects of emergency care that focuses on trauma.

The trauma nurse is thought of as working in the emergency room of large hospitals, which are either Level I trauma centers or Level II hospitals that receive, assess, stabilize, treat, admit or transfer the injured patient. In both settings, the nurses have the same challenges and require similar specialized skills. This book is meant as an orientation to the process of trauma nursing. During the course of this book, the trauma nurse is often referred to in the context of the emergency department in order to illustrate the process of emergency care and treatment.

In order to systematically plan for and carry out the most appropriate care of the trauma patient, the process should begin with gathering information about the injury and the patient. An appropriate assessment, combined with timeliness, enables the patient to be properly triaged to receive the best potential outcome for recovery with the least resulting disability.

# THE TRAUMA NURSING PROCESS

Because trauma situations and emergency departments are often chaotic, the nursing process must be specifically defined to delineate organization and priorities and document the course of action and outcomes.

Six elements of nursing process form an organized structure for providing patient care. They are assessment, nursing diagnosis, planning, decision making, implementation and evaluation.

Nursing diagnosis allows the nurse to act independently and without a physician's order. A relatively recent concept, nursing diagnosis is a clinical diagnosis made describing actual or potential health problems that a professional nurse is licensed to treat. It employs diagnostic reasoning based on assessment data and lists the patient problem, etiology, signs, and symptoms. The nurse is accountable for the outcomes of the actions taken.

Some functions unique to trauma nursing are triage and emergency operations preparedness. Roles are also governed by unique unwritten rules because of the emergent environment and the patient's status (Newberry, 1998). For instance, unplanned situations may require immediate intervention; limited resources must be allocated quickly; the need for immediate care perceived by the patient and others acted upon; there are always unpredictable numbers of patients, and the unknown patient severity, urgency, and diagnosis demand the skills for quick action.

The dynamic nature of the urgent situation, whether in the hospital or another setting, involves broad clinical knowledge and experience, critical thinking skills, physical dexterity, flexibility, the ability to be creative, and ability to improvise. The patient's status may dramatically alter in a moment. Changes in the course of care may be abrupt and frequent.

Excellent management of trauma care is essential. The nurse's role is pivotal for the multidisciplinary team, which consists of emergency nurses; emergency medical and surgical physicians and physician assistants; and pulmonary services, radiology services, laboratory, social services and unlicensed but ancillary staff, such as electrocardiogram (ECG) technicians, cast technicians, nursing assistants, transporters, and so forth.

The accreditation of health care facilities requires accountability in the provision of care. Standards for measuring qualitative and quantitative value identify the distinction between minimally acceptable performance and excellence. The standards are reflected in guidelines for outcome criteria to measure and evaluate performance. The original Standards of Emergency Nursing Practice were developed in 1983 and, since then, have evolved into the 1992 American Nursing Association Standards. These standards are used in such areas as performance evaluations, policies and procedures, standardized care plans, and quality improvement programs. It is these standards that tie the process of clinical application of trauma nursing skills to the assessment of performance and the improvement of the quality of care.

# PATIENT ASSESSMENT

The American College of Surgeons Committee on Trauma determined the four components of the principles of trauma assessment:

1. Rapid and accurate assessment of the patient's condition.

2. Provision of resuscitation and stabilization on a priority basis.

3. Determination of whether a patient's needs will exceed local capability and arrangements for interhospital transfer if necessary.

4. Assurance that optimal care is provided in each step of the treatment process.

*Accurate assessment of the injured person is the critical point for setting the course for immediate and future action and is a deciding factor in the outcome of the patient. Regardless of where the assessment occurs, the principles and methods are the same.*

The onset of the nurse-patient relationship begins the process of care. It usually starts when the nurse and patient meet. At that time, the nurse begins gathering information that lays the foundation for assessment.

When outside the environment of the emergency department, the nurse directly encounters the patient, either at the scene of the injury or another site. In this instance, the nurse has immediate contact and can promptly gather information and begin assessment.

In emergency departments, the trauma assessment process often begins before the nurse even sees the patient, while the patient is en route to the hospital. Information is processed from prehospital EMS personnel, family, those with the patient at the time of the traumatic incident and earlier medical records. Compared to inpatient assessment where comprehensive information is necessary for long-term treatment, emergent assessment of the trauma patient requires the nurse to be selective in the data gathered in order to expedite immediate care.

The skilled use of objective, subjective, verbal, and observation tools reflect the ability to conduct an experienced assessment. These tools guide the nurse in deciding where to focus efforts for the most detailed parts of the evaluation (Peitzman et al., 1998; Soud & Rogers, 1998; Newberry, 1998).

The patient, family and others close to the patient give subjective data. The information describes their perception of the problem and may be affected by their emotional status, culture, and ability to communicate accurately. Often subjective information needs clarification and validation by other tools of the assessment because it is not readily visible to the nurse.

Objective data are observable and measurable. Tools used are inspection, auscultation, palpation, percussion, smell and laboratory and other diagnostic information. The information is considered valid information. Findings direct the attention of the assessment and also serve to validate the subjective information.

In the case of the injured patient, the type of trauma is related to the mechanism of injury. Sometimes there is more than one means of injury, such as in an auto crash where there may be blunt trauma from the steering wheel and penetrating trauma from shards of glass. With experience, the trauma nurse can anticipate the types of injuries to look for based on the trauma incident. This ability enables more selective and rapid evaluation to be conducted.

Continuous reassessment of the patient is necessary to evaluate the effectiveness of the interventions and to determine if new conditions have occurred. This ongoing process provides feedback so that information on the patient's status is always current.

## Primary Assessment

(It is assumed that the reader is certified in cardiopulmonary resuscitation.)

All injured patients, whether coming to the emergency department or in any other situation, should have a rapid primary assessment to determine if there may be a life-threatening condition in progress. The "ABC" mnemonic is used to conduct the initial assessment (Newberry, 1998).

### Airway

Is the airway patent? If not, identify and remove any partial or complete airway obstruction. Position the airway to maintain patency. Have an oropharyngeal airway ready to be inserted. Protect the cervical spine.

### Breathing

Determine the presence and effectiveness of the respiratory efforts. Identify the presence of any irregularities in breathing such as abnormal patterns and sounds. If necessary, assist breathing with oxygen therapy, mouth-to-mouth resuscitation, or bag-valve-mask ventilation. Intubate when necessary.

### Circulation

Evaluate pulse presence and quality, character, and equality. Assess capillary refill, skin color, and temperature. Identify any bleeding or hemorrhaging and treat appropriately. Evaluate for diaphoresis. Initiate chest compressions, medications and/or intravenous fluids as appropriate.

## Secondary (General or Routine) Assessment

**In the trauma patient, always assume that a spinal injury exists until ruled out by a physician.**

As a rule, once the primary assessment has shown that there is not a life-threatening condition and serious injuries are stabilized or ruled out, a secondary assessment is conducted.

Before beginning the secondary assessment, note the level of consciousness, orientation, clarity of speech, and any unusual behaviors.

The purpose of the secondary assessment is to further evaluate the patient for additional injury and medical problems. Included are triage findings; vital signs; chief complaint; physical assessment; systems assessment; current medications; allergies; and a history of illnesses, injuries, and surgeries.

### History

The patient history is an example of subjective information. The questions asked are directed by the presenting complaint, which in the case of trauma, may or may not be evident. The chief complaint is not recorded as a diagnosis but as the patient describes the problem. An example would not be "broken leg," but "I fell down the stairs." The mnemonic "PQRST" (**P**rovoking factors, **Q**uality, **R**egion/radiation factor, **S**everity and **T**ime of onset) is frequently used as a road map for taking the history. Remember that obtaining the patient's name and age not only is part of the history, but a way to determine orientation and alertness.

### Measurements

Each measurement in a trauma patient is essential in the determination of the whole injury picture.

**Vital signs** are indicators of the current status. Sequences of vital signs indicate a trend in the patient's status.

**Temperature** is too often not given enough consideration. Hypothermia and hyperthermia are particularly important to track for indication of unseen factors related to trauma or unidentified medical conditions.

**Respirations** indicate how well the patient is ventilating. Along with the rate, the rhythm and quality of respirations indicate the presence of impairment. Respiratory effort is indicated by tracheal tugging, nasal flaring, the use of accessory muscles and retractions.

**Pulse Oximetry** will help indicate how well the respiratory system is functioning, particularly if there is chest trauma or the patient has a respiratory medical condition. Artificial nails and nail polish alter readings of digital pulse oximetry with a 2% variation.

**Blood Pressure** is affected by a multitude of factors and is an important indicator in trauma regarding volume loss, pain, shock, and other factors. The systolic pressure reflects pump integrity; diastolic pressure is a measurement of the vascular status. Blood pressures vary for many reasons, one of which is being incorrectly taken when done hastily. If there is a possibility of volume depletion, the nurse should measure postural (orthostatic) vital signs. The reason for orthostatic measurement is that compensatory mechanisms such as vasoconstriction can mask volume depletion. Medical history such as hypertension is essential to document.

**Laboratory and other diagnostic** findings should be interpreted relative to other information gathered in the assessment.

*Observation*

Several standard techniques are used in the physical examination. As the nurse gains experience, a routine for efficient and appropriate assessments will develop.

**Inspection** is a key factor because the visual observation of the patient as a whole, along with specific body areas and each system, ties together what the patient says with what is observed. What is the general condition of the patient? Is the general condition related to the trauma? Body movement and posture may reveal pain, areas of injury, degrees of debilitation, and emotional status. If clothes are covering the injury, cut them off for better visualization and attention. Documentation should be specific and related to the injury and system being evaluated.

**Auscultation** is assessment with the stethoscope. Sounds of arteries, organs and tissues are described in terms of pitch, intensity, duration and quality. Presence, absence, or deviation from normal sounds are documented and related to the injury and other findings.

**Palpation** is the use of hands to assess skin temperature, texture, vibrations, and pulsation; masses or lesions; muscle tenseness or rigidity; and deformities. Different areas of the hand and degrees of pressure are used for various kinds of palpation.

**Percussion** allows vibration to be heard when a specific area of the body is struck with the hand or fingers. It outlines the borders of organs, identifies pain and tenderness, indicates fluid in an organ or cavity and aides evaluation of the lung fields for consolidation, fluid or air.

**Olfaction or smell** allows the assessor to identify medical problems such as the fruity aroma of ketosis in the diabetic or possible trauma-related odors of alcohol, gasoline, or marijuana. Other odors indicate infection, gangrene, or poor hygiene. Odors are used with other observations to present the whole picture.

# MAJOR BODY AREAS

In the trauma patient, specific body areas should be evaluated first. Findings will lead the nurse to the systems that need further assessment.

## Head

Because a trauma patient is always assumed to have a spinal injury until it is ruled out by the physician, patients with blunt trauma are transported on a backboard with a Philadelphia collar in place. The head should not be turned or lifted. Observe for lacerations, discoloration, swelling or other signs of injury. Gently palpate for swelling, indentation or other irregularities. Where does the patient describe pain or tenderness? What is the quality of the pain? Is there obvious bleeding or drainage from the surface of the face or head, nose, eyes, ears or mouth? Blood loss from the scalp may not be serious but look dramatic. Do not force open swollen or lacerated eyelids. Do not apply pressure to lacerations of the eyelids; there may be damage to the eye that cannot be seen. Check for damage in the mouth, loose teeth, bleeding, and emesis. Listen to the airway again to ensure that it is patent. Don't try to remove a hairpiece; it may be glued to the scalp. Chapter 5 details management of head trauma.

## Neck

Look for any disfiguring signs. The trachea should be midline. Can the patient speak without physical difficulty? Is there any problem with swallowing? Carotid pulses should be strong and equal on both sides of the neck. Chapter 6 details maxillofacial and neck trauma.

## Chest

Breath sounds should be equal bilaterally. Observe the symmetry of the chest and how it rises and falls with respiration. Palpate for chest expansion, pain, and clavicle or rib fractures. Chapter 9 details chest trauma.

## Abdomen

Observe for discoloration, distortion, or distention. Palpate gently for tenderness or pain. There may be internal injuries. If there is distention or pain, observe for shock and signs of hemorrhage. Signs of hemorrhage require immediate medical attention. Chapter 10 details abdominal trauma.

## Extremities

Obvious deformities indicate a fracture. Identify any break in the skin, especially over a fracture. Compare each extremity with its opposite. Check for distal pulses, equal temperature, discoloration, swelling, numbness and pain. How well does each limb move independently? Do not force movement or try to straighten a limb. Placing a hand on each side of the pelvis and applying pressure will indicate possible fracture if there is pain. Numbness in the hands or toes or lack of sensation in the absence of obvious deformity may indicate a spinal cord injury. Can the patient wiggle his fingers and toes? A conscious and alert patient who cannot move the arms or legs indicates a spinal injury. Be sure to watch the respirations if a spinal cord injury seems likely. Chapter 8 details spinal trauma, and Chapter 13 details orthopedic trauma.

Various trauma scores are used as tools to estimate the severity of injury. For instance, the Champion Sacco Trauma Score *(see Figure 2-1)* grades the patient in terms of cardiopulmonary and neurologic functions. Four categories are totaled to indicate where the patient is on an impairment range in order to help determine the order of care and transport, the level of care needed and for prehospital triage.

The Glasgow Coma Scale (GCS) is used as a standardized objective measurement of neurological function. Painful stimuli may need to be used if the patient does not respond to verbal commands. Numerical values are given to clinical findings that identifies a baseline and then tracks changes in the patient's status. GCS scores are not used by themselves but in conjunction with other clinical assessment findings.

Specific system assessment will be discussed in the chapters discussing the trauma management for that system.

# TRIAGE

Triage is the French word for "sorting." In the emergency medical services system, triage is synonymous with assessment and sorting the patient by the severity of illness or injury. The process is used to make sure the patient is in the right place within the right amount of time. Triage is used in a variety of situations: during mass casualties or disasters, in military operations, before prehospital transport to direct the patient to the proper level hospital, and at the entry point to the emergency department.

The main purpose of an effective triage system is rapid identification of patients with acute, life-threatening conditions. Additional goals include determining the level of care needs for all patients and regulating the patient flow through the emergency department. The patients are not seen in order of appearance but in order of severity of need.

# FIGURE 2-1 *(1 of 2)*
## The Champion Sacco Trauma Score

# THE CHAMPION SACCO TRAUMA SCORE

The Trauma Score is used to give each injured patient a numerical score that can be used to estimate the severity of injury. The patient is graded in terms of cardiopulmonary and neurologic functions. Each category receives a numerical score. A high number indicates normal function, while a low number signifies impaired function. The numbers are totaled to give a Trauma Score. The lowest possible score is 1 (severe impairment). The highest possible score is 16 (normal for all categories).

The use of the Trauma Score can help to determine the order of care and transport, the level of care required, and if transport to a special facility is needed.

Each patient should be scored during the initial assessment and each time that vital signs are taken.

The following is based on the Trauma Score developed by Champion and Sacco. For additional information, see: Champion HR, Sacco WJ, Carnazzo AJ, et al: Trauma Score. *Critical Care Medicine* 9 (9): 672-676, 1981. Note that variations of this procedure have been adopted by some EMS Systems.

WARNING: Follow local guidelines if you are allowed to apply painful stimuli to a patient. Your local protocol should include what actions you may take when the mechanism of injury or state of consciousness indicates possible spinal injury.

## TRAUMA SCORE

| Respiratory Rate | 10-24/min | 4 |
| | 24-35/min | 3 |
| | 36/min or greater | 2 |
| | 1-9/min | 1 |
| | None | 0 |
| Respiratory Expansion | Normal | 1 |
| | Retractive | 0 |
| Systolic Blood Pressure | 90 mmHg or greater | 4 |
| | 70-89 mmHg | 3 |
| | 50-69 mmHg | 2 |
| | 0-49 mmHg | 1 |
| | No Pulse | 0 |
| Capillary Refill | Normal | 2 |
| | Delayed | 1 |
| | None | 0 |
| **Cardiopulmonary Assessment** | | |

## GLASGOW COMA SCALE

| Eye Opening | Spontaneous | 4 |
| | To Voice | 3 |
| | To Pain | 2 |
| | None | 1 |
| Verbal Response | Oriented | 5 |
| | Confused | 4 |
| | Inappropriate Words | 3 |
| | Incomprehensible Words | 2 |
| | None | 1 |
| Motor Response | Obeys Command | 6 |
| | Localizes Pain | 5 |
| | Withdraw (pain) | 4 |
| | Flexion (pain) | 3 |
| | Extension (pain) | 2 |
| | None | 1 |
| **Glasgow Coma Score Total** | | |

### TOTAL GLASGOW COMA SCALE POINTS

| | |
|---|---|
| 14 – 15 = 5 | |
| 11 – 13 = 4 | CONVERSION = |
| 8 – 10 = 3 | APPROXIMATELY |
| 5 – 7 = 2 | ONE-THIRD |
| 3 – 4 = 1 | TOTAL VALUE |

**Neurologic Assessment**

**Total Trauma Score = Cardiopulmonary + Neurologic**

*Reprinted by permission from* Grant, H. D., Murray, R. H., Jr., & Bergeron, J. D. (Eds.). *Brady Emergency Care* (5th ed.). Englewood Cliffs, NJ: Prentice-Hall, 1990.

# FIGURE 2-1 *(2 of 2)*
# The Champion Sacco Trauma Score

# TRAUMA SCORE CONTINUED

## SCORING THE PATIENT

There are four elements to the cardiopulmonary assessment. The numerical values are added together to produce a cardiopulmonary score.

There are three elements to the neurological assessment. These are derived from the Glasgow Coma Score. Each category of the Glasgow Coma Score is given a numerical value. These numerical values are added together to produce a subtotal. This number is then reduced by approximately one-third its value to produce the neurologic assessment score.

The cardiopulmonary assessment and the neurologic assessment scores are added together to give the Trauma Score.

For example, a patient has a respiratory rate of 30 breaths per minute (3), retractive chest movements (0), a systolic blood pressure of 80 mmHg (3), and delayed capillary refill (1). The total score for cardiopulmonary function is 3+0+3+1=7.

This same patient shows no eye opening (1), no verbal response (1), and an extension reaction to pain (2). Added together, the total is 4. Approximately one-third of this number is 1. The cardiopulmonary and neurologic scores are added together (7+1) to give a Trauma Score of 8.

## TRAUMA SCORE DEFINITIONS

### RESPIRATION RATE
The number of respirations (1 inspiration and 1 expiration) in 30 seconds, multiplied by two.

### RESPIRATION EXPANSION
NORMAL — clearly visible chest wall movements that are associated with breathing.
RETRACTIVE — the use of accessory muscles (neck and abdominal muscles) to assist with breathing.

### SYSTOLIC BLOOD PRESSURE
The systolic pressure recorded by auscultation or palpation (see pages 60-61).

### CAPILLARY REFILL
This is determined by pressing a nail bed, the skin on the forehead, or the lining of the mouth (oral mucosa) until there is a loss of normal color (blanching or turning white). The pressure is released and the time for color return is measured. Normal return of color will take place in approximately two seconds (about the time it takes to say to yourself, "capillary refill").
NORMAL REFILL — the color returns within two seconds.
DELAYED REFILL — the color returns sometime after two seconds.
NONE — there is no indication of capillary refill.

## GLASGOW COMA SCALE DEFINITIONS

### EYE OPENING
This test is valid only if there is no injury or swelling that prevents the patient from opening the eyes.
SPONTANEOUS — the patient opens his or her eyes without any stimulation.
TO VOICE — the patient will open his or her eyes in response to your request. Say, "Open your eyes." If the patient's eyes remain unopened, shout the command.
TO PAIN — if the patient does not open his or her eyes in response to your voice command, pinch the back of his or her hand or the skin at the ankles (apply the stimulus to an uninjured limb).

### VERBAL RESPONSE
ORIENTED — an aroused patient should be able to tell you his or her name, where he or she is, and the date in terms of the year and month.
CONFUSED — the patient cannot give accurate responses, but he or she is able to say phrases or sentences and perhaps take part in a conversation.
INAPPROPRIATE WORDS — the patient says one or several inappropriate words, usually in response to a physical stimulus. Often, the patient will curse or call for a specific person. This may happen without any stimulus.
INCOMPREHENSIBLE SOUNDS — the patient mumbles, groans, or moans in response to stimuli.
NO VERBAL RESPONSE — repeated stimulation will not cause the patient to make any sounds.

### MOTOR RESPONSE
OBEYS COMMANDS — this is limited by the apparent nature of the patient's injuries and the injuries that can be associated with the mechanism of injury. The patient is asked to perform a simple task such as moving a specific finger or holding up two fingers.

If the patient does not carry out the command, painful stimuli can be utilized by applying firm pressure to an uninjured nail bed for five seconds or pinching the skin on the back of an uninjured hand or at an uninjured ankle.

LOCALIZES PAIN — the patient reaches to the source of the pain. Often, the patient will try to remove your hand from the pain site.
WITHDRAWS — the patient moves the limb rapidly away from the source of the pain. The arm may be moved away from the trunk.
FLEXION — the patient slowly bends the joint (elbow or knee) in an attempt to move away from the pain. The forearm and hand may be held against the trunk.
EXTENSION — the patient will straighten a limb in an effort to escape the pain. The movement appears slow and "stiff." There may be an internal rotation of the shoulder and forearm.
NONE — the patient does not respond to the repeated application of the stimulus.

NOTE: A special thanks is given to the people at Emergency Health Services, Department of Health, Commonwealth of Pennsylvania for their help in supplying information for this figure.

Primary functions in triage are assessment of the patient, which includes obtaining a brief history; identifying current medications; and conducting a physical assessment including vital signs.

Emergency department triage systems vary greatly. In 1982, Thompson and Dains identified the three most common triage systems. They included Type I, traffic director; Type II, spot checker; and Type III, comprehensive. The comprehensive system may be a single-tiered system where the nurse who has the first contact with the patient conducts the triage assessment, documents the findings, assigns triage acuity and designates the treatment area. This process does not make the patient feel rushed and the nurse has an opportunity to establish rapport. Triage protocols and some interventions are often begun in the triage area. Large-volume EDs may need more than one nurse in the triage area.

Some large EDs use a multitiered system to rapidly identify the patients with high severity and expedite flow. The first triage nurse sees each patient and does a rapid assessment to verify the chief complaint and determine if there is immediate threat to life, limb or vision. A brief interview, visual observation, and tactile examination of the skin and pulse determines acuity. If the patient does not require immediate attention, a chart is completed and the patient is sent to the second tier. Second-tier triage conduct the patient interview, measure vital signs, and, if necessary, initiate triage protocols. With a multitiered system one nurse's time is not taken up with a comprehensive assessment. The nurse is also able to see everyone who enters the area and immediately identify anyone appearing acutely ill or injured (Newberry, 1998).

Regardless of the system used for triage, the nurse should have immediate visual access of the patients entering but not be compromised as far as security of the area.

## Urgency

Patient acuity and the priority of care is identified by urgency categories. Specific criteria is used to classify patients into two or more categories. Most commonly used is the three-level system: Level 1: emergent and needs immediate attention; Level 2: urgent and should be seen within an hour, and Level 3: nonurgent and is seen when ED capability and accessibility permits. A comprehensive triage system uses four classifications.

## Triage Nursing

The triage nurse's function is important to identify if the patient is critically ill or injured, how soon he will be seen, and where in the ED he will be seen. An effective triage nurse must be skilled in rapid assessment and make accurate determinations of the patient's acuity. The triage area can rapidly become hectic with several patients demanding immediate attention at the same time, phone calls, and rescue units coming into the ED. Priorities must be set quickly and people-skills should be well developed.

# SUMMARY

The process of trauma nursing is complex and requires in-depth knowledge and skills. The trauma nurse needs to be efficient and organized because of the nature of the job. Traumatic injury is often a threat to life, limb or vision. Assessment and treatment can take place in many settings and is not limited to a major trauma center hospital. The evaluation of a patient is the critical point for setting the course for immediate and future action, and is a deciding factor in the outcome for the patient. Triage is the process of prioritizing patients to ensure they receive the most prompt and appropriate care. The triage system functions in varied areas such as mass casualties, prehospital and emergency department settings.

# EXAM QUESTIONS

## CHAPTER 2

### Questions 6–10

6. A function unique to trauma nursing is

   a. riding rescue units.

   b. triage.

   c. splinting fractures.

   d. telemetry.

7. Primary assessment is conducted

   a. by the physician.

   b. on all injured patients.

   c. to determine neurological damage.

   d. only in the emergency department.

8. All trauma patients are considered

   a. to need emergent care.

   b. to have kinetic injuries.

   c. to have injuries that can be a threat to life or limb.

   d. to have priority over medically ill patients in the emergency department.

9. Secondary assessment is conducted

   a. in multitiered triage.

   b. on patients who do not have a life-threatening condition.

   c. on patients being admitted to the inpatient unit.

   d. after the patient has received initial care.

10. Triage is considered

   a. a new concept in emergency care.

   b. necessary to assign priority of care to the injured.

   c. an integral part of managed health care.

   d. specifically designed for rescue units.

# CHAPTER 3

# AIRWAY MANAGEMENT

## CHAPTER OBJECTIVE

Upon completion of this chapter, the reader will be able to identify appropriate airway management techniques in the trauma patient.

## LEARNING OBJECTIVES

Upon completion of this chapter, the reader should be able to:

1. Describe the normal human airway and its physiology.

2. Describe the process of assessing the patency of a trauma patient's airway.

3. Identify the causes of the airway being unable to ventilate effectively.

4. Describe the techniques for opening and securing the airway.

5. Identify the differences between pediatric and adult airways.

## INTRODUCTION

Life is dependent upon continuous and adequate breathing. The body does not have any oxygen reserve. When respirations stop, the only oxygen available to the body is that which remains in the lungs and the bloodstream. The heart will soon arrest.

The purpose of respiratory support is to ensure and maintain an open airway, provide any necessary supplemental oxygen and institute positive-pressure ventilation when spontaneous breathing is not adequate or absent.

Management of the trauma patient begins with primary assessment, the ABCs of patient status. The patient's life may depend upon the organization and efficiency in the evaluation of the airway, breathing, circulation and neurologic care. Without sufficient oxygen to the brain, the patient will either have various degrees of brain damage or die.

For the patient breathing spontaneously, supplemental oxygen may prevent cardiac or respiratory arrest. While the patient can make spontaneous respiratory efforts, he may still have inadequate alveolar ventilation because of respiratory depression, fatigue, or obstruction from edema; displacement of the tongue or epiglottis; or a foreign body. For the patient who is not breathing, obstruction can be more difficult to recognize.

It is essential to understand the anatomy and physiology of the airway, how to rapidly and efficiently assess the airway in the trauma patient, know appropriate techniques to use for a particular kind of injury, and how to maintain the airway once it is established.

# BASIC ANATOMY AND PHYSIOLOGY OF THE AIRWAY

The airway is part of the respiratory system, which is made up of structures and organs enabling oxygen to circulate and feed the body's tissues. Normal gas exchange in the lungs depends upon adequate ventilation and perfusion. When the brain functions as it should, it triggers the cycle of inspiration to take in oxygen followed by expiration to rid the body of carbon dioxide waste. If there is head trauma, the breathing pattern may be disrupted or stopped altogether.

## Upper Airways

Upper airways include the nose, mouth, pharynx, and larynx. Their functions are to filter, humidify and warm inspired air and protect the lower airways from foreign objects. Structures include the tongue, hyoid bone, thyroid cartilage, epiglottis, and vocal cords.

Triangular shaped, mostly made of cartilage, the nose is the primary passage to direct air to the lungs. Inside, the lateral walls are formed by three bony projections, the turbinates. They increase the surface area to warm the air and can also hinder the insertion of nasal airways. The interior is very vascular and can bleed profusely with relatively little injury.

The mouth is used to take in food and air and communicate. Dentition functions by chewing. The tongue, which is attached to the floor of the mouth, is freely movable and aids in moving food to the back of the mouth and in speaking. (Chapter 6 discusses maxillofacial and neck injuries in detail.) The hyoid bone is U-shaped and attached to the root of the tongue but not to any bones, which possibly can contribute to airway obstruction.

The pharynx, or throat, channels air into the larynx. It is muscular and includes the nasopharynx, oropharynx and laryngopharynx. Located behind the nasal cavities, the nasopharynx extends from the posterior nares to the uvula. Adenoids and openings to the eustachian tubes are located here. The oropharynx extends downward from the uvula to the epiglottis and contains the palatine tonsils. Continuing down, the laryngopharynx extends from the epiglottis to the opening of the larynx. Constrictor muscles here send food or liquid into the esophagus and also produce the gag reflex when stimulated by the ninth cranial nerve. Opening into the larynx and esophagus, the pharynx may become obstructed with food, foreign bodies or fluids. Lying behind the trachea, the esophagus is a straight, collapsible tube extending from the pharynx to the stomach.

Between the pharynx and the upper end of the trachea is the larynx. Vocal cords at the opening of the trachea are folds of mucous membrane projecting into the larynx. They vibrate to make sound and can close spasmodically, causing laryngospasm or choking, a pulmonary defense mechanism. Closure of the larynx allows for the buildup of air under pressure in the lungs—a function necessary for coughing, another pulmonary defense mechanism. *Note:* Endotracheal intubation robs the patient of this defense, making the caregiver responsible for the protection of the lungs.

During swallowing, the lower airways are protected from foreign substances when the epiglottis closes over the glottis, an opening through the larynx to the lower airways. The epiglottis is a U-shaped piece of floppy mucosa-covered cartilage attached to the thyroid cartilage, also called the "Adam's apple." In unconscious or injured patients, the epiglottis can cover the opening to the trachea and obstruct the airway.

The trachea connects the larynx in the upper airway to the bronchi in the lower airway and is also called the "windpipe." It is the main passage to convey air to and from the lungs. Supported by C-shaped cartilage rings connected by a tough membrane, this is where an external opening can be made to ventilate the lungs when the airway above is obstructed. The trachea branches to the left and right forming the tracheobronchial tree. At the dividing point of the trachea is an important landmark called the carina.

## Lower Airways

Airways channel the air but do not take part in the actual gas exchange. The mainstem bronchi are formed immediately after the trachea divides into the tracheobronchial tree. It is important to remember that the right bronchus is wider and shorter and branches off from the trachea at a lesser angle than the left. Aspirated materials, endotracheal tubes and suction catheters are more likely to enter the right lung than the left.

This portion of the airway conducts air to and from the gas-exchange area of the lungs. During inspiration, the tracheobronchial tree and the lungs expand creating a negative pressure within. During expiration, the airways relax and return to their original size and pressure level.

The bronchial tree holds a residual volume of air that does not reach the lungs. Therefore, approximately 30% of each normal breath is "wasted" ventilation that cannot participate in the exchange of oxygen and carbon dioxide. Consequently, *not all of the air pushed into the patient during CPR can be used for gas exchange, which is one reason why correct compression and ventilation is so important.*

Many more divisions of airways in the bronchial tree end in the terminal or respiratory bronchioles. Beyond this point are 300 million alveoli, air cells within the lungs that are the only structures through which gas exchange occurs.

## Pediatrics

There are very specific anatomic and physiologic differences between the pediatric and adult airways.

In infants and small children, the upper and lower airways are smaller with less developed supporting cartilage, making it easy for mucus and edema to cause obstruction.

In the child, the oropharynx is comparatively small and easily obstructed by the relatively large tongue. The U-shaped epiglottis projects into the pharynx. Adenoids and tonsils are often enlarged. Vocal cords are short and concave. The larynx is easily collapsed if the head is hyperflexed or extended.

Breathing in young children is usually abdominal or diaphragmatic because poorly developed intercostal muscles are not able to move the chest wall adequately in the process of inspiration. During respiratory distress, diaphragmatic breathing and pliable ribs cause the chest wall to move inward or retract with inspiration. Retractions can be suprasternal, supraclavicular, infraclavicular, intercostal, or substernal. A child's chest wall is thin and conducts breath sounds, making assessment more difficult.

Crying children swallow air, causing abdominal distention, complicating respiratory assessment.

Ribs are pliable and do not support the lungs adequately. As a result, blunt trauma to the chest can easily cause pulmonary contusions rather than rib fractures. When there are fractured ribs, severe internal trauma should be suspected. Because the mediastinum is quite movable, there is considerable vulnerablility for great vessel damage from trauma.

Infants and children until age 8 have smaller and fewer alveoli than adults, thus having proportionately less pulmonary reserve. Faster metabolism than adults is accompanied by higher respiratory rates. Oxygen consumption rates are twice as high as in children as in adults. Respiratory failure can occur rapidly.

# INJURY AND OBSTRUCTION

Blunt or penetrating injuries can damage the airways. Direct trauma can cause laryngeal fracture or tracheal collapse. Specific types of maxillofacial and neck trauma are discussed in Chapter 6.

Early preventable deaths often result from delay in or lack of airway control. If any part of the airway is obstructed, immediate assessment and intervention is necessary.

**Remember to protect the cervical spine as the airway is being managed.** However, there should not be any delay in specific airway management due to concern about possible cervical injury (Peitzman, 1998).

The most common cause of airway obstruction in the unconscious patient is the tongue falling to the back of the throat, which obstructs air passage through the pharynx. Other causes are:

• Dentures, avulsed teeth, oral tissue, secretions and blood

• Bilateral mandibular fracture involving anterior attachments of the tongue, which allows posterior collapse of the tongue into the hypopharynx

• Expanding neck hematomas can cause deviation of the larynx and mechanical compression of the trachea

• Laryngeal trauma, such as thyroid cartilage or cricoid fractures can cause submucosal hemorrhage and edema

• Tracheal injury

# ASSESSMENT

For trauma patients, the loss of a patent airway is the most common reason for immediate cardiorespiratory arrest after the injury. Three factors can cause disruption of the airway:

• Occlusion by the tongue or epiglottis

— Loss of tone from central nervous system dysfunction caused by head trauma, hypoxia, stroke, or drugs

— Facial fracture

• Occlusion by a foreign body, particularly from blood, avulsed teeth, or soft tissue and emesis

• Direct traumatic disruption, such as laryngeal fracture or tracheal collapse

Accurate assessment, by looking, listening, and feeling, is essential. If you are with the injured person before rescuers arrive and another person is available, the second person can immobilize the patient's head. If no one else is available, stabilize the head and neck if possible, but not at the expense of delaying airway assessment and management. In rescue vehicle or hospital situations, staff and equipment are immediately available for head and neck stabilization.

## Look

Rapidly look over the entire patient. First note any obvious trauma, skin color and demeanor. A person without good oxygenation develops carbon dioxide buildup in his brain that causes agitation and restlessness. Stand or kneel at the patient's head and watch the chest for movement. The rib cage should rise and fall with each breath, with both sides moving together and with equal expansion. If the movement is unequal, do not rip off, but cut away the clothing so the chest can be visualized. Look for signs of trauma along with noting if there is any change in the chest movement.

## Listen

Leaning closely to the patient's face, listen for sounds of air passing in and out of the nose or mouth. Note any snoring or gurgling sounds that might indicate airway obstruction. If the patient is conscious and is hoarse, there may be damage to the laryngeal structure.

## Feel

Hold the palm of your hand near the nose and lips to feel for the flow of air. Then place palms lightly on each side of the chest over the ribs to determine if both sides are rising equally. Check for the integrity of the rib cage and fractures or displaced areas.

# AIRWAY MANAGEMENT AND STABILIZATION

Information presented here deals only with basic airway management techniques. Advanced methods require special training and certification.

No matter what level of airway management is used, the primary goal with any patient is to ensure that there is a patent airway. However, even if the airway is open, ventilation must be adequate and continuous. If the patient cannot ventilate spontaneously or adequately, it should be done mechanically to whatever extent is necessary.

## Basic Management Techniques

The patient should be supine; the head and neck stabilized with a rigid cervical Philadelphia collar, when available. If no collar is available, another person can stabilize the head and neck.

The 1997 *American Heart Association Advanced Cardiac Life Support Manual* provides the following information on airway management.

### Open the Airway

When there is acute airway obstruction from any cause, opening the airway has the highest priority. Upper airway obstruction in the unconscious person most commonly results from the loss of tone of the submandibular muscles, which directly support the tongue and indirectly support the epiglottis. Displacement of the tongue occludes the airway at the level of the pharynx. Displacement of the epiglottis may occlude the airway at the level of the larynx.

Wear gloves, if possible. Open the mouth and inspect the upper airway for blood or emesis. Use the fingers to sweep the mouth, check for loose or broken teeth or foreign objects. Placing the fingers too far back in the mouth will stimulate the gag reflex and cause the patient to bite down. If there are foreign objects present, remove them by using fingers covered with gauze or cloth. If it is necessary to turn the patient on his side to clear the mouth; pay attention to the stability of the spine and neck. When a rigid tonsil suction tip is available, suction the mouth. Do not use a flexible suction catheter, as it may enter the cranial vault in the patient with a skull fracture.

### Chin Lift Maneuver

**The chin lift method should be used in the conscious or unconscious patient with a suspected cervical spine injury, and it may be used instead of the jaw thrust.** This technique is excellent for relieving anatomical airway obstructions in patients who are breathing spontaneously.

Kneel at the level of the patient's shoulders. Use the fingers of the hand closest to the chest to support the lower jaw. Place these fingers under the bony portion of the chin. The fingertips should bring the chin forward, taking great care not to compress the soft tissue. Grasp the mandible, pulling gently up, which adjusts the displacement of the tongue, lifting it from the back of throat. This technique may be used by itself or with the head tilt maneuver.

### Jaw Thrust Maneuver

**This is the recommended procedure for use on unconscious patients with possible neck or spinal injuries.**

The jaw thrust requires sliding the lower jaw up. The tongue is connected to the floor of the mouth, the mandible. This maneuver may be enough to clear the airway.

To carry out the jaw thrust, kneel at the patient's head facing his feet, and rest your elbows on the same surface as the patient. Carefully reach forward and place one hand on each side of the chin and stabilize the patient's head with forearms. Push the jaw forward, and apply most of the pressure with the index fingers. **Do not tilt or rotate the head.** It may also be necessary to retract the lower lip with your thumb. The airway should open with this maneuver.

This technique should be used for patients who have cervical spine injuries and respiratory compromise. The jaw thrust maintains a neutral position of the cervical spine while resuscitation continues.

If the airway remains obstructed after the chin lift and jaw thrust maneuvers, then the head tilt may be added slowly and gently until the airway is open.

**These maneuvers should be attempted before any airway adjunct is used. If the patient is capable of breathing spontaneously, proper positioning may remedy the airway problem.**

In some cases, an oropharyngeal or nasopharyngeal airway is necessary to maintain airway patency.

### Head Tilt Maneuver

The basic maneuver for opening the airway is the head tilt. This technique may be used when spinal, neck, or head injury is *not* suspected. If these injuries are suspected, use the chin lift or jaw thrust technique. However, all unconscious patients should be treated as though they have a spinal injury.

The most efficient position for the single rescuer is to kneel at the level of the shoulders. The head-tilt procedure is a simple repositioning of the head. If the patient is conscious and seated, lift the

head so it does not flex forward on the chest. When the conscious patient is lying down, place your hand nearest to the top of his head on the forehead. Use the palm of the hand to apply gentle, firm, backward pressure to tilt the head. The fingers of the hand closest to the patient's chest support the lower jaw. Place these fingers under the chin against the bony part of the jaw, not into the soft tissue under the chin.

To open the airway, try to lift the tongue away from the back of the throat. Check to ensure there is adequate air exchange by positioning your head close to the patient's face and then *Look, Listen, and Feel.*

If this is not successful, use the jaw thrust or chin lift technique to raise the epiglottis away from where it may be obstructing the trachea.

### Head Tilt-Chin Lift Maneuver

This maneuver should not be used with patients who have a suspected neck or spinal injury.

The head tilt-chin lift provides maximum opening of the airway and may be used on conscious or unconscious patients needing breathing assistance. It is one of the best methods for clearing obstruction by the tongue and works well for people with loose dentures.

Kneeling at the patient's shoulders, place the palm of the hand closest to the top of the head on the forehead. Apply gentle, firm backward pressure on the forehead to tilt the head. At the same time, place the fingers of the other hand under the jaw at the chin's bony portion, not compressing the soft tissue. Use the fingertips to lift the chin, moving it forward to a point where the lower teeth are nearly touching the upper teeth while supporting the lower jaw, which also helps to tilt the head. The mouth should *not* be completely closed. To maintain an adequate opening of the mouth, it may be necessary to pull back the lower lip. Keep the thumb out of the mouth.

Most of the head tilt occurs from the gentle pressure on the forehead, being sure to apply the pressure backward, not by pushing down on the forehead.

## Mechanical Methods For Airway Control (Airway Adjuncts)

When basic manual techniques do not clear the airway, a mechanical airway is used in the unconscious or semiconscious patient. Specific training is necessary for professionals to be able to properly place these airways.

Some devices used for maintaining an open airway are an oropharyngeal airway, nasopharyngeal airway, esophageal obturator airway (EOA) and endotracheal (ET) tube. Some are more effective than others, because they separate the trachea from the esophagus.

### Oropharyngeal Airway

Probably the most commonly used airway, the oropharyngeal device holds the tongue forward in order to maintain an open airway while ventilating a nonbreathing or unconscious patient who has no gag reflex.

Care should be taken when inserting the airway not to push the tongue into the pharynx and further obstruct the airway. Complications include vomiting and aspiration when the gag reflex is present. This airway is not beneficial in laryngectomy patients.

### Nasopharyngeal Airway

The main advantage of this airway is that it is usually well tolerated by patients who have a gag reflex. If there is resistance in one nostril, the other can be used. Do not use if there is excessive resistance on insertion.

A possible complication is nasal trauma, and in a few patients, the airway will trigger the gag reflex. This airway is also not beneficial in laryngectomy patients.

### Esophageal Obturator Airway (EOA)

EOAs should only be used in unconscious apneic patients without gag reflexes, particularly those with spinal cord injuries.

Complications involve unrecognized misplacement into the trachea, pharyngeal and esophageal perforations, and severe vomiting when the device is removed. These airways are contraindicated in patients with known esophageal disease, severe facial injuries, and those who have ingested caustic agents. EOAs are not beneficial in laryngectomy patients or children.

### Endotracheal Airway

Endotracheal intubation is the most desirable way to control the airway in an unconscious patient and is an advanced technique. In trauma patients without a gag reflex, either an oral or a "blind" nasal route can be used. This maneuver is contraindicated in cervical injuries.

Complications include unrecognized intubation of the esophagus, and insertion too far, becoming lodged in the right mainstem bronchus and only ventilating the right lung. Auscultation of the chest and epigastrium must be done immediately after intubation to verify adequate and bilateral breath sounds.

### Surgical Airways

Severe head or maxillofacial trauma can make securing the airway impossible or contraindicated.

Air flow is established via an invasive procedure. Needle cricothyroidotomy uses a large-bore 14-gauge plastic intravenous catheter that is inserted through the membrane between the cricoid and the thyroid cartilages. The procedure uses a high-flow, high-pressure jet principle of oxygen delivery. The needle is removed, leaving the catheter in place, which is connected to a jet ventilation device.

# NURSING STRATEGIES

In most cases, the nurse has the ability to open and maintain the patient's airway, using only basic trauma nursing skills. The nursing focus is opening and maintaining the airway within the scope of training and skills. Some relevant nursing strategies for the trauma patient with airway compromise include identifying:

* Inadequate airway clearance related to obstruction or injury

* Unstable breathing patterns related to airway trauma

* Alteration of oxygen levels related to gas exchange impairment or decreased blood pressure

* High risk of aspiration related to decreased level of consciousness

# SUMMARY

The airway is the part of the respiratory system that channels the air to the gas exchange areas of the lungs. When trauma or obstruction prevents the gas exchange, sufficient oxygen cannot circulate to the brain and the body, causing either severe damage or death. No place in the body stores extra oxygen.

Early preventable deaths often result from delay in or lack of correct airway management. Even though the patient can make spontaneous respiratory efforts, he still may have inadequate gas exchange.

Blunt and penetrating injuries can damage the airways, but the most common cause of an ineffective airway is obstruction. The most common cause of obstruction in the unconscious patient is the tongue falling to the back of the throat and obstructing the pharynx.

Assessment must be accurate. It should be assumed that every unconscious patient has a cervical spine injury until cleared by the physician. The cervical spine should be stabilized, but not at the expense of a delay in ensuring a patent airway with adequate ventilation. The "Look, Listen, and Feel," process gives a rapid assessment of the patient's airway and injuries.

Before any trauma stabilization is initiated, the airway must be open and able to ventilate effectively.

# EXAM QUESTIONS

## CHAPTER 3
### Questions 11–15

11. The most common cause for the unconscious patient to have inadequate ventilation is

    a. tracheal collapse.

    b. maxillofacial trauma.

    c. obstruction from the tongue.

    d. foreign body obstruction in the pharynx.

12. For trauma patients, the loss of a patent airway is the most common reason for immediate

    a. unconsciousness.

    b. cardiopulmonary arrest.

    c. snoring.

    d. aspiration.

13. Management of the trauma patient begins with

    a. calling 911.

    b. immobilizing the cervical spine.

    c. immobilizing the injury.

    d. Look, Listen and Feel.

14. The recommended airway technique for use on unconscious patients with a possible neck or spinal injury is

    a. head tilt.

    b. chin immobilization.

    c. oropharyngeal airway.

    d. jaw thrust.

15. Where is the body's oxygen reserve located?

    a. There is no reserve

    b. The alveoli

    c. Tracheobronchial tree

    d. The lower airway

# CHAPTER 4

# SHOCK AND CARDIAC ARREST

## CHAPTER OBJECTIVE

Upon completion of this chapter, the reader will be able to describe the principles of managing shock and cardiac arrest.

## LEARNING OBJECTIVES

Upon completion of this chapter the reader should be able to:

1. Describe what a body system is and the purpose of the circulatory system.

2. Describe three factors involved in hemodynamic balance.

3. Relate the causes of inadequate perfusion to shock.

4. Recognize at least three major types of shock and their consequences.

5. Identify at least three causes of cardiac arrest in the trauma patient.

## INTRODUCTION

The body performs many complicated functions. One of the most essential is keeping its internal environment constant, which is known as homeostasis.

The body's means for balancing fluids, chemistry, and physical properties is sensitive. The controlling mechanisms work within narrow limits, affecting functions such as dilation and constriction of blood vessels; metabolism; body temperature; concentration of chemicals and waste products; and levels of acids, oxygen, carbon dioxide and electrolytes.

Usually, the body automatically responds to disturbances in its balance. If the adjustments fail or are inadequate, however, problems occur.

A body system is a group of organs having specific functions. All the systems have their own functions but are also interrelated in what they do. Understanding the different systems' functions is important when trying to determine the extent of injury or the nature of a medical emergency.

The circulatory system comprises the heart and blood vessels. Its purpose is to move blood, carry oxygen and nutrition to the body's cells and tissues, and remove waste.

Other systems include the respiratory, digestive, urinary, reproductive, nervous, special senses, endocrine, musculoskeletal, integumentary and the immune system.

## SHOCK

Shock is a clinical syndrome, a series of reactions to mental or physical upset of the body's internal balance. It is a group of signs and symptoms related to changes in a patient's condition. Sudden emotional or physical trauma, allergic reaction, poisoning, infection, dehydration, myocardial infarction, hemorrhage and reaction to drugs can cause shock.

Because there are so many causes of shock, it is usually described by which essential component is affected:

**Hypovolemic:** An alteration in circulating volume, consisting of either fluid loss or redistribution

**Cardiogenic:** A loss of ventricular effectiveness, contractility or decreased cardiac output

**Distributive or vasogenic:** Overall reduction in systemic vascular resistance (SVR) and vasodilation. Blood volume is normal, but the circulating volume is decreased by massive vasodilation and decreased SVR. Three types are

- Neurogenic
- Septic
- Anaphylactic

**Obstructive or flow obstruction:** An obstruction decreases circulating volume by preventing the myocardium from mechanically emptying during systole or filling during diastole.

**Other Types of Shock**

- Metabolic
- Psychogenic

## Physiology

One control for keeping the internal environment constant is hemodynamic balance (the forces involved in circulating blood through the body). Normal circulation and cellular perfusion occur when the "cardiovascular triad" is functioning properly. The triad includes heart rate, cardiac pumping action/output and circulating blood volume/vascular resistance. Alteration to any one of these factors affects cellular perfusion and oxygenation *(see Table 4-1).* Think of rate, pumping and volume.

The heart pumps to circulate oxygenated blood to all of the body's cells and tissues and remove the waste products. Every part of the body and every tissue does not receive the same blood supply all the time.

The heart, brain, central nervous system, lungs and kidneys are basic to life, requiring a constant supply of blood or their tissues die. Normally, the body contains just enough blood to fill the entire system of the heart and blood vessels, which in a 150-pound adult is about 6 liters. Adequate perfusion means there is enough circulation of blood within an organ or tissue to keep it alive and healthy. Any condition causing inadequate exchange of nutrition and oxygen for waste products in every part of the body sets up a situation for shock.

While there are many causes for shock, a specific hemodynamic problem can induce shock in three ways: rate, pumping or volume, and each one affects the other. Shock is seen when a situation prevents the heart from performing proper pumping action, loss of blood or other bodily fluids; or dehydration resulting in insufficient volume for perfusion. It is also seen when the amount of blood being pooled or shunted away from central circulation is great enough to prevent adequate filling of the system.

In each situation, the results are the same—the internal environment loses its relative balance and the body does not have enough nutrients brought to the tissues and waste carried away. All local bodily processes are affected.

## Recognizing Shock

Sometimes, in a prehospital situation, shock can have such a rapid onset that the patient is in critical condition before emergency responders can arrive on the scene. Other times, shock can sneak up on the patient while basic assessment and care is being initiated.

## TABLE 4-1
## The Cardiovascular Triad

| Rate Problems | Pump Problems | Volume (Includes Vascular Resistance) Problems |
|---|---|---|
| *Too slow* | *Primary* | *Volume loss* |
| • Sinus bradycardia | • Myocardial infarction | • Hemorrhage |
| • Type I and II second-degree heart block | • Cardiomyopathies | • Gastrointestinal loss |
| • Third-degree heart block | • Myocarditis | • Renal losses |
| • Pacemaker failures | • Ruptured chordae | • Insensible losses |
| | • Acute papillary muscle dysfunction | • Adrenal insufficiency (aldosterone) |
| | • Acute aortic insufficiency | |
| | • Prosthetic valve dysfunction | |
| | • Ruptured intraventricular septum | |
| *Too fast* | *Secondary* | *Vascular resistance* (Vasodilatation or redistribution): |
| • Sinus tachycardia | • Drugs that alter function | • Central nervous system injury |
| • Atrial flutter | • Cardiac tamponade | • Spinal injury |
| • Atrial fibrillation | • Pulmonary embolus | • Third space loss |
| • PSVT | • Atrial myxomata | • Adrenal insufficiency (cortisol) |
| • Ventricular tachycardia | • Superior vena cava syndrome | • Sepsis |
| | | • Drugs that alter tone |

Reproduced with permission. *Advanced cardiac life support,* 1997. Copyright American Heart Association.

Never assume that an apparently stable patient is not likely to go into shock. Signs and symptoms usually develop in a specific order, but not all are present at the same time. In most cases, the following order of events occurs:

• The patient becomes restless or combative. Anxiety is apparent while the body is trying to adjust to the onset of shock. The patient appears fearful and has a feeling of impending doom.

• Pulse pressure narrows. The pulse pressure is the difference between the systolic and diastolic pressures. For instance, in the case of hemorrhage, the pressure narrows as the body tries to maintain organ perfusion by increasing the diastolic pressure.

• Pulse rate increases. The heart pumps increasingly faster as the body attempts to compensate for the loss of blood, plasma and/or other fluids or other conditions of inefficient circulation. Unlike the rapid pulse seen in patients experiencing stress and fear, this rate will not slow and may rise significantly when the patient is standing or sitting. Tachycardia develops as the result of the body's effort to meet oxygen and perfusion needs. *Note:* As severe shock progresses and hypoxia develops, the heart rate will begin to slow and eventually stop. Bradycardia in a hypoxic shock patient is a critical warning sign.

• Respirations usually increase. When shock is developing, perfusion throughout the body is diminished, causing decreased oxygenation and an increase in carbon dioxide. If the airway is patent and other injuries have not caused changes in the respiratory drive that originates in the brain, tachypnea develops to combat the imbalance in oxygen and carbon dioxide.

- Capillary refill time increases. The skin becomes pale, appears ashen, and feels cool and moist to the touch. Lips, nail beds and oral membranes become cyanotic. Eventually, diaphoresis occurs while the skin feels cool.

- Thirst, weakness and nausea often occur.

- Hypotension does not occur initially but happens later in shock development as an indication the body cannot compensate or as a response to blood loss.

- Circulatory failure increases, and it becomes increasingly more difficult for the body to compensate. Consequently, the pulse becomes more rapid, weak and thready, and the respirations become increasingly labored and weak.

- Inadequate brain perfusion causes changes in the level of consciousness, which may be continuous or intermittent. Signs may be confusion, disorientation, lethargy or unconsciousness. As the oxygen decreases and carbon dioxide increases in the brain, the patient may become combative.

Other responses may also occur:

- Vasoconstriction: Blood vessels supplying the skin, muscles and internal organs begin to constrict in order to increase central blood flow and divert it to the heart, brain and kidneys.

- Changes in cardiac output: Output may rise at first because of stimulation from stress, but cardiac output inevitably falls as blood volume falls.

- Oliguria: Occurs in advanced shock when the kidneys succumb to inadequate perfusion.

- Metabolic changes: Occur when the cells and tissues do not receive enough oxygen and shift to anaerobic metabolism. This shift increases the production of lactic acid, which can lead to

metabolic acidosis and eventually death if not corrected.

# TYPES, ASSESSMENT AND MANAGEMENT OF SHOCK

## Hypovolemic (Low Volume) Shock

Hypovolemic shock is a hemodynamic problem of body fluid loss or redistribution resulting in insufficient volume for perfusion.

Hypovolemic shock triggered by fluid or blood loss, such as burns or crush injuries, is also known as hemorrhagic shock and is the most common type of shock seen in trauma patients. Other causes are dehydration from vomiting, diarrhea, profuse sweating, peritonitis, or pancreatitis. Bone fractures, especially pelvic and long bones, can cause significant blood loss from crushing and tearing blood vessels and tissues.

### Class I

Hemorrhage with a loss of up to 15% blood volume, about 750 ml. Most adults can lose this amount without showing signs or symptoms because the body is able to compensate adequately.

### Class II

Volume loss of 15–30%, about 1,500 ml. Signs and symptoms are increased heart and respiratory rates; narrowed pulse pressure; restlessness; anxiety; slow capillary refill; and pale, cool skin.

### Class III

Volume loss of 30–40%, about 2 liters in an adult male. Signs of inadequate perfusion are hypotension, tachycardia, tachypnea and an alteration in mental status.

### Class IV

Volume loss of greater than 40%, a critical situation where the patient is likely to die. The pulse is rapid, respirations shallow, skin cold and clammy,

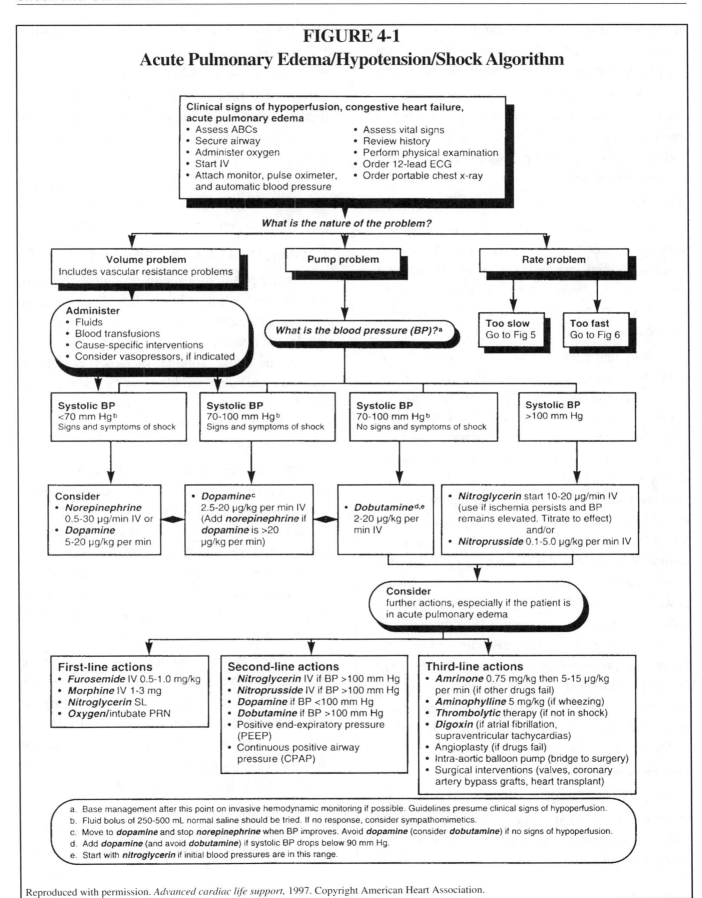

## FIGURE 4-1
## Acute Pulmonary Edema/Hypotension/Shock Algorithm

**Clinical signs of hypoperfusion, congestive heart failure, acute pulmonary edema**
- Assess ABCs
- Secure airway
- Administer oxygen
- Start IV
- Attach monitor, pulse oximeter, and automatic blood pressure
- Assess vital signs
- Review history
- Perform physical examination
- Order 12-lead ECG
- Order portable chest x-ray

*What is the nature of the problem?*

**Volume problem**
Includes vascular resistance problems

**Pump problem**

**Rate problem**

**Administer**
- Fluids
- Blood transfusions
- Cause-specific interventions
- Consider vasopressors, if indicated

*What is the blood pressure (BP)?*[a]

**Too slow**
Go to Fig 5

**Too fast**
Go to Fig 6

**Systolic BP**
<70 mm Hg[b]
Signs and symptoms of shock

**Systolic BP**
70-100 mm Hg[b]
Signs and symptoms of shock

**Systolic BP**
70-100 mm Hg[b]
No signs and symptoms of shock

**Systolic BP**
>100 mm Hg

**Consider**
- *Norepinephrine* 0.5-30 µg/min IV or
- *Dopamine* 5-20 µg/kg per min

- *Dopamine*[c] 2.5-20 µg/kg per min IV (Add *norepinephrine* if *dopamine* is >20 µg/kg per min)

- *Dobutamine*[d,e] 2-20 µg/kg per min IV

- *Nitroglycerin* start 10-20 µg/min IV (use if ischemia persists and BP remains elevated. Titrate to effect) and/or
- *Nitroprusside* 0.1-5.0 µg/kg per min IV

**Consider**
further actions, especially if the patient is in acute pulmonary edema

**First-line actions**
- *Furosemide* IV 0.5-1.0 mg/kg
- *Morphine* IV 1-3 mg
- *Nitroglycerin* SL
- *Oxygen*/intubate PRN

**Second-line actions**
- *Nitroglycerin* IV if BP >100 mm Hg
- *Nitroprusside* IV if BP >100 mm Hg
- *Dopamine* if BP <100 mm Hg
- *Dobutamine* if BP >100 mm Hg
- Positive end-expiratory pressure (PEEP)
- Continuous positive airway pressure (CPAP)

**Third-line actions**
- *Amrinone* 0.75 mg/kg then 5-15 µg/kg per min (if other drugs fail)
- *Aminophylline* 5 mg/kg (if wheezing)
- *Thrombolytic* therapy (if not in shock)
- *Digoxin* (if atrial fibrillation, supraventricular tachycardias)
- Angioplasty (if drugs fail)
- Intra-aortic balloon pump (bridge to surgery)
- Surgical interventions (valves, coronary artery bypass grafts, heart transplant)

a. Base management after this point on invasive hemodynamic monitoring if possible. Guidelines presume clinical signs of hypoperfusion.
b. Fluid bolus of 250-500 mL normal saline should be tried. If no response, consider sympathomimetics.
c. Move to *dopamine* and stop *norepinephrine* when BP improves. Avoid *dopamine* (consider *dobutamine*) if no signs of hypoperfusion.
d. Add *dopamine* (and avoid *dobutamine*) if systolic BP drops below 90 mm Hg.
e. Start with *nitroglycerin* if initial blood pressures are in this range.

oliguria develops, and the patient may become comatose. The heart will slow and is likely to stop if rapid assessment and intervention does not occur.

Redistribution of blood, plasma or other body fluids from the intravascular compartment to the interstitial space due to changes in capillary permeability or capillary fluid pressures can also cause hypovolemic shock.

### Assessment

Internal hemorrhage is difficult to recognize, although occasionally blood flows from the mouth or anus. Nothing can be done outside the hospital environment to control internal bleeding. However, it is critical to recognize the situation and report it immediately.

When fluid volume is lost, less blood is able to return to the heart, decreasing cardiac output. In an attempt to compensate, the pulse rate increases. A good estimation is that if the pulse rate increases by more than 20 beats per minute when the patient is elevated from lying down to sitting, the volume deficit is approximately 1 unit of blood. A systolic pressure less than 70 mm Hg with a pulse greater than 130/minute indicates there may be as much as a 40% blood volume loss. When the blood pressure cannot be obtained in the arm, a rough guide is: if a carotid pulse can be felt, the systolic pressure is probably at least 60 mm Hg; if a femoral pulse is palpable, the systolic pressure is probably at least 70 mm Hg; and if a radial pulse can be felt, then the systolic pressure is probably at least 80 mm Hg. *Note:* Pulse rate and blood pressure alone may not give enough information for management decisions. The entire clinical picture must be looked at in determining patient care.

### Management

Hypovolemic shock requires volume replacement, usually normal saline or lactated Ringer's intravenous solutions. If there is massive hemorrhage with profound volume loss, more than one IV line with a large-bore needle running wide open is necessary.

Depending on local rescue protocols, the patient will probably arrive at the emergency department with pneumatic antishock garments. They provide the equivalent of an instant 2-to-4 unit transfusion.

Ensure that the patient does not aspirate any blood or vomit. The severely volume-depleted patient will require advanced life support skills.

## Cardiogenic (Low Output) Shock

Cardiogenic shock can be caused by any hemodynamic situation in which the heart is unable to work adequately. The heart fails to pump as it should, the rate decreases, and most likely, so does the cardiac stroke volume. Increased peripheral resistance puts more workload on the left ventricle, thereby raising its oxygen requirements. Even if the blood pressure elevates to nearly normal, the cardiac output remains low.

Trauma to the heart, such as a steering wheel contusion to the chest, may cause cardiogenic shock. However, there does not necessarily have to be specific damage to the heart itself for cardiogenic shock to occur. The cardiac output can decrease due to a malfunction of the heart, as in a myocardial infarction, cardiac arrhythmia, chronic progressive heart failure, pericardial tamponade or pulmonary emboli.

In a myocardial infarction, if the heart cannot increase its oxygen supply to meet the greater demand, the area of infarction may increase. If chronic obstructive pulmonary disease (COPD) is associated with this condition, oxygenation of the blood as it passes through the lungs may be more decreased, further aggravating the cardiogenic shock.

Although cardiogenic shock is not as common as hypovolemic shock in trauma patients, it should be considered when there is no evidence of blood loss but the patient shows evidence of shock.

### Assessment

Usually there are no injuries, but there may be chest pain. Blood volume loss does not occur. However, the physiologic effects are similar to those in hypovolemic shock. The pulse is often irregular and weak, blood pressure low. There may be jugular distention, which is almost always a sign of cardiogenic shock. Capillary bed refill response resembles vasogenic shock. Cyanosis is usually seen around the lips and nail beds and skin color may be pale and grey. Often there is difficulty breathing. There may be wheezing. Rales can be heard due to a backup of fluid the heart is unable to pump out of the lungs. The patient is often anxious and fearful.

### Management

Recognition of cardiogenic shock may be difficult, but it is absolutely necessary to identify and aggressively treat as soon as possible. Eighty to 100% of these patients will die. Quickly administer high-flow oxygen.

Unless there are traumatic injuries with volume loss, there is usually no requirement for fluid replacement, elevation of the legs, or pneumatic antishock garments. Some forms of cardiogenic shock can be managed with small boluses of fluid replacement, particularly in the case of right heart failure. **This is an advanced life support procedure.**

Positioning is important to make breathing easier and the patient more comfortable. The patient will tell you which position is the most comfortable. Frequent vital signs, monitoring cardiac rhythm, and maintaining body temperature should be carefully conducted and documented.

## Distributive or Vasogenic Shock

Distributive shock occurs when the volume is adequate and the cardiac function is normal but the distribution is impaired. Extreme vasodilation causes a maldistribution of intravascular volume to the circulatory network and interstitial spaces. There are three types of vasogenic shock: neurogenic, septic and anaphylactic.

### Neurogenic Shock

Neurogenic shock is a complex phenomenon. Fibers traveling from the brain stem's cardiovascular centers to the sympathetic centers (that accelerate the heart, constrict blood vessels and raise blood pressure) in the thoracolumbar spinal cord are interrupted. There is a loss of sympathetic responses, including cardiac stimulation and vasoconstriction, especially in large veins and arterioles. The sympathetic system is unable to react to the parasympathetic system's slowing of the heart rate and vasodilatation. Without control of vasodilatation, the blood vessel diameter becomes so large that there is not enough blood in the system to meet the expanded volume need. Hypotension develops. Additionally, vagus nerve (tenth cranial nerve) stimulation causes bradycardia. Cardiac output and blood pressure drop. When the blood pools in the extremities, the skin is pink and dry and there is a backup in the cardiovascular system. The pooling quickly creates hypothermia due to the radiation of peripheral heat.

While a head injury seldom causes shock, spinal cord injury and spinal anesthesia can produce neurologic shock. Neurologic and neurovascular diseases, including diabetes, may cause a loss of autonomic or involuntary nervous system control. Neurogenic shock can be transient and easily correctable in some forms, such as fainting and hypotension due to gastric distention.

### Assessment

The ABCs are important in assessing neurological damage. With a high cervical injury, the patient may not be breathing.

Immobilize the head manually, which ensures better observation and evaluation than a cervical collar. Look, listen and feel. Especially look for bradycardia, pink, warm and dry skin, which indicates poor cardiac output and peripheral pooling of blood.

Check for neurological deficits: equality of pupil size and reaction; level of consciousness; response to commands; and any flaccid paralysis, tingling, or numbness in the extremities. Observe for any absent reflexes or decreased mobility distal to the spinal injury. Suspect neurogenic shock in any trauma patient who has paralysis and who has hypotension without accompanying tachycardia. Note where there is tenderness and pain or absence of feeling. Observe for bladder or bowel dysfunction.

## Management

Clear and stabilize the airway and maintain sufficient ventilation. Give supplemental oxygen and assist ventilation, if necessary. The spine must be immobilized. Monitoring of vital signs, cardiac rhythm and level of consciousness should be done on a continuous basis.

### Septic Shock

The most common cause of septic shock is untreated infection. Signs of infection are warm and pink or ruddy skin, rather than cool and clammy. When patients have bacteria or bacterial toxins in the bloodstream, septic shock develops. Sepsis occurs when the body fights off infection, the bacteria die and endotoxins are released. The endotoxins interfere with cell metabolism, damaging the surrounding tissues. Histamine dilates the blood vessels, increasing pressure on the capillaries, causing them to leak outside the vascular space, producing edema and relative hypovolemia.

Unless treatment is delayed or the trauma causes contamination of the abdominal cavity from intrusion of the gastrointestinal system, septic shock is seldom a concern in the initial management of trauma patients.

## Assessment

Septic shock is subtle and may appear to just be nonemergent flu. Don't forget septic shock is a form of distributive shock. Early systemic infection signs, called the "warm stage," are when the patient has chills and fever; flushed, warm and moist skin; the pulse may be bounding and rapid; and the blood pressure normal or slightly hypotensive. This stage lasts from 30 minutes to 16 hours.

If septic shock is not recognized and treated, the "cool stage" may develop. Characteristics are tachypnea; tachycardia; pale, clammy and cool skin; normal or slightly decreased blood pressure; thirst; peripheral edema and congested lungs. These signs may be brief, followed by severe hypotension, thready pulse and respiratory failure. Toxic shock syndrome presents with fever; diffuse rash; systolic pressure below 90 mm Hg; and a scaling or loss of skin, particularly on the hands.

## Management

Ask for a specific illness history. Check circulatory status and give support oxygen. If breathing is not too difficult, keep the patient flat. Circulatory status, cardiac rhythm, vital signs, and level of consciousness should be frequently assessed and documented. Normal body temperature should be maintained. Intravenous fluids will be ordered if the patient is hypotensive.

### Anaphylactic Shock

Anaphylactic shock is the most severe type of allergic reaction, and may be life-threatening. What should be a normal protective response of the body to exposure to a foreign protein or drug, in anaphylaxis, becomes a profound allergic hypersensitive reaction.

Oddly, the reaction does not happen on the first contact with a potential antigen (a foreign element that causes the formation of antibodies, which are defender chemicals). On the first exposure, the antibodies form. Subsequent exposures to the antigen make the body overreact and go into anaphy-lactic shock.

A mild allergic reaction can become critical, even beyond 30 minutes after contact or ingestion. In such cases, prehospital care may truly be life-saving.

Common causes are insect stings; ingested substances including foods such as nuts, spices, berries, fish, and shellfish; inhaled substances including dust, pollens, and chemicals; injected antitoxins and drugs; and chemicals absorbed through the skin.

**Assessment**

Response to the antigen is rapid dilation of the blood vessels and hypotension. Tissue lining the respiratory tract may swell, obstruct the airway, and lead to respiratory failure. Symptoms include itching; burning skin, especially on the face, back, and chest; painful constriction in the chest with dif-ficult breathing; dizziness; restlessness and anxiety; nausea, abdominal cramping, or pain; vomiting and diarrhea; severe headache; and rarely, temporary loss of consciousness.

Careful interviewing is essential. Determine if the patient has any known allergies or has experi-enced a severe allergic reaction before. Find out if the patient has a "vial of life" or other prescribed medication for allergic reactions. Look for any type of medical-information devices.

Conduct the ABCs. The airway may be obstructed and there may be wheezing or respira-tory rales. Check the level of consciousness and look for restlessness or syncope. Note the blood pressure pattern; it may go from high and drop to shock level. Also note the pulse rate and quality; skin color; blotches, rashes, hives and swelling, particularly around the eyes, face, tongue, wrists and ankles. There may be cyanosis of the lips and paleness around the mouth and tongue.

**Management**

Keep the airway open and stable and maintain ventilation. CPR may be necessary. Provide basic shock care. Place the patient in a supine or semi-Fowler's position. Immediate action is necessary because anaphylactic shock can be life threatening.

## (Flow) Obstruction Shock

When the ejection of blood from the heart is impaired, so is the circulating volume, and flow obstruction shock may develop. The obstruction may be mechanical, or caused by compression of the great veins, pulmonary arteries, aorta, or the myocardium. When the obstruction interferes with the myocardium emptying during systole or filling during diastole, there is inadequate cardiac output and tissue is not perfused adequately.

Causes also may be pathologic changes such as embolism or heart disease. A pulmonary embolus that obstructs a large part of the pulmonary artery prevents the right ventricle from emptying. Incomplete right ventricular emptying causes decreased cardiac output, right ventricular failure and increased right atrial pressure. In the trauma patient, flow obstruction shock is most often caused by injuries such as cardiac tamponade (accumulation of excess fluid in the pericardium, resulting from pericarditis or injury to the heart or great blood vessels). Pericardial tamponade pre-vents atrial and ventricular filling during diastole.

The clinical picture varies, depending on the cause of the obstruction. Frequently seen is pain in the chest or back, dyspnea, tachypnea, tachycar-dia, profound hypotension, cyanosis, and diaphoresis. Management is aimed at resolution of the obstruction and support of the airway, breath-ing, and circulation.

## Other Types of Shock

### Metabolic Shock

Metabolic shock is frequently seen in patients who have been either ill for a long time or have experienced an extremely severe brief illness. Failure of the adrenal, thyroid or pituitary glands may also lead to metabolic shock. Excessive loss of fluid from vomiting, diarrhea and polyuria can cause dehydration and changes in body chemistry, including sodium and acid/base balance.

### Psychogenic Shock

Psychogenic shock is a nervous system reaction often caused by fear, upsetting news, the sight of something horrifying, blood or injury. Sudden dilation of the blood vessels causes momentary interruption of the blood flow to the brain and the patient experiences syncope. Usually the condition is brief and resolves quickly. However, if injury has also occurred or the patient remains confused, suspect a head injury.

# NURSING STRATEGIES FOR THE PATIENT IN SHOCK

Prevention can be as complex as the shock itself. Shock cannot be seen. It is a syndrome and has many indicators. Every tissue in the body must have adequate perfusion or it cannot survive.

The brain and spinal cord are damaged after 4 to 6 minutes without any blood supply, as are the kidneys after 45 minutes. Skeletal muscle and the gastrointestinal system can last for nearly 2 hours lacking blood supply without serious damage.

The best management for shock is prevention. Recognizing the probable causes of shock is critical to beginning appropriate treatment. Specific principles of initial treatment can be applied to all shock patients. The goal is to either replace or maintain enough blood in the system for adequate perfusion.

Prompt patient management must be appropriate and effective, or the patient may die.

The specific actions used may depend upon where the caregiver is located, prehospital or in the hospital.

- When there is doubt that the patient is in shock, after ensuring a clear airway and stabilizing the cervical spine, if the patient is unconscious, administer a high concentration of oxygen before doing anything else. Full ventilatory support should be given if necessary. If blood volume is down, oxygen may be lifesaving.

- Note the level of consciousness for the best indication of brain perfusion. If the patient is alert, he is adequately perfused. Agitation, restlessness, or combativeness may indicate the patient is hypoxic and perfusion is decreasing.

- Hypotension is when the systolic blood pressure is less than 90 mm Hg.

- Do not wait for the blood pressure to drop before shock is suspected and treated. Falling blood pressure is a late sign of shock, especially in patients over 55 and under 5 years of age. It signals the collapse of compensatory mechanisms, and the patient may be near death. Blood pressure in the arm only gives information about perfusion in the arm, not the vital organs.

- If a carotid pulse can be palpated, the systolic blood pressure is estimated to be at least 60 mm Hg; the femoral pulse, 70 mm Hg; the radial pulse, 80 mm Hg.

- If the patient has a distended or tender abdomen, fractured long bones in the arm or thigh, bleeding from body orifices, penetrating trauma of the torso, or hematemesis, it is best to assume that there is internal hemorrhage.

- Patients with hemorrhagic shock should have aggressive fluid resuscitation and early use of blood products.

- Active, obvious bleeding should be controlled by applying direct pressure (wearing gloves and using a sterile, dry dressing), elevation or using pressure points, splints, a blood pressure cuff or tourniquet. Do not remove any previously placed dressings as bleeding could exacerbate.

- Only use a tourniquet if trained to do so and it is absolutely necessary, such as with traumatic amputation. Never apply on the elbow or on the knee.

- Watch for bleeding from the mouth and vomiting. Prevent aspiration.

- Do not apply direct pressure to bleeding from an injured eye; it could cause loss of vision or the eye, itself.

- Prevent loss of body heat with a blanket over and under the patient, particularly if the patient is lying on the ground. However, if the patient has a suspected head, neck, or spine injury, do not attempt to put a blanket under him. Do not overheat the patient.

- Do not give the patient anything by mouth, including ice. Oxygen will make the patient's mouth dry but anything by mouth can cause vomiting.

- If the patient is not in the hospital, he should be immediately transported to the nearest facility that provides the appropriate level of care. If also indicated, and trained staff and equipment are available, a pneumatic antishock garment should be used.

# EXAMPLES OF NURSING DIAGNOSES RELATED TO SHOCK

- Potential fluid volume deficit related to trauma

- Impairment in tissue perfusion related to hypovolemia

- Decreased cardiac output related to hypovolemia

- Anxiety and fear related to decreased oxygen in the brain

- Anxiety and fear related to the hospital environment

- Impaired gas exchange related to inadequate perfusion

# BASIC CARDIOVASCULAR ANATOMY AND PHYSIOLOGY

## Heart

The heart *(Figure 4-2)* is a muscle with four chambers through which the body's blood is pumped. Between each chamber is a valve that prevents the backflow of blood as it is pumped through the heart.

Deoxygenated venous blood enters the right atrium through the inferior and superior vena cavae, flows into the right ventricle, and then the pulmonary artery. After the blood is oxygenated, it enters the left atrium through the pulmonary veins. The heart is the only place in the body where deoxygenated blood flows through an artery (the pulmonary artery) to pick up oxygen and the oxygenated blood returning from the lungs flows through veins (pulmonary veins). From the left ventricle, the blood is pumped into the body through the aorta and the arterial system. The heart muscle is perfused by the right and left coronary arteries. These arteries lie on the surface of the heart and fill during ventricular diastole, or relaxation.

A unique characteristic of the cardiac tissue is its intrinsic ability to initiate electrical activity. The heart has its own electrical conduction system that initiates its mechanical functioning, called systole and diastole. Systole is the contraction part of the heart cycle. Approximately 60% of the cardiac cycle is diastole, the period when the ventricles are filling, referred to as the relaxation period.

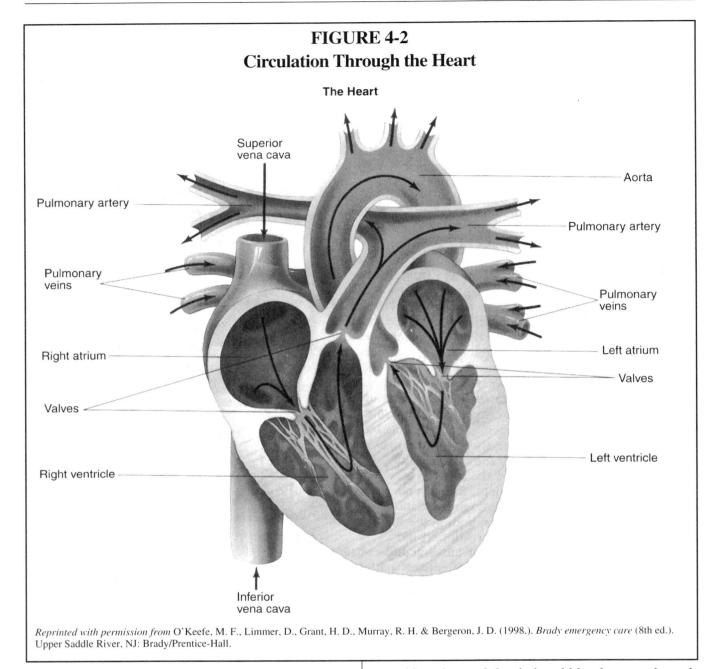

**FIGURE 4-2**
**Circulation Through the Heart**

*Reprinted with permission from O'Keefe, M. F., Limmer, D., Grant, H. D., Murray, R. H. & Bergeron, J. D. (1998.). Brady emergency care (8th ed.). Upper Saddle River, NJ: Brady/Prentice-Hall.*

## Vessels

Blood vessels carry the body's blood to and from the heart for the purpose of replenishing its oxygen supply and getting rid of waste products. The arteries convey bright red oxygenated blood from the heart through the body. Arterial blood pulsates because of the heart's pumping action. The arteries become progressively smaller, finally branching into microscopic capillaries, where the oxygen is given up to nourish the cells and tissues. The waste products of metabolism are accumulated at this point, and the dark red blood passes through more capillaries to the veins. The blood then flows back to the heart for circulation through the lungs to replenish the oxygen and release the carbon dioxide waste for elimination.

The blood vessels have the ability to constrict or dilate, depending upon physiological factors. The major vessels are:

• **Aorta,** or the great vessel, exits from the left ventricle of the heart, forms a large arch and

**TABLE 4-2**
**Blood Volumes**

| *Subject* | *Total Blood Volume* | *Lethal Blood Loss If Not Replaced (Rapid)* |
|---|---|---|
| Adult male (154 lb, 70 kg) | 5.0–6.6 L | 2.0 L |
| Adolescent (105 lb, 48 kg) | 3.3–4.5 L | 1.3 L |
| Child (early to late childhood; depends on size) | 1.5–2.0 L | 0.5–0.7 L |
| Infant (newborn, normal weight range) | 300+ ml | 30–50 ml |

*Note*: One liter equals about 2 pints. One milliliter is about the same as 20 drops from a medicine dropper.

*Reprinted with permission from* Grant, H. D., Murray, R. H., Jr. & Bergeron, J. D. (Eds.). (1990). *Brady emergency care* (5th ed.). Englewood Cliffs, NJ: Prentice-Hall.

then, as the descending aorta, travels down the length of the chest and torso. Just above the legs, the aorta divides to bring blood to the lower extremities. The upper extremities are supplied by three vessels exiting from the arch of the aorta.

- **Pulmonary artery** exits from the right ventricle of the heart to channel the venous blood returning from the body to the lungs for oxygenation.

- **Vena cavae:** The superior and inferior vena cavae enter right atrium, bringing the venous blood to the heart. The superior vena cava brings venous blood from the head and upper extremities and the inferior vena cava brings venous blood from the trunk and legs.

- **Pulmonary veins:** Four veins that carry oxygenated blood from the lungs to the left atrium. While they are not called the "great" vessels, they are essential to cardiovascular circulation.

## Lungs

Essential to life, the lungs are the major respiratory organ. It is here that the blood picks up oxygen that has been pulled in through inspiration and gets rid of carbon dioxide waste through expiration. Blood enters the lungs from the right ventricle through the pulmonary artery, which subdivides and becomes progressively smaller vessels until they reach the alveoli for gas exchange. There, carbon dioxide is removed from the blood, the oxygen is replenished and the blood returns to the left atrium in order to circulate through the body again.

## Blood

Blood is a suspension of red blood cells (erythrocytes), white blood cells (leukocytes), platelets and other particles in an aqueous colloid solution. Half the blood's volume is made up of straw-colored plasma liquid, which is where the exchange takes place between the fixed cells in the body and the external environment. Nutrients, including oxygen, are transported to the cells and tissues, while cellular waste such as nitrogen are removed. Other essential functions of the blood include regulation of pH, temperature, and cellular water; prevention of fluid loss through coagulation; and protection against toxins and microbes.

# INJURY, THE HEART AND CARDIAC ARREST

When a blunt or penetrating force strikes the body, that energy is absorbed and causes damage to the tissues. A consequence of the trauma can be shock, which results from the failure of the cardiovascular system to sufficiently nourish all the vital tissues of the body.

Hemorrhagic shock from blood loss due to injury may be obvious or initially not seen. Blunt trauma often causes internal bleeding that may be hard to detect and not as rapid as penetrating damage. Penetrating trauma that fractures bones or lacerates internal organs also may cause internal hemorrhage. The internal bleeding ranges from being minor, such as a bruise from a bump on the skin, to massive hemorrhage from internal organs, leading to death. **Early detection is critical and may not be related to being able to see the hemorrhage.**

Areas of internal hemorrhage include

- **Abdominal trauma:** The liver, spleen, or other abdominal organs can be severely damaged from blunt or penetrating trauma. Bleeding causes the abdomen to become distended and very tender. If not detected, the results may be fatal.

- **Aortic rupture:** If the aorta is torn, ruptures, or dissects, shock occurs rapidly, with death following in a matter of minutes. If immediately detected and the patient survives the initial injury long enough for stat access to an operating room, it is possible for the patient to survive.

- **Cardiac tamponade:** The heart is surrounded by a fibrous, fluid-filled sac called the pericardium. The fluid in the pericardium lubricates the heart and prevents friction when the heart contracts. Blunt or penetrating trauma may cause bleeding into the pericardial sac. When the excess fluid causes pressure that constricts the heart, it results in cardiac tamponade. A consequence may be pericarditis, injury to the heart or great vessels, or obstructive shock.

- **Myocardial contusion:** Blunt trauma, such as from a steering wheel, may bruise the heart to the point that it is unable to effectively contract, resulting in pump failure and shock.

- **Bone fracture:** When the femur, humerus or pelvis are fractured, considerable bleeding may occur at the site of the fracture. Up to 1 liter of blood can be lost from a fractured femur, even from a closed fracture with the skin intact. If both femurs are fractured at the same time, the blood loss may be life threatening.

# CONSIDERATIONS REGARDING RESUSCITATION

Professionals who deliver health care outside the hospital work under protocols defined by the system in which they work. Nurses working in the hospital setting take their direction from the physician or defined protocols. However, a nurse who comes upon a severely injured person in a trauma situation is not functioning under any protocols, and often must make decisions rapidly.

The American Heart Association in 1994 made the following suggestions regarding a trauma patient in cardiac arrest outside the hospital setting.

- Start resuscitative efforts when the patient appears to have a chance of survival.

- Do not attempt resuscitation of:

---

## FIGURE 4-3
## Causes of Cardiac Arrest Associated with Trauma

- Severe central neurologic injury with secondary cardiovascular collapse.

- Hypoxia resulting from neurologic injury, airway obstruction, large open pneumothorax, or severe tracheobronchial laceration or crush.

- Direct and severe injury to vital structures such as the heart or aorta.

- Underlying medical problems that led to the injury, such as sudden ventricular fibrillation.

- Severely diminished cardiac output due to tension pneumothorax or pericardial tamponade.

- Exsanguination leading to hypovolemia and severely diminished delivery of oxygen.

- Injuries in a cold environment (e.g., fractured leg) complicated by severe hypothermia.

---

— A person in cardiac arrest who has total body burns, hemicorporectomy (removal of the lower half of the body), or decapitation, or

— A person who has obvious severe trauma and has no vital signs, no pupillary response, and no shockable electrical cardiac rhythm.

- People with deep penetrating cranial injuries or with penetrating cranial or truncal wounds associated with asystole and a transport time of more than 15 minutes to a definitive care facility are unlikely to benefit from resuscitative efforts.

- Chances of survival are inversely proportional to the period of pulselessness and time spent conducting basic CPR.

- Minimize delays in getting the patient to a hospital with a fully equipped resuscitation team.

- Even when an advanced life support rescue vehicle is rapidly available, administration of cardiac medications and chest compressions in trauma patients are of uncertain value.

When trauma causes cardiac arrest, the outlook is grim. Survival depends upon rapid access to a trauma center. The age and health status of the victim are also crucial factors.

# SUMMARY

One of the most essential body functions is homeostasis. The balance of fluids, chemicals and physical properties is very delicate. The controlling mechanisms work within narrow limits.

Shock is a clinical syndrome that has different reactions to interference in the body's internal stability. Causes include myocardial infarction, sudden physical or emotional trauma, hemorrhage, infection and dehydration, poisoning, allergic reactions, and reaction to drugs.

However different the responses are, a common denominator of shock is failure of the body to maintain adequate organ perfusion. When the body's organs are not adequately perfused because of ineffective cardiac pumping action/output, circulating blood volume/vascular resistance, or heart rate malfunction, a shock response occurs.

Trauma can cause a variety of shock responses, depending upon the type and location of the injury. Cardiac arrest may be a consequence of trauma, and usually, the treatment is different than when the arrest is the primary problem. In all cases, the essential goal is to regain or maintain enough oxygenated blood to the body to keep all the organs adequately perfused.

It is essential to assess, identify and treat shock as soon as possible.

# EXAM QUESTIONS

## CHAPTER 4
### Questions 16–20

16. Which three factors maintain hemodynamic balance?

    a. Heart rate, circulating blood volume, cardiac pumping action/output

    b. Circulating blood volume, cardiac pumping action/output, cell temperature

    c. Cardiac pumping action/output, cell temperature, heart rate

    d. Heart rate, circulating blood volume, cell temperature

17. In most cases, the first noticeable sign of shock is

    a. restlessness.

    b. decreased pulse pressure.

    c. tachycardia.

    d. tachypnea.

18. What type of shock is caused by bodily fluid loss?

    a. Cardiogenic

    b. Neurogenic

    c. Septic

    d. Hypovolemic

19. A good indicator that the brain is adequately perfused is

    a. pupillary response.

    b. level of consciousness.

    c. skin temperature.

    d. blood pressure.

20. The cause of cardiac arrest related to trauma is

    a. syncope.

    b. severe central neurologic injury with secondary cardiovascular collapse.

    c. seat belt contusion.

    d. epistanis.

# CHAPTER 5

# HEAD INJURY

## CHAPTER OBJECTIVE

Upon completion of this chapter, the reader will be able to describe the principles of proper management of head injuries.

## LEARNING OBJECTIVES

Upon completion of this chapter, the reader should be able to:

1. Identify the major areas of the head and their functions.

2. Describe the most frequent causes and types of head injuries.

3. Describe the type of damage associated with a specific kind of head injury.

4. Recognize the importance of the Glasgow Coma Scale (GCS) in the assessment of a patient with a head injury.

5. Relate the assessment priorities to why they are important.

## INTRODUCTION

What matters in a head injury is damage to the brain.

Traumatic brain injury (TBI) is the leading cause of trauma deaths. Two million people a year in this country have traumatic brain injuries. The cost in terms of death and dis-abilities, along with medical, rehabilitative, loss of productivity and psychosocial impact is tremendous. The paradox of the emergency medical services (EMS) system is that because of improved training and technology, more traumatic head and spine injury victims are able to be kept alive, but there are also now more severely disabled people who require costly extensive rehabilitation and life-long maintenance and care.

Most of the victims of traumatic head injuries are between the ages of 16 and 30 years who have been involved in motor vehicle crashes. To further complicate the injuries, often the patient has alcohol or drugs, legal or otherwise, on board. Although the mandatory use of seat belts and campaigns against drunk driving have decreased the traffic fatalities by an estimated 25%, the incidence of penetrating injury to the brain and spinal cord is increasing. Gunshot wounds play a major part in penetrating trauma. Other leading causes of head trauma are recreational injuries and falls.

The faster a head injury is identified, assessed, and interventions begun, the better the patient's potential for survival with minimized disabilities.

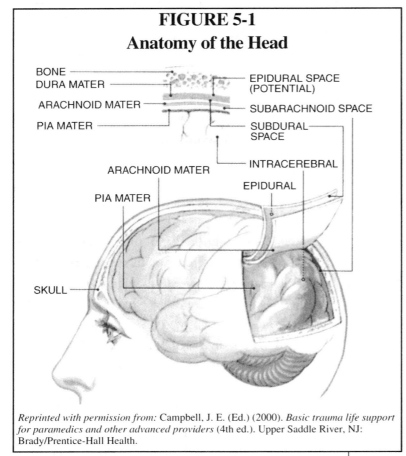

**FIGURE 5-1**
**Anatomy of the Head**

BONE
DURA MATER
ARACHNOID MATER
PIA MATER

EPIDURAL SPACE (POTENTIAL)
SUBARACHNOID SPACE
SUBDURAL SPACE
INTRACEREBRAL

ARACHNOID MATER
PIA MATER
EPIDURAL
SKULL

*Reprinted with permission from:* Campbell, J. E. (Ed.) (2000). *Basic trauma life support for paramedics and other advanced providers* (4th ed.). Upper Saddle River, NJ: Brady/Prentice-Hall Health.

# ANATOMY AND PHYSIOLOGY

The severity of head injuries is high because there is little support or protection for the head. Understanding the basic anatomy and physiology of the head and brain is essential for the most appropriate assessment and initial interventions for head injuries.

## Scalp

The scalp is the thickest layer of body covering but thins with age and balding. It provides spongy protection for the skull. There are five layers: skin, subcutaneous tissue, galea aponeurotica, ligaments, and periosteum. The tissue is very vascular, and it does not take a large laceration to result in a lot of bleeding. Uncontrolled bleeding can result in significant blood loss. Direct pressure can usually control the bleeding.

## Skull

The skull, or cranium, functions as a container to hold and protect the brain. It is composed of the frontal, parietal, temporal, and occipital bones. Cranial bones join with the facial bones to form the cranial vault, which is a rigid cavity. An opening called the foramen magnum allows the spinal cord to pass through.

Other important areas are the depressions in the interior base of the skull called the anterior, middle and posterior fossae. The anterior fossa contains the frontal lobe, which coordinates voluntary movements and controls judgment, affect, and personality. The parietal, temporal and occipital lobes are in the middle fossa. The parietal lobe controls sensory interpretation; the temporal lobe controls hearing, behavior, emotions, and dominant-hemisphere speech; and the occipital lobe is responsible for vision. The brain stem and cerebellum are in the posterior fossa.

The temporal area is especially thin, making it very vulnerable. The base of the skull is rough and has irregularities that can bruise and lacerate the brain when the head is jarred suddenly or in rapid deceleration. The solid structure of the adult skull makes it unable to tolerate expansion of the brain or increase in volume without serious problems.

## Meninges

Inside the skull there are three very vascular layers of membranes, the meninges, that surround and protect the brain and spinal cord. The outer layer is the dura and is the thickest and toughest of the three layers. The meningeal arteries are located in a space between the skull and the dura called the epidural space.

Lying under the dura is a weblike transparent serous membrane called the arachnoid.

The third layer, the pia, is attached to the brain and the arachnoid in some areas.

## Brain

Made up of billions of nerve cells, the adult brain weighs about 3 lb and occupies approximately 80% of the intracranial space. Brain tissue is the most energy-consuming tissue in the body and receives about 20% of the body's oxygen supply. Brain cells cannot go more than 4–6 minutes without oxygen before irreversible damage occurs, unless they are in a hypothermic state and the metabolism is drastically slowed.

The brain has three distinct parts: the cerebrum, brain stem, and cerebellum. The cerebrum, about 90% of the brain's weight, is divided into two hemispheres, the left and right. Each hemisphere has lobes named for their corresponding part of the skull. They control specific intellectual, sensory, and motor functions.

The brain stem joins the spinal cord, serving as a key reflex and relay center for the central nervous system. Consciousness, breathing, heart rate, and "vegetative functions" are controlled here.

The cerebellum surrounds the brain stem in the posterior fossa and coordinates activities below the level of consciousness, such as posture and equilibrium.

Inside the brain are a series of four interconnected cavities called ventricles. Cerebrospinal fluid (CSF) is produced here. It bathes the outer surface of the brain and acts as a shock absorber between the brain and the skull, along with serving as a blood-brain barrier against harmful substances.

## Cranial Nerves

Twelve pairs of cranial nerves originate in the brain stem, with each separate nerve having a name and a Roman numeral identifier. These nerves have unconscious control over sensory, motor, or both activities. Functions and areas they affect are important to recognize because they are instrumen-

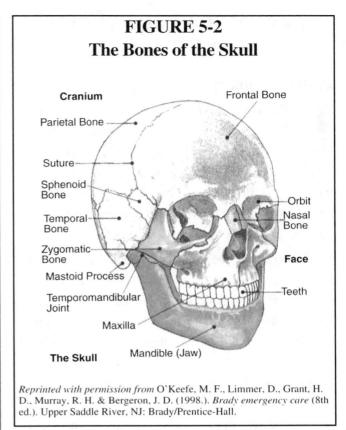

**FIGURE 5-2**
**The Bones of the Skull**

*Reprinted with permission from* O`Keefe, M. F., Limmer, D., Grant, H. D., Murray, R. H. & Bergeron, J. D. (1998.). *Brady emergency care* (8th ed.). Upper Saddle River, NJ: Brady/Prentice-Hall.

tal in the accurate assessment of damage from a head injury since they are indicators of brainstem activity and neurologic function.

The most important cranial nerve for assessment of a head injury is the third, or oculomotor, nerve that controls pupillary constriction. In a patient with an altered level of consciousness, a nonreactive or sluggish pupil indicates damage or pressure to the third nerve. This nerve is frequently injured in head trauma.

## Pediatric Differences

The anatomy and physiology of the child has a bearing on the greater incidence of TBI during childhood and the particular types of traumatic brain injury that occur (Soud & Rogers, 1998). The child's head is disproportionately large for the body size, and the neck is comparatively weak. The cranial bones are thinner, and the brain tissue is thinner, softer, and more fragile than an adult's. Consequently, there is a greater chance that cerebral edema will develop in a child than an adult.

# CONDITIONS OF HEAD INJURIES

## Pathophysiology

Unconsciousness stems from either the cerebral cortex or the reticular activating system in the brain stem. Because the brain is in an enclosed box, as pressure increases in the head, it causes the cerebral blood flow and oxygen to decrease, which in turn, causes the level of consciousness to diminish.

If there is a swelling in one part of the brain, it compresses another area because the head cannot expand. If the whole brain swells, or there is a rapidly growing hematoma, it takes up the limited cranial space, compressing the blood vessels. Along with the decrease in blood volume able to circulate in the head, the cerebrospinal fluid cannot get into the head.

The pressure in the arteries of the skull is considerably higher than the pressure in the head. When the pressure inside the head increases enough to equal the pressure in the skull's arteries, the vessels are squeezed, further restricting the arteries. The body reads the decrease in blood flow and the resulting drop in blood pressure. The sympathetic response is to increase the blood pressure. Additionally, the pulse slows because of the pressure on the vagus (X cranial) nerve. Respiratory response alters the breathing pattern.

**The triad of rising blood pressure, slowing pulse rate and changing respiratory pattern is a hallmark of increasing intracranial pressure (ICP).** The increasing pressure causes an alteration in the level of consciousness leading to unconsciousness, deficits in vital functions and can lead to brain death from inadequate cerebral perfusion. If the response to the ICP becomes exhausted, the brain begins to shift and can herniate into the tentorium above the cerebellum, causing death.

## Specific Head Injuries

Trauma is physical injury to the body from an external force, severe enough to endanger limb or life. The mechanism of injury may be either blunt or penetrating.

Most brain injuries are caused by blunt trauma to the head, especially in motor vehicle crashes. When a vehicle hits an object, it stops but the occupant continues forward, crashing into the interior of the vehicle. As the person hits the interior of the vehicle and stops, the brain continues to move forward, striking the skull. As the brain hits the skull during the deceleration injury, it absorbs energy and rebounds to the opposite side of the skull. The first contact of the brain with the skull is called the *coup* and the rebound collision with the skull is called the *contrecoup*.

Penetrating injuries enter through the skull. Usually a fracture occurs, and the projectile may drive bone fragments along with a foreign body into the brain, causing damage along the way. Intracranial bleeding and structural damage result. When impalement is the source of the penetrating injury, the object lodged in the head should be left in place and stabilized while the patient is being evaluated. Removal could worsen the effects from the injury.

Any trauma, blunt or penetrating, can cause swelling of the brain or bleeding from damage to the blood vessels. In either case, pressure increases in the head.

Head injuries fall into two groups: focal and diffuse. Focal injuries have a specific area of involvement and diffuse injuries involve the entire brain.

# FOCAL INJURIES

## Scalp Laceration

As stated earlier, the scalp is vascular and bleeds profusely, even with a small laceration. While a laceration may cause a considerable amount of blood loss, it is not likely to be life threatening. Direct pressure will usually initially control the bleeding, followed with wound repair.

## Skull Fracture

A skull fracture may or may not be immediately obvious. The clinical picture directly correlates to the type of fracture, area, and structures damaged. If there is no occurrence of associated brain injury, CSF leak, hematoma, or subsequent infection, skull fractures are not of serious consequence to the patient.

A linear fracture is caused by blunt trauma, is nondisplaced, and usually has minimal neurological deficit. Eighty percent of skull fractures are linear. Supportive care is generally all the patient needs.

If the impact has enough force, the fracture may be depressed, with bony fragments being driven into the brain. The depressed fracture will require surgical intervention if bone fragments become lodged in the brain tissue. When the damage to the skull causes an open wound or laceration, surgical repair is urgent to control bleeding and pressure in the brain and manage the risk of infection.

Basilar fractures may result from an extension of a linear fracture to the floor of the skull. Most commonly, these fractures occur through the floor of the anterior cranial fossa from craniofacial injuries, and may cause enough damage for the CSF to leak through either the nose or ears (Peitzman et al., 1998). Carotid artery and cranial nerve injuries are also frequently seen with basilar fractures, in particular, the facial nerve (cranial nerve VII).

Basilar fractures may not be visualized on an x-ray or CAT scan, so positive clinical findings may have to be relied on for the diagnosis. Bleeding can cause dramatic distinguishing changes in the appearance of the patient. When blood leaks into the intraorbital tissue, it causes what is known as "Raccoon's eyes." Another characteristic is "Battle's sign," the ecchymosis behind the ears seen 12 to 24 hours after the initial injury. Other clinical signs of fracture are CSF leaks from the nose or ears. Neurologic changes with a basilar fracture range from slight alteration in mental status to agitation or severe combativeness.

## Contusion

When the brain hits against the cranium it becomes bruised, particularly in acceleration-deceleration trauma. Usually these are coup and contrecoup injuries. Depending upon the size and location of the contusion, neurological deficit may or may not be evident. Increased intracranial pressure will result from a large contusion. Symptoms include alteration of consciousness, nausea, vomiting, visual and speech difficulties, and weakness.

## Epidural Hematoma

Epidural hematomas result from a direct strike to the head, causing an arterial bleed between the skull and dura mater. Often the injury is from a slow-velocity blow such as in a fight or from a baseball. Patients with an epidural hematoma do not always have a skull fracture. If the middle meningeal artery is torn, a hematoma can form and rapidly become large. These patients have a morbidity and mortality rate of more than 50%, even if the hematoma is quickly detected.

Signs of a rapidly growing hematoma and increasing intracranial pressure are loss of consciousness (LOC) followed by a lucid period (usually a hallmark of an epidural bleed), followed by

## FIGURE 5-3
## Epidural and Subdural Hematomas

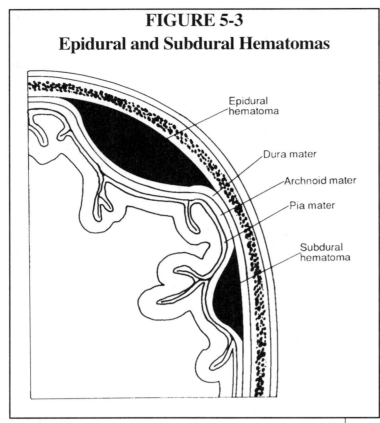

Epidural hematoma

Dura mater

Archnoid mater

Pia mater

Subdural hematoma

another LOC period; developing hemiparesis; and a dilated and fixed pupil on the side of impact. The triad of increasing blood pressure, slowing pulse rate, and changes in respiratory patterns warns of elevated ICP.

### Subdural Hematoma

Occurring more frequently than other intracranial injuries, subdural hematomas have the highest morbidity and mortality of all cranial hematomas. They are usually the result of venous bleeding between the dura and the brain and frequently are associated with brain tissue damage.

Subdural hematomas are classified as acute, subacute and chronic. Acute hematomas are often caused by high-velocity impact injuries and have a grave prognosis because of the underlying brain injury. Even with immediate surgical intervention, more than 50% of the patients will not survive the damage. Clinically, the patient has LOC; hemiparesis; and fixed, dilated pupils.

A subacute hematoma, also from high-impact trauma, develops more slowly, from 48 hours to 2 weeks. The patient experiences a progressive decline in the level of consciousness proportionate to the growth of the hematoma. Because the brain is able to compensate for the gradual collection of blood, the neurologic functions deteriorate slowly. These patients have a better prognosis than those with acute hematomas.

In the chronic hematoma, months after what seemed like a minor head injury, blood has slowly accumulated in the subdural space or between the layers of the dura. Since the causative injury happened quite a while previous to the symptoms becoming evident, the actual incident may have been forgotten. The elderly frequently have this type of injury. Their brain decreases in size due to atrophy, thus allowing more blood to collect in the increased intracranial space before symptoms become noticeable. Although it takes more time to recognize the chronic subdural hematoma, the mortality rate is almost as high as that of the acute subdural hematomas.

### Other Focal Injuries

Intracerebral clots and intraventricular hemorrhages are also focal injuries. Depending upon the size of the clot and the source of bleeding, surgical evacuation is necessary to manage the intracranial pressure.

# DIFFUSE INJURIES

Diffuse, or axonal, brain injuries are associated with widespread disruption of neurologic function. The damage can cause diffuse (scattered, spread about) disruption of both the function and structure of the brain.

In less severe injuries, the axonal injury is functional in character. As the trauma increases in severity, so does the amount of diffuse physical disruption. When severe, the injuries can result in coma, not from compression of the brain, but from direct damage to the brain stem or cerebrum.

Diffuse injuries usually are not visible lesions, as with focal lesions, but are injuries to many microscopic axons of the brain.

Several categories of diffuse brain injuries are recognized: mild concussion; classic cerebral concussion; and mild, moderate or severe diffuse axonal injury (DAI).

## Concussion

A concussion occurs from a direct blow or acceleration-deceleration injury where there is a temporary loss of consciousness and associated memory deficiency without underlying brain damage. Injury is not severe. There may be temporary amnesia. Headache, nausea, vomiting, and visual disturbances are also likely to be experienced. It is important to determine any incidence and length of LOC, neurologic status, and memory deficits.

Postconcussional syndrome will exhibit headache, memory loss, and diminished activities of daily living. The symptoms can last for as long as a year after the injury.

## Diffuse Axonal Injury (DAI)

This type of injury, usually the result of acceleration-deceleration forces from blunt trauma, causes shearing and disruption of the brain's microscopic neuronal/axonal structures. Widespread shear-strain lesions are frequently multiple and bilateral.

Whether mild, moderate or severe in designation, all diffuse axonal injuries are distinguished by a coma greater than 6 hours in duration, which is the result of diffuse, rather than focal damage.

Prognosis varies with the degree of primary injury and the associated damage. The patient may be unconscious from 6 hours to a prolonged period of time. Decerebrate or decorticate posturing may

last for a brief period of time until the patient awakens, or the brain stem impairment may not resolve.

# PATIENT ASSESSMENT

Assume there is a spinal injury until the physician declares otherwise. Immediately immobilize the head and neck. Before any further physical assessment is conducted, the standard ABC plan should be followed (see chapter 2, "Primary Assessment.")

The evaluation after the ABCs is to determine the baseline status of the patient from which stabilization and management of his injuries begins.

*All patients with head injuries should be continuously monitored to determine if the status is constant, improves or deteriorates. Change may occur on a minute-to-minute basis.*

**Neurologic assessment** of consciousness is to determine the highest level of response with the least stimulus. Even the most subtle change from the initial assessment is the earliest indication of deterioration or improvement in the patient's condition.

The Glasgow Coma Scale (GCS) is a component of the neurologic assessment intended as a clinical index to evaluate the degree of impaired consciousness. A number value is given to eye opening ability, best motor response, and best verbal response to provide immediate recognition of these specific clinical values. Current status and trends can be quickly identified. It is key to determine the GCS as early as possible and then continuously. Degree of consciousness is an important indicator of traumatic brain injury. However, the GCS is not an indicator in and of itself. It is to be used along with other clinical findings and history obtained in order to form the whole picture.

Normally, the pupil will constrict with direct-light examination, and a constriction of the opposite pupil should occur. Compression of the third cranial nerve will cause dilation of one pupil, but about 20% of the population has unequal pupils (Sheehy, 1998), so the dilated pupil should be evaluated for its ability to react. If the pupils are dilated and fixed, it is an indication of impending herniation of the brain.

Posturing and unequal motor responses indicate brain damage. Specific movements indicate where in the brain the damage has occurred.

The oculocephatic reflex, or "Doll's eye" examination can be conducted after the cervical spine is cleared for injury. It is an indicator of brain stem integrity. The head is quickly rotated to the right or left. An intact brain stem will cause the eyes to deviate away from the direction the head is turned. If the brain stem is damaged, the eyes will either remain midline or will not move with the rotation.

In the ice water caloric test, the practitioner injects ice water into the ear of the unresponsive patient. The response should be conjugate movement of the eyes. Dysconjugate, asymmetrical or lack of movement indicates a disturbance in the functional connection between the medulla and midbrain. A conscious or semiconscious patient will have severe vomiting and dizziness, which makes this test prohibited for these patients. The test should not be conducted on a patient with a tympanic membrane rupture.

Other reasons for unconsciousness, aside from, or along with, the head injury, may be ingestion of substances, hypotension, hypothermia, seizure disorders, complications from diabetes, toxicity from uremia, tumors, stroke, infections, or psychiatric disorders.

**Respiratory patterns** usually change with head trauma. Rates may slow or become rapid, uneven, noisy or the patient may develop respiratory embarrassment or arrest. Changes may indicate increased intracranial pressure, other injuries, hypovolemia, or metabolic abnormalities.

**Blood pressure** elevation without a medical reason may be part of the triad indicating increasing ICP: rising blood pressure, slowing pulse rate and changing respiratory pattern. Pain, anxiety, or preexisting hypertension can also contribute to the blood pressure rising. The onset of hypotension generally indicates a terminal situation in head injuries. There may be bleeding elsewhere in the body.

As previously discussed, the development of bradycardia may reflect increased ICP. Bradycardia with hypertension can be due to a rapidly expanding hematoma. The **pulse rate** is an important factor to be evaluated with other assessment data to determine if it is related to the head injury.

It cannot be emphasized too often that continuous assessment and recording of results are essential in the management of the patient's care. Included in the assessment is communication with the conscious patient and any others who have information about the patient prior to the injury or about the injury itself.

# NURSING STRATEGIES FOR THE HEAD INJURY PATIENT

Whether you are in the prehospital or hospital setting, the principles of trauma management for the patient with a possible head injury are the same.

The first goals of stabilization are ventilation, oxygenation, maintenance of blood pressure, restoration of circulating volume, and prevention of further injury.

Once the ABCs are complete, the patient's neck and spine are stabilized until the physician clears them.

The head-injury patient is likely to vomit. Care must be taken to prevent aspiration. Activate suction equipment and have available for use at any time. If the patient is still on a backboard, be sure he is adequately immobilized in case he needs to be turned quickly to prevent aspiration. Do not insert any tubes into the nose unless directed by the physician to do so.

At this point, any bleeding should be controlled. Since scalp vessels bleed profusely, it may be difficult to visualize the site. Probing through the laceration or wound to observe depth or search for foreign bodies should not be done. The vessels are easily compressed with gentle, continuous direct pressure. Obvious deformity, palpable bony defects or instability, should not have direct pressure, but pressure around the wound can be gently applied, taking care to exert pressure only on stable bone.

Be sure to watch for signs of shock, especially in children, as considerable blood can be lost from the face and scalp. If the patient shows signs of shock without obvious excessive bleeding from the face or scalp, it is not due to brain injury, unless it is a terminal event. Internal injuries may be the cause. As with any patient in shock, if there are multiple injuries, intravenous (IV) fluids will be ordered to ensure adequate perfusion of the brain. The flow rate should be monitored carefully, and signs of increasing ICP immediately reported and documented.

Hypotension is rarely caused by a head injury. More likely, hypotension is caused by hemorrhage in another area of the body. If the patient has hypotension with a normal pulse rate and without pallor, it may be an indication of neurologic shock associated with a spinal cord injury.

Additionally:

- The patient with an isolated head injury without extreme bleeding, should be fluid restricted in order to minimize cerebral edema.

- The pupils are checked for size, equality and activity as part of the continuous assessment of the patient.

- Any bleeding or CSF coming from the nose or ears should be immediately reported to the physician.

- Monitor blood gasses as ordered, and report abnormal levels to the physician.

- Continuously monitor and report any changes in the level of consciousness and neurologic status.

- Regardless of the patient's level of consciousness, be careful about discussing his status or other aspects of his injury in his presence. Always assume the patient is able to hear what is being said.

## EXAMPLES OF NURSING DIAGNOSES RELATED TO HEAD INJURY

- Ineffective airway clearance related to decreased level of consciousness

- Alteration of breathing related to trauma

- Impairment in gas exchange related to ineffective respiration or poor oxygen supply

- Possibility of additional injury related to seizure activity

- Possibility of aspiration related to altered level of consciousness and blunted reflexes

- Pain related to trauma

- Decreased tissue perfusion in the brain related to head injury

- Impaired mobility due to brain trauma

- Restlessness due to hypovolemia from trauma

- Anxiety related to fear from head injury

## SUMMARY

Injuries to the head are the leading cause of traumatic deaths and significant disabilities. Motor vehicle crashes involving people between the ages of 16 and 30 years are the predominant cause of these injuries.

Knowledge of the anatomy and physiology of the head along with the dynamics of head injuries is fundamental to identifying types of head injuries and conducting effective initial and secondary assessments. All patients with potential or obvious head trauma need to be continuously monitored because of the potential for a rapid change in status.

The faster the head injury is identified, assessed and interventions initiated, the better the patient's potential for minimized injuries and sur-

# EXAM QUESTIONS

## CHAPTER 5
### Questions 21–25

21. Head injuries are severe because

    a. the scalp provides only a thin protection.

    b. the cranial nerves are easily damaged.

    c. there is little support or protection for the head.

    d. the brain is so large.

22. Focal head injuries

    a. are more severe than diffuse injuries.

    b. are more likely to be caused by motor vehicle crashes.

    c. involve a specific area of the brain.

    d. usually penetrate the skull.

23. Indicators of a severe head injury are

    a. coup and contrecoup.

    b. concussion and blinking.

    c. dystonia and listlessness.

    d. rising blood pressure, slowing pulse rate and changes in respiratory patterns.

24. All patients with head injuries

    a. have a loss of consciousness.

    b. have obvious damage to the head.

    c. should be continuously assessed during treatment.

    d. have increased intracranial pressure.

25. The Glasgow Coma Scale serves to

    a. identify where the injury is located.

    b. determine if there is swelling in the brain.

    c. provide an important component of neurologic assessment.

    d. identify increased intracranial pressure.

# CHAPTER 6

# MAXILLOFACIAL AND NECK TRAUMA

## CHAPTER OBJECTIVE

Upon completion of this chapter, the reader will be able to recognize the causes and management of maxillofacial and neck trauma.

## LEARNING OBJECTIVES

Upon completion of this chapter, the reader should be able to:

1. Identify the anatomical structures and related functions of the face and neck.

2. Describe frequent causes and types of maxillofacial and neck trauma.

3. Relate assessment priorities to why they are important.

4. Describe methods of stabilization and airway management in maxillofacial and neck trauma.

5. Recognize basic nursing strategies for maxillofacial and neck trauma.

## INTRODUCTION

Maxillofacial and neck trauma is frequently seen in the emergency department. Motor vehicle crashes are the most common cause, but physical assaults, personal altercations, and handguns are increasing contributors to facial and neck trauma. Falls are also a frequent cause of these injuries in the elderly and children.

The area involved includes the facial bones, neurovascular structures, skin, subcutaneous tissue, muscles, glands, and the upper airway. It takes significant force to fracture the midface or maxilla, and as a result, multisystem injuries usually accompany these types of fractures. When there are multiple injuries, maxillofacial trauma is a complicating factor.

Assessing even a severe facial injury does not take priority over recognition and treatment of life-threatening injuries. As in every injury, rapidly checking the ABCs of airway, breathing and cervical spine stabilization come first. Maxillofacial and neck trauma may appear severe, but usually is not critical unless the airway is compromised. Patients with trauma to the neck can be high risk because the airway, carotid vessels, jugular vessels, and cervical spine are all contained in this compact area. Specific head and spinal injuries are discussed in other chapters.

## ANATOMY AND PHYSIOLOGY

### Facial Structures

The skull functions as a rigid container. There are two specific areas, the cranial vault and the 14 facial bones. The structures of the face, jaw, and neck form part of the upper airway.

The main facial bones are the frontal, nasal bone, maxilla, zygoma, and mandible. All of the facial bones touch the maxillae.

The **frontal** bone or forehead joins to the frontal process of the maxilla, the nasal bone, and laterally to the zygoma.

The **orbital complex** is a bony pyramid-shaped cavity in the skull that contains and protects the eyes. It is comprised of the frontal bone, zygoma, and maxilla. Posteriorly is the optic foramen, a groove for the optic nerve and ophthalmic artery at the orbit's apex.

The **maxilla,** also called the midface, are two bones that meet in the midline of the face. They form the skeletal base of most of the upper face. Included are most of the orbital floor, sides of the nasal cavity, the upper jaw, and the roof of the mouth, which also houses the upper teeth.

The **sinus cavities** in the midline of the face lighten the weight of the bony structure and act as resonating chambers. They develop from the nasal cavities, communicate with them, are filled with air and beyond that, their specific function is not known.

The **nose** is made up of a pair of bones that form the bridge, is mostly made of cartilage, and protrudes from the face, making it vulnerable to injury. The nasal cavity is divided by the septum.

The **zygoma** forms the cheek and the lateral wall and floor of the orbital cavity. The zygoma articulates with the maxilla, frontal bone, and zygomatic process of the temporal bone to form the zygomatic arch.

The **mandible** is horseshoe shaped, lies horizontally, and is the only movable bone in the face. It is the strongest bone and anchors the lower teeth. The mandible articulates with the temporal bone to form the temporomandibular joint.

## Cranial Nerves

The **facial nerve** (cranial nerve VII) gives sensory and motor innervation to the side of the face. It originates in the brain stem and then subdivides into six branches, leading to the scalp, forehead, eyelids, facial muscles for expression, cheeks, and jaw. Injuries to the facial nerve produce a paralysis to the facial muscles; a possible loss of taste; and a disturbance in the secretion of the lacrimal and salavary glands, depending on the part of the nerve involved.

Other nerves that can be affected by facial trauma are the **oculomotor** (cranial nerve III), **trochlear** (cranial nerve IV) and **abducens**, (cranial nerve VI), which innervate the ocular muscles. Injuries can produce blurred vision; diplopia; deviation of the eyeball; impair ocular movements; ptosis, or inability to open the eye; and affect the ability of the pupil to constrict. The **trigeminal** (cranial nerve V) is the largest of the cranial nerves. Trauma can cause paralysis of the muscles used to chew; inability to clench the jaw; loss of ability to feel light tactile, thermal and painful sensations to the face; and loss of the corneal and sneezing reflexes.

## Upper Airway

The upper airways are the nose, mouth, pharynx, and larynx. Here, air is filtered, warmed, and humidified, and the lower airways are protected from foreign objects. Structures include the tongue, hyoid bone, thyroid cartilage, epiglottis, and vocal cords.

The **mouth** takes in food and air and is used to communicate. It contains the teeth and the tongue. The tongue is freely movable, attached to the floor of the mouth; aids in speech; and moves food to the back of the mouth. It can fall to the back of the throat and obstruct the airway, and in the unconscious patient, it is the most common cause for airway obstruction.

The **teeth** are essential for chewing and emerge from the maxilla and mandible. They also maintain the shape of the lower face. When they are missing, it is more difficult to ventilate a patient. Trauma can dislodge the teeth and obstruct the airway.

The **hyoid bone** is U shaped and attached to the base of the tongue. It does not touch any other bone. Because of its attachment to the tongue, it is likely to obstruct the airway.

The passages from the nose and mouth meet at the **pharynx** or throat. The pharynx begins at the base of the skull and opens into the esophagus and the larynx. It is muscular and is divided into the nasopharynx behind the nasal cavities, containing the adenoids and openings to the eustachian tubes; the oropharynx extending from the uvula to the epiglottis and containing the palatine tonsils; and the laryngopharynx, which extends from the epiglottis to the opening of the larynx. Here, constrictor muscles send food and liquid into the esophagus. The gag reflex and swallowing is controlled by the glossopharyngeal nerve (cranial nerve IX). The pharynx may become obstructed with food; liquids; or foreign bodies, such as teeth.

From the pharynx, the **larynx** extends down to the upper end of the trachea. A leaf-shaped structure just behind the root of the tongue and attached to the thyroid cartilage is the **epiglottis**. It covers the entrance to the larynx during swallowing, allowing food to go down the esophagus and keeping food, liquid, and foreign objects out of the airway. Although the larynx assists in speech, it mainly functions as an air passage opening into the trachea or the "windpipe." Vocal cords project into the larynx from the trachea, and when they spasm, they cause choking. The larynx can close, allowing for air buildup in the lungs, which can be forcefully expelled, known as a cough.

Extending from the upper airway, the **trachea** is the main passage to convey air from the upper airway in and out of the lungs. It is supported by C-shaped cartilage connected by a tough membrane, through which an opening can be made for artificial ventilation during upper airway obstruction or a crushing injury of the neck.

**Major Vessels**

**Carotid arteries** run alongside the trachea on either side of the neck, arise from the aorta, and are the principal blood supply to the head and neck. Both the right and left carotids divide to form the internal and external carotid arteries. Chemoreceptors in the arteries respond to changes in blood chemistry, such as hypoxia, and cause reflex increases in pulse rate, blood pressure, and respiratory rate. If the blood supply to the head is interrupted, brain damage will occur. When a carotid pulse can be palpated, the systolic blood pressure is at least 60 mm Hg.

**Jugular veins:** The external jugular vein receives blood from the exterior of the cranium and the deep parts of the face. It lies superficially to the sternocleidomastoid muscle as it descends the neck to join the subclavian vein. The internal jugular vein receives blood from the brain and superficial parts of the face and neck. It runs alongside the internal carotid artery and joins the subclavian vein to form the innominate vein.

Laceration or a tear of the carotid arteries or jugular veins can rapidly lead to exsanguination. Air can also be drawn into the venous vessels and form a fatal air embolus.

# MECHANISM OF INJURY

Blunt maxillofacial or neck trauma can range from an uncomplicated nasal fracture to a major head injury or the collapse of the upper airway. Frequently, rapid deceleration and forceful impact with a hard surface are the mechanism for trauma to the face or neck. Motor vehicle crashes, sports accidents, falls, or impact from assault are the most frequently seen sources of these injuries.

Penetrating trauma of the face is most often caused by a projectile. One or multiple lacerations, impalement or puncture wounds, particularly of the cheek and eye, may be caused by a sharp implement, such as a knife, shards of glass, or a missile such as a bullet. An associated injury in the neck, such as severance or a tear of a major vessel, is a critical situation.

Many times there is a combination of blunt and penetrating trauma, with multiple lacerations and injuries of various severity, such as seen in vehicular crashes, assaults and falls. Injuries can cause distortion of the face and copious bleeding. Foreign objects and blood can obstruct the airway, which presents a problem when there is a fracture of the mandible. Because the head, face and neck are involved, it should be assumed there is a head and cervical injury until the patient is cleared after assessment.

# MAXILLOFACIAL AND NECK INJURY

## Soft-Tissue Trauma

Contusions are a frequent result of blunt trauma that does not alter the integrity of the skin. Pain, swelling, and discoloration is the result of extravasation of blood into the damaged tissue. Around the eyes, a contusion may indicate an orbital fracture.

Animal or human bites are highly contaminated because of the bacteria and debris in the mouth. Extensive or gaping wounds present infection and cosmetic problems, along with the possibility of foreign bodies.

Road rash and friction injuries have the potential problems of tattooing or epidermal staining. Gunpowder can also cause permanent discoloration and cosmetic disfigurement, along with

burns to the epithelial and collagen layers while penetrating the skin. Glass fragments are often embedded in the skin after the head has gone through a windshield.

Soft-tissue injury from air bags can cause minor abrasions to the face, neck, and upper chest. Occasionally, air bags cause scleral or corneal injury and lacerations to the eyebrows and eyelids. Ear injuries and deafness can also occur.

Lacerations are open cuts caused by a shearing force through the layers of the skin. They range from simple to deep cuts and are associated with crush injuries and fractures. For cosmetic reasons, lacerations of the face require special attention.

Lacerations of the lips require the skills of a plastic surgeon so the vermilion borders can be perfectly matched and step-off deformities of the lip do not develop.

Intraoral injuries often have debris, crushed tissue and tooth fragments. Gaping intraoral lacerations frequently develop ulcerations and infections because of the contamination in the mouth. The tongue may be lacerated from the teeth.

Ear injuries are classified as hematomas, lacerations, and avulsions. Hematomas that are not drained can result in a "cauliflower ear," which is a scar deformity. Cartilage may be lacerated along with the skin. Avulsion injuries are more involved than simple lacerations and require skin preservation so grafting from other body areas is not required.

Deep cheek lacerations may involve the parotid gland, parotid duct and branches of the facial nerve, which controls facial expression. Indicators are disruption to forehead symmetry, inability to fully close the eyelids, inability to purse the lips, and inability to lower or depress the lower lip. Facial nerve injury can be overlooked if the patient is unconscious or has multiple facial bandages. Facial paralysis from blunt trauma, rather

## FIGURE 6-1
## Complications of Facial Fracture

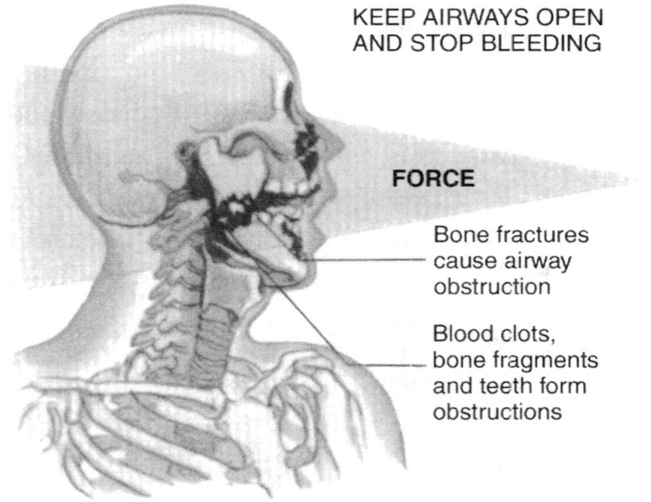

KEEP AIRWAYS OPEN
AND STOP BLEEDING

FORCE

Bone fractures
cause airway
obstruction

Blood clots,
bone fragments
and teeth form
obstructions

*Reprinted with permission from* O`Keefe, M. F., Limmer, D., Grant, H. D., Murray, R. H. & Bergeron, J. D. (1998.). *Brady emergency care* (8th ed.). Upper Saddle River, NJ: Brady/Prentice-Hall.

than laceration, has a good chance of recovery if the damage is not extensive.

An avulsion is the tearing of a flap of skin from the body surface. It may be completely removed or stay partially attached to the body. The injury usually causes a lot of bleeding, requiring immediate direct pressure. When there is head trauma and the scalp is torn from the skull, it may indicate a skull fracture and neck injury. Degloving injuries are severe avulsion injuries, usually involving subcutaneous tissue and underlying skeletal structures.

Blunt or penetrating trauma to the neck may cause tracheal injury and close the airway. Hypoxia and death rapidly follow.

## Major Vessel Injury

Penetrating trauma to the neck is a serious emergency. Laceration of a great vessel can cause hemorrhaging; air can get sucked in and cause an embolus. It is difficult to stop the hemorrhaging because of the pressure in the vessels.

The carotid arteries are the major neck arteries and suppliers of blood to the head. They supply the blood for perfusion and oxygenation of the brain.

Bright red, spurting blood in a pulsating flow from an open neck wound indicates a carotid artery may be damaged, which is an extreme emergency.

Dark red venous blood streaming from an open neck wound is an acute emergency because of the potential volume loss and possibility of air entering the venous system, producing an air embolus.

## Fracture

### Nasal Fracture

Because the nose is the most prominent facial feature and offers the least resistance, it is the most common facial fracture. The mechanism is usually blunt trauma. If left untreated, deformity can result, along with airway obstruction. When the overlying skin is broken, the fracture is open.

Direct blunt trauma to the front of the nose can cause posterior displacement of the bones, damaging the ethmoid and frontal sinuses, lacrimal duct, and orbital margins. Damage to the cribriform plate can tear the dura, causing the cerebrospinal fluid to leak from the nose. A septal hematoma presents as a bluish, bulging mass. Emergency aspiration of the hematoma is required to prevent airway obstruction, septal necrosis, and a permanent deformity. A blow from the side of the nose can cause lateral displacement. Bleeding from nasal trauma can be profuse, being intranasal as well as in the pharynx. If a fracture involves the nasal mucosa of the lacrimal system, blowing the nose can cause intracranial air or subcutaneous emphysema that may subsequently become localized infection or meningitis.

### Mandibular Fracture

The second most frequent type of facial fractures are mandibular. A forceful blow from motor vehicle crashes, sports or altercations are the usual mechanism of injury. Loss of bony support, in a

## FIGURE 6-2
### Signs of Facial Fracture

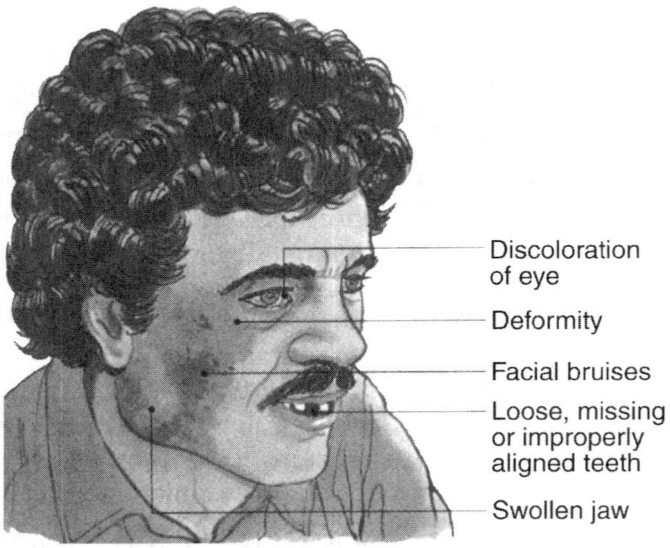

- Discoloration of eye
- Deformity
- Facial bruises
- Loose, missing or improperly aligned teeth
- Swollen jaw

*Reprinted with permission from O'Keefe, M. F., Limmer, D., Grant, H. D., Murray, R. H. & Bergeron, J. D. (1998.). Brady emergency care (8th ed.). Upper Saddle River, NJ: Brady/Prentice-Hall.*

mandibular fracture can be life threatening if it displaces posteriorly and blocks the airway. Malocclusion is the most prominent symptom, but symptoms vary with the location of the fracture. The face may be asymmetric with swelling and ecchymosis. Sublingual hematoma can compromise the airway. There may also be tears in the external canal of the ear or the tympanic membrane.

### Maxillary Fracture

It takes great force to cause a midface fracture, and usually there are other fractures involved. There are three different types of maxillary fractures:

LeFort I is a lower-third fracture that is horizontal, where the body of the maxilla is separated from the base of the skull above the palate but below the zygomatic process attachment. Separation may be unilateral or bilateral, and the maxilla may or may not be displaced. The hard palate and the upper teeth are loose.

LeFort II is a middle-third fracture including the central maxilla, nasal area and ethmoid bones. The nose, lips and eyes are usually edematous; subconjunctival hemorrhage and epistaxis fre-

quently occurs. Cerebrospinal fluid rhinorrhea suggests skull fracture.

LeFort III is an orbital complex fracture causing total cranial facial separation. The nose and dental arch move without frontal bone involvement accompanied by massive edema, ecchymosis, epistaxis and malocclusion. Ocular injuries are secondary to the swelling. Airway obstruction, likely from hemorrhage and cervical spine fracture, should always be considered.

### Zygoma Fracture

Zygomatic fractures occur in two patterns: zygomatic arch and tripod. Fracture of the cheeks most often occurs from blunt trauma to the front or side of the face. If there is also a fracture of the orbital floor, the situation may become critical.

### Orbital Blowout Fracture

Orbital blowout and zygoma fractures can occur separately, but are often found together. The orbital blowout is caused when pressure from a traumatic force causes the globe to "blow out"—fracture—one or more of the bones of the orbital wall. The weakest part of the orbit is the floor.

Increased pressure can cause the orbit's contents to prolapse into the maxillary sinus, causing entrapment of the inferior rectus muscle, inferior oblique muscle, infraorbital nerve, orbital fat and connective tissue. The globe may also become entrapped.

This fracture is seen in sports-related injuries and altercations. Golf balls are so small that they can go through the protective orbit and rupture the globe. When the globe is perforated, blowing the nose or manipulating the eyes can cause intraorbital air. If there is subcutaneous orbital emphysema, a fracture of the sinus arch should be suspected. Nose blowing, coughing, sneezing, vomiting, and straining can force air from the sinuses through the fracture into the orbital space. If there is bulging of the eye and limitation of

## FIGURE 6-3
## Signs of Basilar Skull Fracture: Battle's Sign and Raccoon Eyes

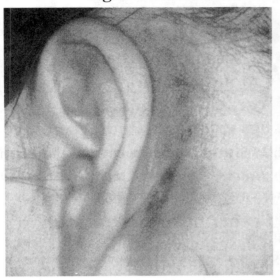 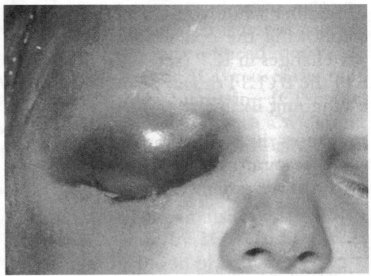

*Reprinted with permission from:* Campbell, J. E. (Ed.) (2000). *Basic trauma life support for paramedics and other advanced providers* (4th ed.). Upper Saddle River, NJ: Brady/Prentice-Hall Health.

motion, ocular involvement is a consideration. Double vision, pupil asymmetry, sunken appearance of the globe, anesthesia of the cheek and upper lip or drooping of the lid are all indicators of a blowout fracture.

# ASSESSMENT

## Primary Assessment

As with any head or neck injury, particularly if the patient is unconscious, the primary assessment assumes there is a cervical fracture. Stabilization of the neck, a clear airway, and adequate oxygenation are the first priorities.

There are many causes for airway obstruction in cases of head and neck injury. When the facial structures are damaged or the tongue is left without support, occlusion of the airway is likely. Foreign objects, such as avulsed teeth or dentures, can also obstruct the airway. A fracture of the nasoorbital complex compromises the airway due to hemorrhage. A gunshot wound may cause hemorrhage or a hematoma. Altered mental status or

injury may decrease the gag reflex, leaving the airway unprotected.

Identify serious injuries that threaten life or limb and control any profuse bleeding.

## Secondary Assessment

Once the neck is stabilized, the airway open, the patient adequately ventilated, and hemorrhage contained, the secondary assessment should be conducted.

Maxillofacial injuries seldom are life threatening unless there is a compromised airway. However, there are likely to be other associated fractures.

- Respond immediately to hemorrhaging from the major arteries or veins in the neck, this is an acute emergency.

- Conduct visual evaluation of the head and face for contusions, abrasions, lacerations, hemorrhage, asymmetry or defects of the bones, and abnormalities of the eyes, eyelids, mouth, mandible, and ear.

- Lightly palpate the face and skull, before edema or hematomas obscure landmarks, to identify crepitation, deviation, depression, or abnormal movement. Check inside the mouth for lacerations, loose or broken teeth or bleeding.

- Facial swelling may be extensive, often accompanied by discoloration and deformities.

- Be aware that Raccoon eyes (black eyes or discoloration under the eyes) and Battle's sign (ecchymosis over the mastoid area), are indicators of a fracture at the base of the skull.

- A nasal septal hematoma must be identified and reported to the physician for immediate evacuation to prevent a saddle nose deformity.

- Blood or clear fluid (cerebrospinal) may drain from the nose or ears.

- Assess for loss of vision, double vision, pupil reaction and symmetry, and extraocular movements.

- The teeth may be misaligned or the patient may have difficulty speaking or moving his jaw.

- Check for loss of sensation of the lips, drooping of the face, and other indications of nerve injury.

- Visually evaluate the neck for contusions, abrasions, lacerations, and larynx deformity, which may indicate additional injuries. Bruises or deformities directly over the trachea may indicate a serious or impending airway obstruction due to tissue swelling or the acute emergency of a ruptured trachea.

- Palpate for tracheal, pulmonary, or laryngeal subcutaneous emphysema and deviation of the trachea from the midline.

- Check for laryngeal fracture, typically indicated by the triad of laryngeal crepitus, hoarseness, and subcutaneous emphysema.

- Carefully palpate the cervical spine for tenderness which may indicate injury.

- Assess the pain level.

# NURSING STRATEGIES FOR THE MAXILLOFACIAL AND NECK TRAUMA PATIENT

Although maxillofacial injuries, especially those associated with other injuries, may be life threatening, most of them are not. They frequently have a lot of bleeding and are frightening to the patient. Careful assessment along with good communication with the patient can make treatment easier and ease the patient's fears. As in all patient care situations, the nurse should let the patient know what is being done and why.

- Stabilize the head and neck.

- Do not remove a Philadelphia cervical collar until cleared by the physician, even if the patient complains it is uncomfortable.

- Maintain the airway, breathing and circulation. Damaged facial structures can cause airway obstruction. If there is airway compromise, the *only recommended procedure* for use on the unconscious patient with a potential cervical fracture is the jaw thrust. If there is no cervical damage, the chin lift/head tilt method can be used.

- Contain hemorrhage.

- Have a suction device assembled and ready for use. If the patient is alert, he can self-suction with a tonsil tip catheter, which leaves the nurse free to manage other problems.

- Do not lift or move the head to further examine the patient or apply bandages until the physician has cleared the patient. Additionally, do not let the patient eat or drink until cleared in case surgery is immediately indicated.

- If the patient is conscious, once the cervical neck has been cleared by the physician and there are no other contraindicated injuries, elevate the head of the gurney or bed to reduce swelling, bleeding, congestion and to promote drainage.

- Do not try to force the eyelids open to check the pupils; there may be damage to the globe or other ocular injuries.

- Remember nasal fractures and mouth injuries usually bleed a lot, much of which drains into the stomach, causing nausea and vomiting. If the patient is able to help, give him some gauze pads or a suction device to absorb drainage and keep the blood from running down the throat.

- Malocclusion is an important clinical sign of mandibular or maxillary fracture.

- Carefully suction blood and emesis to prevent filling the pharynx and blocking the airway or draining into the stomach. Be careful not to obstruct the flow of blood, which can result in airway obstruction or increased intracranial pressure in the case of a skull fracture.

- Ice packs and direct nasal pressure help control swelling and bleeding from the nose.

- Use pulse oximetry to help monitor oxygen saturation levels.

- Excessive bleeding and swelling in the facial structures and the mouth, along with being unable to clear the airway effectively, calls for aggressive intervention. Supplemental oxygen should be provided. Intubation may be required, which is an advanced life support skill.

- Never insert a nasogastric tube or nasal airway in a patient with a suspected midface or skull fracture; it could penetrate the cranium and enter the brain.

- Remember facial injuries rarely cause shock from bleeding. If the patient develops hypotension, it is most likely from injuries in the chest, abdomen, retroperitoneal space, or bones.

- Control facial bleeding with direct pressure, which should be applied with a sterile dressing, except where there is an obvious fracture, a ruptured or penetrated eyeball, leaking cerebrospinal fluid, or exposed brain tissue.

- **Do not** attempt to remove an object impaled in the head, even if it is in the brain or eye. If in a prehospital situation, stabilize the object with padding and bandages, and transport the patient immediately. The **only** exception is if the object is obstructing the airway. Remove the object as a matter of life or death. Be prepared for hemorrhage control as bleeding will increase. *Note*: When a drop of bloody drainage from the nose or ear is placed on white paper and a bull's eye or halo forms, the fluid is considered positive for cerebrospinal fluid.

- Degloving injuries usually involve subcutaneous tissue and underlying skeletal structures. Because the tissue is viable, debridement should be careful, and not deep.

- To prevent avulsed tissue from drying out or getting contaminated, lay sterile dressings moistened with saline over the tissue.

- If possible in the prehospital scene, retrieve avulsed tissue, such as an ear; cover with a sterile, moist dressing, wrap in plastic, label and bring it to the emergency department.

- Save loose or dislodged teeth, when time permits. Put them in moist gauze or a container with saline or milk, and label with the time and patient's name. They may possibly be reimplanted if done quickly.

- When applying pressure to bleeding from the neck, be sure to restrict blood loss but not to occlude the airway. If bleeding is severe, administer oxygen and look for shock. Keep in mind the potential of air being sucked into the jugular vein and the formation of an air embolus. Keep the wound covered with a wet, sterile dressing.

- Never shave the eyebrows of a patient with facial trauma. They usually do not grow back and are needed as landmarks for repair.

# EXAMPLES OF NURSING DIAGNOSES RELATED TO MAXILLOFACIAL AND NECK INJURIES

- Ineffective airway clearance related to trauma and foreign objects
- Suffocation related to hemorrhage, trauma to the airway, airway compromise
- Risk for infection related to open injuries, debris, and contamination
- Impaired skin integrity related to trauma, lacerations, avulsions, and degloving injuries
- Anxiety and loss of self-image related to disfigurement from injury
- Impairment of breathing related to nasal fracture, disfigurement, and blockage
- Fear and anxiety related to the potential of continued injury from abuse
- Impairment in verbal communication related to maxillofacial trauma
- Cosmetic disfigurement of the face related to lacerations, tattooing, or epidermal staining

# SUMMARY

Maxillofacial and neck injuries are the most frequent types of injuries seen in the emergency department. Maxillofacial injury can be very dramatic in appearance, often because of hemorrhaging or disfigurement from fractures. Although usually not life threatening, the involvement of facial bones, neurovascular structures, skin and subcutaneous tissue, and glands can be complicating factors in the management of multiple injury patients.

Neck trauma can be high risk because of potential damage to the airway, carotid arteries, jugular veins and cervical spine. Blunt or penetrating trauma to the neck can bring about rapid death from hemorrhage or airway obstruction.

The mechanism of injury can be blunt or projectile trauma. Often severe facial injuries are seen in conjunction with other forceful injuries.

Motor vehicle crashes are the most common cause of facial trauma, but guns, assault and falls are becoming major factors in these injuries.

Assessment must be rapid and organized. It should be assumed that a person with facial, head or neck trauma has a cervical spine injury, and trauma management cannot proceed until the airway is open and the patient is getting adequate oxygen, the neck is stabilized and profuse bleeding is controlled.

# EXAM QUESTIONS

## CHAPTER 6

**Questions 26–30**

26. A person with maxillofacial trauma who is unconscious should be assumed to have

    a. been injured from blunt trauma.

    b. an airway obstruction.

    c. a cervical neck injury.

    d. cranial hemorrhaging.

27. An indication of a mandibular fracture is

    a. Battle's sign.

    b. malocclusion.

    c. carotid artery involvement.

    d. LeFort's Syndrome.

28. A patient is brought into the emergency department with maxillofacial trauma. He is showing rapid development of airway obstruction. What may have happened?

    a. Bleeding and tissue swelling

    b. Bone fragments entering the trachea

    c. Loss of cerebrospinal fluid through the nose

    d. Delayed response to fracture

29. A passenger involved in a motor vehicle accident went through the windshield and lacerated his neck. When he comes into the emergency department, he is rapidly losing consciousness and has dark red blood flowing from a laceration in his neck. It is likely that he has

    a. hypoglycemia.

    b. a rupture of the zygoma.

    c. a laceration of a jugular vein.

    d. a severe cranial injury.

30. A nasal septal hematoma is important to identify because

    a. it is so disfiguring.

    b. the patient can be left with a buckle nose deformity.

    c. it indicates a midface fracture.

    d. immediate evacuation is necessary to prevent saddle nose deformity.

# CHAPTER 7

# OCULAR TRAUMA

## CHAPTER OBJECTIVE

Upon completion of this chapter, the reader will be able to identify appropriate strategies for recognition and management of eye trauma.

## LEARNING OBJECTIVES

Upon completion of this chapter the reader should be able to:

1. Identify important structures and functions of the eye.

2. Describe common causes and types of ocular trauma.

3. Relate assessment priorities to why they are important.

4. Recognize appropriate basic nursing strategies for the patient with ocular trauma.

5. Identify concerns and means used to preserve the vision of patients with ocular trauma.

## INTRODUCTION

Eye injuries are frightening because of the fear of resulting vision defects or loss. Injuries may be obvious, as with penetrating trauma, or difficult to detect, particularly in an unresponsive patient who has multiple injuries. True traumatic emergencies of the eye are quite rare, even more rare to be life-threatening. When a true traumatic emergency does occur, it is most often urgent and a serious threat to the patient's eyesight.

Most acute eye problems are medical in nature, such as in angle-closure glaucoma or retinal artery occlusion. Nonemergent eye injuries are frequent and must have prompt evaluation and treatment to prevent visual defects. Children are more likely than adults to sustain a traumatic injury of the eye.

Typical eye injuries seen in the emergency departments are corneal or conjunctival foreign body, conjunctivitis, and corneal abrasion. While these injuries are uncomfortable, they usually do not cause significant damage to the eye.

## ANATOMY AND PHYSIOLOGY

The eye, shaped like a globe, is approximately 1 inch in diameter, about 80% of which sits in a bony structure of the skull called the orbit. The orbital structure protects the eye and is made up of the frontal, zygoma and maxilla facial bones. The optic foramen is a groove in the posterior part of the orbit through which the optic nerve and ophthalmic artery pass. Six oculomotor muscles move the eye and are innervated by cranial nerves IV and VI.

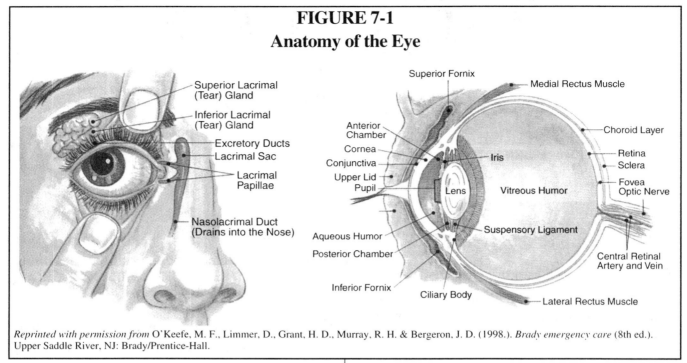

**FIGURE 7-1**
**Anatomy of the Eye**

*Reprinted with permission from* O`Keefe, M. F., Limmer, D., Grant, H. D., Murray, R. H. & Bergeron, J. D. (1998.). *Brady emergency care* (8th ed.). Upper Saddle River, NJ: Brady/Prentice-Hall.

The eyelids protect the eyes. Their inner surfaces are moistened with tears produced by the lacrimal (tear) glands. Every time the eye blinks, the lids cover the exposed surface to clean away dirt and other irritants and bathe it with tears. The tears are then drained through the lacrimal duct, which leads to the nasal cavity.

The white of the eye is the **sclera**. It is a semi-rigid capsule made up of fibrous tissue surrounding the globe that helps to maintain its shape and contain the fluids within the eye.

The colored portion of the external eye, the **iris**, is a contractible membrane suspended between the lens and the cornea. The iris is often used as an identifier of people by its color, and it surrounds an adjustable opening called the **pupil**.

The pupil regulates the amount of light that enters the interior of the eye. In bright light, the pupil constricts, to decrease the amount of light entering the eye. Dim light causes the pupil to expand and let more light into the eye. Constriction of the pupil is controlled by the oculomotor or third cranial nerve. A sluggish pupil indicates damage to the nerve.

A clear portion of the sclera, the **cornea**, lies over the iris and pupil as protection. It helps to keep the fluids in the eye and plays an important part in focusing light.

Covering the sclera, the cornea and lining the surfaces of the eyelids is the **conjunctiva**. It lubricates the tissues that make contact with the air. When the tiny vessels in the conjunctiva become swollen with blood, the eyes look pink or "bloodshot."

The interior of the eye is divided into an anterior and posterior chamber. The anterior chamber is located between the cornea and the lens. It is filled with a clear, watery fluid, the **aqueous humor,** which circulates through the anterior and posterior chambers. If the aqueous fluid leaks and is lost through a penetrating injury, it will replace itself with proper treatment.

The colorless **lens** is enclosed in a capsule and is suspended behind the iris and the pupil. As light rays pass through the cornea and the aqueous humor, they bend, which is the beginning of the focusing process. The light continues through the transparent lens. Muscle action changes the shape of the lens to make it thicker or thinner, which controls how the light reaches the retina.

The lens is the dividing structure between the anterior and posterior chambers. The entire posterior cavity is located behind the lens and is filled with a transparent jelly-like substance called the **vitreous humor.** The vitreous humor is important in maintaining the shape and length of the globe. It exerts a degree of pressure on the lens so that the lens is able to function properly. Vitreous humor cannot be replaced, and it cannot regenerate itself. If the vitreous humor is lost, the eye is lost.

During the process of the image being focused, it is inverted so that it is upside down on the **retina**. The retina is the innermost lining of the eyeball and totally lines the interior of the eye. It extends from where the optic nerve (cranial nerve II) enters at the back of the globe to the margin of the pupil. The retina is light sensitive where the rays focus to receive the image formed by the lens. The cells of the retina convert light into electrical impulses that are conducted through the optic nerve to the vision center (occipital lobe) at the back of the head. As the brain processes the information it is receiving, it corrects the image so that it is perceived as being upright.

# MECHANISM OF INJURY

Disease or injury may cause ocular emergencies. Injury to the eye may indicate other head trauma that can have a broad range in severity. There may also be an injury to the cervical spine. Assume there are serious head injuries if there are indications of fractures around the orbit, the sclera is red due to bleeding, one or both eyes cannot move, one pupil is larger than the other, both pupils are unresponsive, or the eyes cross or turn in different directions (O'Carroll, 1990).

Blunt trauma to the eye may be caused by motor vehicle crashes, assault, a fall or other direct blow to the eye. Injuries range from minor corneal abrasions or contusions to retinal detachment or the loss of an eye. Most often, the injury is to the orbit rather than the eyeball. An example of an incident causing blunt injury to the globe is where an object, such as a golf ball, is small enough to strike the eye by passing through the orbital rim.

Projectiles, such as a knife or a missile, cause most penetrating injuries to the eyeball. Injury may affect the surface of the eye or the globe. Damage includes laceration, impalement, or puncture, any of which threaten vision or the eye, itself. Many times these injuries occur due to the lack of protective eyewear.

Burns also cause ocular trauma and are an immediate threat to vision. Burns can be chemical, from a heat source, or radiation.

# OCULAR INJURIES AND INTERVENTIONS

## Periorbital Injury

Injury includes the eyelid and the periorbital tissue. Since the area is so close to the globe, the globe may be involved and should be evaluated. Damage may cause a contusion, laceration, or avulsion of tissue. Treatment includes early closure of a wound before edema develops, with careful approximation of the edges. If tissue is avulsed and missing, plastic surgery is recommended. The eyelid has an excellent blood supply, so trauma in this area usually does not develop infection.

## Foreign Body

Foreign bodies most often are very small particles, such as pieces of dirt, dust, or metal shavings. All foreign bodies in the eye are considered contaminated. The particle may be seen on the surface of the cornea with the naked eye, or it may require a magnifier, such as a slit lamp, to be identified. Because the patient is extremely uncomfortable when there is a foreign body in the eye, even if the object can't be immediately visualized, it is safe to assume one is there. Organic foreign bodies are more likely to cause infection, and metallic objects will leave a rust ring unless removed within 12 hours.

The patient will have pain, especially when the eyelid is opened and closed; copious tearing; and sensitivity to light. The pain is similar to that of a corneal abrasion. The foreign body must be located and identified, which may require local anesthesia for effective examination. Children may need conscious sedation or general anesthesia. Removal can be done with a cotton swab and saline irrigation or a 25 or 27-gauge needle. If the foreign body is large or imbedded, an ophthalmologist is required for removal and follow up. The object may leave an abrasion or a rust ring if it is metal. Antibiotic ointment and patching follows removal of the foreign body.

With a history of a high-speed projectile, there is a good possibility of an intraocular foreign body. Metal fragments and other small projectiles can enter the eye at a high rate of speed, ending up in the posterior chamber. Intraocular foreign bodies are easily overlooked because ordinarily they are so small. The entry site may be hard to locate because of the small size. There may or may not be a change in the visual acuity. The patient feels only slight discomfort. The pupil may take on the same shape as a cat's eye.

An intraocular foreign body is an ocular emergency. The amount of damage depends on the size, makeup, and shape of the object. Early intervention is necessary to save the vision. Plain radiographs identify the position and number of foreign bodies. It may be necessary to use a CT scan for a clearer identification of the object. Surgery is indicated in

most cases to prevent additional damage secondary to hemorrhage, infection, or a detached retina.

## Contusion

An ocular contusion is a closed injury, most often to the orbit. The eyelid may or may not be damaged. The patient usually has pain. If he complains of visual disturbance or double vision, the damage could be acute. The eye may appear swollen or red. If the iris is not visible or there is blood between the cornea and the iris, immediate treatment is necessary.

A patient may want a cold pack to the eyes to relieve his pain. This remedy is contraindicated if there are any indications of more serious eye damage or a head injury. In this case, it is not desirable to cause rapid changes in circulation. A cold pack will rapidly constrict the blood vessels and change the circulation. If cold is applied, pressure should not be.

## Corneal Abrasion

A scratch or scrape to the cornea is likely to be caused by a foreign object and is a common occurrence. Contact lens scratches are frequent. Normally, the cornea appears smooth, clear, wet, and moist. An abrasion is rarely visible to the naked eye without fluorescein staining. Injury can abrade or denude the epithelium and expose the superficial corneal nerves, which causes pain, tearing, and eyelid spasms.

Antibiotic ointments are applied, and the eye should be patched for 24 hours. Patching prevents eyelid movement and further irritation to the eye.

## Corneal Laceration

Small lacerations are considered abrasions and treated as such. Larger lacerations may be accompanied by lid wounds that can affect the movement of the lid or injure the lacrimal system. There may also be involvement with the sclera or the conjunctiva. If the laceration is deep enough to enter the anterior or posterior chamber and allow the aqueous and/or vitreous humor to leak, it is an emergent situation.

Pressure on the globe can cause the vitreous humor to leak out through a deep laceration into the posterior chamber. Unlike aqueous humor, vitreous cannot regenerate or be replaced. Loss of vitreous humor is likely to lead to blindness. To preserve the vitreous, the injured eye is closed, and either a donut ring or a non-Styrofoam cup is placed over the eye. The ring or cup is then secured with roller gauze until an ophthalmologist can evaluate and treat the patient. Surgery may be indicated to preserve the intraocular contents.

If the eyelid is bleeding, a pressure dressing should **not** be applied unless it is certain there are no lacerations to the globe. If the globe is also bleeding, loose dressings over the lid aid in clotting and help prevent contamination.

If the globe is bleeding but there are no open wounds to the lid, loose dressings to **both** eyes should be applied.

## Conjunctival Laceration

Laceration to the conjunctiva causes bleeding and swelling from the conjunctiva, which covers the sclera, cornea, and the lining of the lids. Fingernails and hairbrushes are the most common perpetrators of these lacerations. Small lacerations are treated like abrasions. Larger lacerations require an ophthalmology consult and may need surgical repair.

Lacerations less than 5 mm are generally treated with antibiotic ointment, patching, and observation. A larger than 5-mm injury requires suturing.

## Subconjunctival Hemorrhage

A dramatic situation, the bright red subconjunctival hemorrhage is not as serious as it may appear. It might involve a small area or the entire conjunctiva. The cause can be blunt trauma, sneezing, coughing episodes, or Valsalva's maneuver. In the case of blunt trauma, there is always the danger of another ocular injury. The hemorrhage is likely to be painless, benign and heal spontaneously. Rarely, a hyphema may develop as a secondary condition.

After other ocular injuries are ruled out, the patient can be assured the condition will resolve in 2 to 3 weeks.

## Avulsion

If the eyelids are torn or torn away and the eyeball is protruding, pulled from the socket, or pulled out of the socket, it is considered an avulsion and can be very serious. The condition rarely happens.

If the eyelid is severely lacerated or torn off, careful protection with dressings is required. A completely avulsed lid should be retrieved, packaged, and transported with the patient, just as any amputated part would be.

The eye should not be forced back into the socket.

## Hyphema

Blunt trauma causing a bleed into the anterior chamber of the eye is referred to as hyphema. The size of a hyphema ranges from small to complete involvement of the anterior chamber. "Eightball hyphema" is total involvement that has started to clot. A complication is a blocked flow of aqueous humor, causing increased intraocular pressure. The sclera may appear bloody. Blood in the anterior chamber may be seen in persons with light-colored eyes, but in those with dark eyes, it can be extremely difficult to see.

The injury is painful and may cause photophobia and blurred vision. Watch for an altered level of consciousness and a head injury. Patients with bleeding disorders; receiving anticoagulant drug therapy; or kidney, liver, or sickle cell disease should be carefully monitored because of the potential for increased bleeding complications. Rebleeding within 2 to 5 days, and up to 14 days, is the most common complication. Corneal blood staining, secondary glaucoma, and loss of vision or the eye can also occur.

Management varies and is controversial. Activity ranges from complete bed rest to quiet activity. There is also a difference of opinion as to whether the patient should be hospitalized or have the eye patched. Pharmacological management is also used.

## Iris Injury

It may be difficult to tell an iris injury from a microhyphema. The hyphema is characterized by red blood cells in the anterior chamber, whereas the iris injury, or iritis, result in white blood cells in the anterior chamber. Traumatic iridocyclitis is an inflammation of the iris after a contusion of the eye. The injury causes pain, photophobia, and asymmetry in pupil size. The pupil in the affected eye does not contract as well as the unaffected pupil.

Complications include recession of the eyeball into the orbit and loss of the eye. Treatment includes topical use of cycloplegic agents and topical or systemic steroid medication.

## Lens Injury

Injury to the lens can cause partial or full dislocation, opacification or cataracts. Surgery is required but not emergent unless leaking aqueous humor causes acute angle-closure glaucoma.

## Retinal Detachment

Retinal detachment is not truly a detachment where the entire retina separates from the choroid (a vascular layer between the sclera and the retina). Instead, the pigment layer of the retina remains attached to the choroid and the rest of the retina detaches from it. The detachment may or may not have a tear. When there is a tear, the vitreous seeps between the layers. Additionally, with a tear, the loss of blood and oxygen supply makes the retina unable to see light and disrupts impulses to the

optic nerve. A detachment can occur from various medical causes, a hole or break in the inner sensory layer, or can be precipitated by trauma.

The condition is disturbing to the patient who sees floaters, flashing lights and has the sensation of a curtain moving across the field of vision. Loss of vision depends on the site of the detachment and whether the macula is involved.

Treatment includes possible laser repair or scleral buckling for a torn retina, bed rest and patching both eyes.

## Burn Injury

Burns to the eyes can be caused by chemicals, heat or radiation. The delicate tissues of the eye are easily damaged permanently. Burns are an immediate threat to sight and very painful.

### Chemical Burns

The most urgent of all ocular emergencies, chemical burns can occur almost anywhere. Chemical burns can be caused by acid, alkali, or another type of irritant.

Acid burns immediately damage the cornea by denaturing the tissue, which makes the tissue look white and opaque. Damage stops after the initial contact because the denaturing process neutralizes the action of the acid.

Alkaline substances, such as lye and drain cleaners, also cause the cornea to become opaque. However, alkaline chemicals in particular are very destructive because, unlike acids, they continue to eat into the tissue until thorough irrigation completely removes the chemical. It should be remembered that automobile air bags have alkaline powder in them, and when they are deployed, serious eye burns can result.

The only emergency treatment for chemical burns is flushing the eye with sterile water or normal saline. However, if nothing else is available, tap water should be used. Copious irrigation takes priority over everything, including assessment. The eye may have to be held open so that it can be adequately flushed. Irrigation should be gentle and not forceful to prevent increased pain or further damage to the tissue. If the other eye is not burned, it must be carefully protected during irrigation to prevent the chemical from being flushed into it. Hopefully, the patient's eye was continuously irrigated during transportation to the emergency department.

With alkaline burns, irrigation should continue for at least 30 minutes or until the ocular pH reaches 7.4. In acute situations, irrigation may continue from 2 to 4 hours until the pH reaches the necessary level. The eyelid also should be rolled back so the interior can be swabbed and irrigated. Careful observation should be made for contaminated foreign bodies that could continue to burn the eye.

An ophthalmologist should evaluate, treat and follow through as soon as possible.

### Thermal Burns

When the face is burned with fire, reflex causes the eyes to quickly close because of the heat. The eyelids may also get burned because they are also exposed to the fire. Globe burns usually don't occur, as they are protected by the eyelids. If the situation involves an explosion, steam, hot metal, or gasoline, the globes are more likely to be burned.

The patient should arrive at the emergency room with the eyelids covered with moist sterile dressings.

Burned eyelids may develop contractures that are disfiguring and affect vision.

### Light/Radiation Burns

Exposure to extreme light conditions can endanger vision. The rays of light pass through the lens and focus on the retina, severely damaging the sensory cells.

Laser rays burn the retina, which may not be painful but are very damaging. Burns from infrared rays, such as from looking directly into the sun or directly at an eclipse, are more severe than ultraviolet radiation burns. Permanent loss of vision is secondary to the absorption of infrared rays by the iris and the increased lens temperature, which precipitate cataract formation. Protective eyewear has reduced the occurrence of this type of burn.

Ultraviolet rays, from a welding unit (flash burns), sunlamp, or prolonged snow glare (snow blindness), cause a superficial burn of the eyes. The ultraviolet radiation is absorbed by the cornea. Not painful at first, the patient may be initially unaware that his eyes have been burned. Within 6 to 10 hours, severe pain, photophobia and corneal irregularity develop. The pain is considered the most severe of all ocular burns. Acute conjunctivitis, keratitis, redness, swelling and tearing occur. Visual acuity is diminished.

The patient should be protected from bright light, and moist dressings over the eyes help to alleviate pain.

Topical ointments and patching for 24-hours are used for treatment. There may be some residual decreased vision.

## Perforation or Rupture of the Globe

Blunt or penetrating force can cause this major ocular emergency.

Penetrating trauma perforating the eye or rupturing the globe may cost the loss of an eye. Perforation with a sharp object will penetrate the globe. Blood, aqueous and vitreous humor may seep out, ensuring the loss of the eye.

Blunt force may cause the globe to rupture secondary to an abrupt rise in the intraocular pressure. Rupture will occur at a point of weakness in the eye, often at the insertion point of the extraocular muscles or the corneoscleral junction.

Globe rupture results in an unusually deep or shallow anterior chamber, altered light perception, hyphema, and possibly, vitreous hemorrhage. The pupil will take on a teardrop shape, with the point toward the rupture site.

Manipulation of the eye should be avoided. If there is an impaled object, it must be secured and the eyes patched to limit movement and prevent further damage. If the eye has not been eviscerated, the object will need to be surgically removed. When vitreous humor is lost along with damage to the lens and ciliary body, enucleation may be necessary.

Detailed examination or assessment should be delayed until an ophthalmologist is able to conduct it. General anesthesia may be necessary to properly examine the eye.

Eyedrops should not be used when a global rupture is suspected. Other treatment includes keeping the patient NPO for surgery and to prevent nausea and vomiting. Antibiotics, tetanus prophylaxis and corticosteroids are given as ordered.

## Orbital Fracture

Orbital fractures involve the orbital floor and the rim. A fracture of the orbital floor is serious and usually the result of blunt trauma. A blowout fracture results from direct impact to the orbit, because the orbit is full of fluid, it can not compress. The floor of the orbit and the medial orbital wall are weak and collapse from the pressure. The orbit may herniate into the maxillary or ethmoid sinus, trapping the inferior rectus muscle.

Orbital fractures are not a true emergency unless the vision is impaired or the globe has been injured.

Diagnosis is made from the history and by the observation of periorbital hematoma, subconjunctival hemorrhage, and periorbital edema. When the inferior rectus and oblique muscle is trapped in the fracture, there is enophthalmos (sunken eye), an upward gaze, and the patient complains of diplopia. Facial x-rays or CT scans are used to confirm the diagnosis. Symptoms resolve without

needing surgical intervention in 85% of the patients.

The patient should be warned against doing Valsalva's maneuver or blowing his nose to prevent herniation of the globe.

## Contact Lenses and Prostheses

Four types of contact lenses are widely used. Hard lenses cover the cornea and are about the size of a shirt button. Soft lenses cover the entire cornea and part of the sclera and are slightly larger than a dime. Extended-wear lenses are similar to soft lenses and appear to be the same. Scleral lenses cover the cornea and a large part of the sclera and are about the size of a quarter.

There are several common problems associated with wearing contact lenses. When hard or soft lenses are worn too long, they are difficult to remove because they adhere to the cornea. Lubricating drops will loosen the lens for easier removal.

Other problems include losing a contact under the eyelid and getting chemicals or dirt particles under the lens and irritating the cornea. Contact lenses should be removed when there is ocular trauma or the patient has a change in mental status.

When the contact is lost in the eye, the upper lid should be reverted and the lens removed. If the lens cannot be seen, the cul-de-sac should be swept with a moistened swab to catch the lens. If the lens is still not visualized, fluorescein stain should be used.

The cornea can have an abrasion and feel as though the lens is still in the eye. When a foreign body gets under a contact lens, the lens should be removed and cleaned. Force or pressure should not be used when removing a contact lens. Special suction cups are available to remove hard lenses. If the lens can be seen but not easily removed, it should be slid on to the sclera until the ophthalmologist can remove it.

If the globe is perforated, the lens should not be removed because the pressure of removing the contact lens on the eyeball can worsen the leaking of vitreous humor.

In rare situations, the patient has an artificial eye. If the pupil does not respond, the eye moves separately from the other eye's movement, or it has a similar, but different appearance than the other eye, ask the patient if he has an artificial eye. Verification should be noted so that there is no misleading or incorrect information about the condition of the eye.

# ASSESSMENT

Following the ABC assessment, ensuring the airway, breathing, and circulation are stable, the patient is assessed to determine if there is an immediate danger of vision loss or the loss of an eye. In the triage process, only a patient with the possible loss of life is seen ahead of the patient whose vision is threatened.

Traumatic ocular emergencies threatening vision and requiring immediate attention are globe penetration and acute chemical burn. With a history of trauma:

- Identify the mechanism of injury and tetanus immunization status.

- Determine how long ago the injury occurred.

- Find out if the injury occurred in a motor vehicle crash and if the airbag deployed. Alkaline powder may be burning the eyes.

- Ask about the use of protective eyewear, glasses, or contact lenses.

- Obtain the past ocular history, including injury; disease, such as diabetes or glaucoma; trauma; and surgery.

- Determine the patient's visual acuity and light perception before the trauma and if it is changed now.

- Examine the patient's visual acuity, pupil reaction, position of the globe, ocular motility, and external appearance.

- A physician may need to perform a slit-lamp examination, fluorescein stain, intraocular pressure measurement, and direct ophthalmoscopy.

Note immediate signs and symptoms:

- Secure a penetrating object so it will not cause further damage.

- Is there obvious leaking of the vitreous humor, a jellylike substance; or any bleeding?

- Note if the globe is ruptured or there is a change in the shape or contour.

- Note if the eye has been burned, what type of burn, if the cornea is white and opaque, and the lids are burned.

- Is there a subconjunctival hematoma or a hyphema, redness and swelling of the conjunctiva or copious tearing?

- Look for indications of an orbital fracture or blowout fracture, including: enophthalmos, periorbital edema, subconjunctival hemorrhage, and if the patient complains of diplopia.

The following signs indicate serious head injury or brain damage:

- The pupils are unequal in size or do not react to light.

- One or both eyes protrude.

- One or both of the orbits are fractured.

- Blood is in the sclera.

- One or both of the eyes cannot move.

- The eyes cross or turn in different directions independent of each other.

# NURSING STRATEGIES FOR THE PATIENT WITH OCULAR TRAUMA

The goal is to maintain vision and prevent the loss of the eye. Almost all ocular trauma management includes the removal of any contact lens, irrigation, patching, and the use of ocular medication. Medications are meant to decrease pain, provide antibiotic therapy, change pupil size, reduce allergic reactions and clean the eye.

Always inform the patient what is being done and why, to prepare him and allay fears.

- Stabilize any other injuries until the eye emergency is treated.

- Vision screening should be conducted prior to treatment in non-critical injuries.

- The patient should be supine and keep his eyes still to prevent further injury.

- Instillation of eyedrops or ointments should have attention taken to prevent contamination, and be observed for any untoward effects.

- Patients with cardiovascular diseases may develop adverse systemic effects from eyedrops.

- Either saline or lactated Ringer's solution may be used for irrigating foreign bodies, chemicals, or other substances. Dextrose solutions should not be used.

- Do not irrigate if the globe is ruptured.

- If there is a chemical burn, the eyes must be immediately irrigated. In the case of chemical burns, the contact lenses should be removed so the chemical is not trapped under the lens. Eyes should be flushed from the inner canthus to the outer canthus. Do not attempt to neutralize the chemical with any solution other than flushing with saline or lactated Ringer's.

- Ordinarily, contact lenses should be left in place and reported to the physician for further direction.

- The nurse should not try to remove a foreign body from the cornea.

- As discussed before, do not attempt to push a protruding globe back into the orbit.

- A sterile dressing may be gently placed over the injured eye to reduce further contamination or absorb blood. **DO NOT** use pressure on the dressings; it could rupture the globe or squeeze out vitreous humor.

- Sterile patches over both eyes might alleviate pain and discomfort until the physician can treat and medicate the patient. Patching minimizes ocular stimulation by reducing movement and limiting light exposure. The reason for patching both eyes is that it simulates total blindness; patching one eye alters depth perception.

- When a patient is discharged with one eye patch, discharge instructions should include information about altered vision and the hazards of driving or using machinery.

- The nurse should never attempt to remove an impaled object. Stabilize the object if it has not been done in the rescue unit.

- Provide a quiet environment and reassure the patient. Elevating the head of the bed reduces swelling and congestion in the eye, if other injuries do not prohibit this position.

- If a patient is unconscious, close his eyes whether or not there is ocular trauma. Unconscious patients cannot blink. If the eyes will not stay closed, they can be gently taped shut.

- Unless the injury is very superficial, an ophthalmology consult should be requested.

- The patient should be NPO until after being seen by the physician, in case surgery is necessary.

# EXAMPLES OF NURSING DIAGNOSES RELATED TO OCULAR TRAUMA

• Anxiety related to unfamiliarity with the treatment being used and fears of loss of vision or the eye

• Risk of further injury related to impaled objects, protruding globe, and other trauma

• Pain related to ocular injury

• Altered sensory perception related to ocular injury or an eye patch

• Risk of infection related to the trauma

• Knowledge deficit related to fears from the trauma and the trauma management

• Alteration of body image due to observable trauma to the eyelid or globe

# SUMMARY

Although most ocular injuries are not life threatening, they can be disfiguring and debilitating. Most injuries are not true emergencies, and although painful, are treatable without permanent damage. Other than imminent death for another patient, the serious eye injury takes top triage priority in the emergency department. Accurate assessment of the patient by the emergency room nurse has a major bearing on the immediacy and outcome of treatment.

The mechanism of ocular injury can be blunt or penetrating trauma or burns. Ocular injury may indicate head or neck trauma, especially when the orbit is involved.

Eye injuries cause anxiety because of the pain, disturbance in vision, threat of the loss of an eye, and the potential for disfigurement and alteration in lifestyle.

Vision cannot be replaced; eyes cannot be transplanted, only parts of them, such as the corneas. Proper management of ocular trauma is essential and has to begin the moment of injury.

# EXAM QUESTIONS

## CHAPTER 7
### Questions 31–35

31. A part of the eye that cannot be replaced is the

    a. aqueous humor.
    b. cornea.
    c. avulsed eyelid.
    d. vitreous humor.

32. A blowout fracture is when

    a. the globe is blown out of the socket due to trauma to the back of the head.
    b. the vitreous humor is blown out through a penetrating wound to the globe.
    c. direct impact to the orbit collapses the floor of the orbit and medial orbital wall.
    d. the intraocular pressure is so great that the lens is blown out through the pupil.

33. A patient comes into the emergency department with a piece of metal protruding out of the globe. The object has a cup over it, held in place with roller gauze. As soon as possible, the nurse should

    a. irrigate the eye to get rid of any foreign objects.
    b. call the ophthalmologist for stat consult and reassure the patient.
    c. under sterile conditions, gently remove the metal object, followed by patching both eyes.
    d. make sure both eyes are patched.

34. The one and only emergency treatment for chemical burns of the eye is

    a. continuous flushing of the eye with sterile saline or water.
    b. patching both eyes.
    c. securing non-Styrofoam cups over both eyes.
    d. getting an immediate thorough history from the patient to determine what kind of chemical is involved.

35. A patient fell and struck the back of his head two days ago. He has had a headache since that time, along with seeing bright flashes on the periphery of his eye and dark spots that seem to float across his line of sight. It is likely that he has

    a. traumatic glaucoma.
    b. retinal detachment.
    c. an intraorbital contusion.
    d. ocular inversion.

# CHAPTER 8

# TRAUMA TO THE SPINE

## CHAPTER OBJECTIVE

Upon completion of this chapter, the reader will be able to relate the proper procedures for managing spinal injuries.

## LEARNING OBJECTIVES

Upon completion of this chapter, the reader should be able to:

1. Describe the relationship between the peripheral and the central nervous systems.

2. Identify frequent causes of spinal cord trauma.

3. Describe frequently seen spinal cord injuries.

4. Relate assessment priorities to basic nursing strategies for the spinal cord trauma patient.

5. Describe some of the personal and monetary costs of spinal cord injuries.

## INTRODUCTION

Every year, more than 10,000 people in the United States are affected by spinal cord trauma. Sixty percent of the injuries occur in people between the ages of 16 and 30 years old, and 82% are males (Peitzman et al., 1998). Half of the injuries involve the cervical spine, and nearly half of those result in quadriplegia. The financial cost alone to society is more than 4 billion dollars a year.

The most common cause of spinal injury is the motor vehicle crash: head-on collisions, rollovers, ejection and collisions with pedestrians. These injuries make up at least 49% of the acute cases. Falls, direct blows to the head or neck, sports injuries such as football and diving, and penetrating wounds from guns or knives make up a large portion of the rest of the injuries. As recreational and technological opportunities expand, the means for spinal cord injury increase. In recent years, in-line skating, extreme skiing, snowboarding and bicycling have added to the mechanisms of injury. Upper cervical injury is increasingly identified as a cause of death in cases of child abuse, particularly infants. "Shaken baby" trauma causes acceleration-deceleration damage to the brain. Because the infant's head is relatively large and heavy and the neck is weak, the brain bounces back and forth in the cranium, causing eventual tearing of the cortical veins, along with cervical injury.

Since the development of emergency medical services as a system in the early 1970s with advanced prehospital and emergency department care, more people sustaining spinal cord injuries survive and many survive in better condition. The rapid advanced medical interventions along with spinal cord rehabilitation systems across the country have decreased complications and brought about better recovery potential for those injured. However, because more survive, more people are left with seriously debilitating and crippling injuries.

Today, society has become more knowledgeable and accepting about adapting to, and including, those with spinal cord injuries in the workforce, sports, and the social world.

# ANATOMY AND PHYSIOLOGY

## Overview

A "system" is a combination of interrelated parts forming a complex or unitary whole. The body's nervous system is a perfect example of a complex unitary whole having several components or interrelated systems. It literally controls all activities of the body.

### Anatomical

Anatomically, the nervous system has two divisions: the central nervous system (CNS) and the peripheral nervous system (PNS).

The **central nervous system** is the brain and spinal cord. The brain is the controlling organ of the body, serving as the center of consciousness, directing voluntary and involuntary activities, perceiving one's surroundings, and controlling reactions to those surroundings. It receives and sorts information and directs the body's response. It is the brain that enables us to experience thought and feelings. Three major subdivisions of the brain are the cerebrum, cerebellum, and brain stem. The brain stem is the continuous portion of the brain that joins with the spinal cord and functions as an important relay and reflex center. It is the most primitive part of the central nervous system, and controls all the body functions necessary for life.

The spinal cord is the part of the central nervous system that transmits messages back and forth between the brain and the body. As in the brain, the spinal cord has cell bodies, but it is mostly made up of nerve fibers extending from the brain to just below the brain stem where it forms the spinal cord. Many nerve cells in the CNS have long fibers that continue outside the system to form cables of nerve fibers linking the CNS to various organs in the body.

The linking cables of nerve fibers reaching outside the CNS make up the **peripheral nervous system.** This system includes the nerves that enter and leave the spinal cord and those that connect the brain and organs without passing through the cord, such as the optic nerve. There are 31 pairs of peripheral nerves, called spinal nerves, and 12 pairs of cranial nerves.

The cranial nerves arise from the brain stem, each having a name and corresponding Roman numeral and pass directly through holes in the skull to their innervations. They may be sensory nerves, motor nerves, or both. Mostly, cranial nerves are specialized and have particular functions in the head and face.

The 31 pairs of spinal nerves provide pathways for responses to specific stimuli. Each nerve has paired roots that extend from either side of the spinal cord to transmit sensory and motor impulses. The paired nerves correspond to specific segments of the spinal cord and are: 8 cervical, 12 thoracic, 5 lumbar, 5 sacral, and 1 coccygeal nerve.

Three categories of peripheral nerves are sensory, motor and connecting nerves. Sensory nerves carry messages sent from the body to the central nervous system. Sensory nerves are complex, being made up of many types of cells, such as those in the retina, ear, skin, muscles, joints and the body's organs. They do as the name implies and detect sensations of heat, cold, position, motion, pressure, light, hearing and balance, taste, smell and many others. Each cell has distinctive nerve endings that only perceive one type of sensation and send only one type of message. Cranial sensory nerves go directly to the brain and do not pass through the spinal cord.

The nerves sending messages from the central nervous system to the muscles are motor nerves. Each muscle in the body has its own motor nerve. An impulse in the motor strip of the brain's cerebral cortex is sent along the spinal cord to a cell body. The receiving cell body in the spinal cord then transmits the impulse to the motor nerve of the specific muscle it causes to contract.

In the brain and spinal cord are cells, the connecting nerves, with short fibers that connect the sensory nerves with the motor nerves. Some connect directly in the spinal cord without having to go through the brain, allowing the nerves to transmit impulses between nerves within the CNS. Connecting nerves in the spinal cord form a **reflex arc** between sensory and motor nerves of the extremities. When an irritating stimulus is transmitted from the sensory nerve along the connecting nerve directly to the motor nerve, immediate response occurs, even before the information can be sent to the brain. Examples of reflex reactions are the responses that occur when one touches something very hot or when the physician taps the patellar tendon.

### Functional

Aside from the anatomical divisions of the nervous system, there are functional divisions: the somatic and autonomic nervous systems.

Activities that are voluntary and which one has control over, such as walking and writing, are controlled by the **somatic nervous system.** The peripheral nerves send sensory information to the brain for interpretation. The brain then responds to the voluntary muscles to act.

In the involuntary or **autonomic nervous system,** one has no conscious or deliberate control over the functions it governs such as digestion, dilation and constriction of blood vessels, and perspiring.

Some of the cells forming the autonomic system are inside the CNS and others lie alongside the spinal cord near the point where the spinal nerve roots exit. There are two branches of the autonomic system: the **sympathetic** and the **parasympathetic**.

Along the vertebral column, a chain of ganglia (a collection of nerve-cell bodies) form the main sympathetic trunks that extend from the base of the skull to the coccyx. They are supplied by the thoracolumbar portion of the spinal cord nerve roots. The sympathetic system responds to stress and threatening situations by causing the pupils to dilate, blood vessels to constrict, stimulating sweating, increasing the heart rate, causing sphincter muscles to constrict and preparing the body to respond to stress.

The parasympathetic system is the other side of the sympathetic coin, the balancing side. The parasympathetic nerve cells are found in the brain stem and the sacral area of the spinal cord. They cause the pupils to constrict, blood vessels to dilate, slow the heart rate, relax the sphincters and other responses.

Autonomic functions include slowing or increasing the heart rate and strength of contractions, dilating or constricting blood vessels in skeletal muscles and abdominal organs, changing bronchial diameter, relaxing or contracting the urinary bladder, dilating or constricting the pupils, and increasing or decreasing saliva and digestive juices. Any injury interfering with the function of the autonomic system can be life threatening.

To summarize, the nervous system *anatomically* is divided into the central nervous system and the peripheral nervous system. *Functionally,* the nervous system is made up of the somatic and autonomic components.

# THE SPINAL CORD

The purpose of the spinal cord is to transmit nerve messages, or impulses, back and forth between the brain and the body in order to control functions and movements. Impulses are electrical, moving along nerve fibers within the cord.

Nerve fibers in the spinal cord are grouped together in tracts. Sensory input from the body to the cord is received by the ascending tracts and brain commands for body motor functions travel through the descending tracts. While it is not necessary to know the names of all the tracts, it is important to know that the functions of three tracts relate to position sense, pain sense and movement, and should be checked after an injury.

The base of the skull has an opening, the foramen magnum, through which the spinal cord exits to enter the spinal canal down to the lumbar vertebrae. Meninges covering the brain continue down to surround the cord, which is about 1 cm in diameter. Fluid that bathes and cushions the brain also surrounds the cord, which is why it is called cerebrospinal fluid (CSF).

The spinal cord is housed in the spinal column. Here, it is well protected by 33 vertebrae, aligned by strong ligaments that connect, support, provide stability and prevent excessive flexion or extension of the vertebrae. The vertebrae support the head and body, allowing man to walk upright. Segments of the vertebrae are: 7 cervical, 12 thoracic, 5 lumbar, 5 fused sacral and 4 fused coccygeal.

Between each of the cervical, thoracic and lumbar vertebrae are broad, flat, intervertebral discs made of fibrocartilage. They act as shock absorbers for the vertebrae.

The vascular supply is the vertebral artery and spinal rami arteries entering between the vertebrae. Different from other areas of the body, spinal arter-ies cannot develop an adequate collateral blood supply when they are injured or obstructed.

# MECHANISM OF INJURY

The spine can normally withstand forces up to 1,000 foot pounds. High-speed travel and contact sports can cause forces well above that level. The body of an unrestrained 150 lb passenger flying upward and forward in a low-speed accident can easily place 3,000–4,000 foot pounds of force against the spine as the head suddenly meets the windshield. Similar force encounters a skier as he collides with a tree.

The major causes of adult spinal trauma in order of occurrence are car crashes, shallow water diving/swimming, motorcycle crashes and all other falls and injuries. Rapid forward deceleration during a motor vehicle crash and rapid vertical deceleration from a fall are the two primary causes of injury to the spine. Patients over 45 years old have more spinal injuries from falls than motor vehicle accidents.

Pediatric patient frequency and injury patterns are quite different. Most pediatric spinal injuries are the result of falling, either from a height or bicycle; being struck by a car; diving accidents or sports-related injuries.

Trauma to the spinal cord is from primary, or direct, injury and secondary injury, a consequence of the initial trauma. Secondary injury is a physiologic consequence from damage to the spinal cord. Primary mechanisms of injury can be blunt or penetrating forces, or movement that pushes the spine beyond its normal limits of motion or weight-bearing ability. The majority of spinal injuries are closed and not directly visible.

Types of injuries to the spine include:

- Fracture, with or without bone displacement
- Dislocation

## FIGURE 8-1
### Anterior Ligament Rupture Caused by Hyperextension and Posterior Dislocation of the Vertebrae

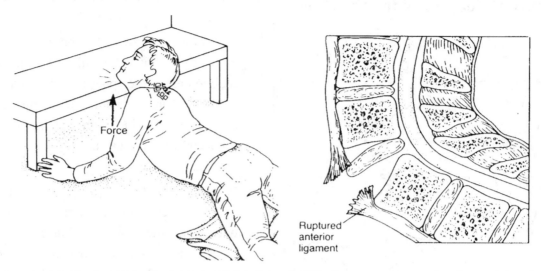

Force

Ruptured
anterior
ligament

*Reprinted with permission from Kitt, S., Selfridge-Thomas, J., Proehl, J. & Kaiser, J. (1995). Emergency nursing: A physiologic and clinical perspective (2nd ed.). Philadelphia: Saunders.*

- Subluxation

- Ligament strain

- Disk injury, including compression

- Shearing

The following basic types of movement can injure the spinal cord (Newberry, 1998):

**Hyperextension:** The head is forced back, and the cervical vertebrae are moved to an overextended position *(see Figure 8-1).*

**Hyperflexion:** The head is forced forward and the cervical vertebrae are moved to an overflexion position *(see Figure 8-2).*

**Over rotation:** The head turns to one side and the cervical vertebrae are forced beyond their limits; vertebrae can shatter and be forced into the spinal cord.

Violent or excessive flexion, extension, or rotation can cause bone damage and tearing of muscles, ligaments, and the spinal cord.

**Axial loading:** A severe blow to the top of the head, or when the weight of the body is driven against the head, causes a blunt downward force on the spinal column and vertebrae. For example, axial loading with compression occurs when a patient falls from a substantial height and lands standing, forcing the weight of the head and thorax down against the lumbar spine, while the sacral spine is driven upward.

**Lateral bend:** The range of lateral bending is more limited than flexion or extension. The head and neck bent to the side beyond the normal range of motion, or a sudden lateral thrust can cause damage to the cervical spine as the head tries to stay in place while the body is pushed from beneath.

**Compression:** Forces from above and below compress the vertebrae, can cause the vertebrae to shatter and force bone fragments into the spinal cord *(see Figure 8-3).*

**Distraction:** Opposite of compression, distraction pulls the spine apart which easily can cause stretching and tearing of the spinal cord. Hanging, either by suicide or when a child's chin is caught on a crossbar in a playground, are the most common causes, which result in

## FIGURE 8-2
## Posterior Ligament Rupture Caused by Forward Dislocation of the Vertebrae

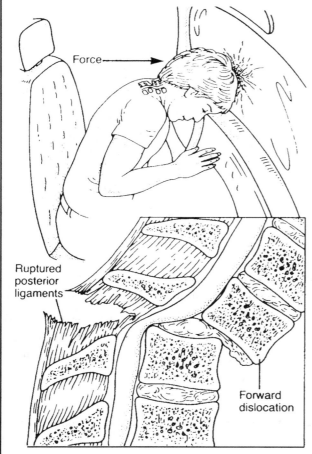

*Reprinted with permission from* Kitt, S., Selfridge-Thomas, J., Proehl, J. & Kaiser, J. (1995). *Emergency nursing: A physiologic and clinical perspective* (2nd ed.). Philadelphia: Saunders.

the body's weight being abruptly borne by the head.

Injury can occur to either the spinal cord, column or both at the same time. Ligament sprains usually are uncomplicated and heal without problems. Trauma to the spinal column does not always affect the cord or the nerves. Not all vertebral injuries are fractures. Trauma to the spine severe enough to injure the cord is usually severe enough to make the spinal column unstable. If injury to the spinal column makes it unstable, it can no longer protect the cord. Dislocations and displaced fractures can be severe, with the entire column becoming unstable, compressing the cord and leading to

paralysis *(see Figure 8-2)*. Even with a slight displacement of 1 mm, a vertebra can pinch or shear the cord, the difference between normal function and permanent paralysis.

Some parts of the spine are more vulnerable than others. The cervical vertebrae are the most mobile part of the spine in order to allow the head to turn and are the point of most injury. In the child, cervical spine injuries are uncommon. When they do occur, they are usually associated with multiple trauma.

The second most frequent site of injury is the flexible juncture of the thoracic and lumbar vertebrae. Since the thoracolumbar spine supplies ganglia of the sympathetic nervous system, injury to the spinal cord in this area not only can cause voluntary system paralysis, but also can affect the sympathetic segment of the autonomic system. When the sympathetic nerves are damaged, reflex vasoconstriction cannot occur; blood may pool in the vascular system due to the loss of vascular tone; there is an associated fall in blood pressure, and all the signs of neurogenic shock appear.

It is safe to assume that when there is soft tissue damage to the face, head or neck due to a sudden deceleration injury, there is accompanying spinal cord damage. Spinal injury can be associated with trauma to the head, neck or back, and sometimes is associated with trauma to the chest, abdomen, pelvis, or extremities.

When projectiles or other penetrating forces enter the spinal cord, they can cause shearing. Structure and function can be disrupted or ended. Bone fragments may be driven into the cord with the penetrating force, causing further damage.

Bleeding or a hematoma at the trauma site can compress the cord; and loss of blood supply can bring about irreversible damage.

If damage is severe enough, the patient will have partial or complete loss of bodily sensation or function. Loss starts at the site of the injury and

## FIGURE 8-3
### Compression Force Causing Wedging and Crush-type Injury of the Vertebrae

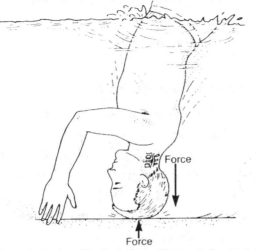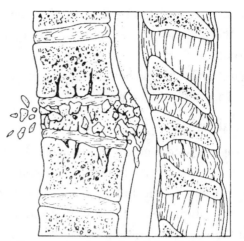

*Reprinted with permission from* Kitt, S., Selfridge-Thomas, J., Proehl, J. & Kaiser, J. (1995). *Emergency nursing: A physiologic and clinical perspective* (2nd ed.). Philadelphia: Saunders.

continues downward. If the injury is high level and severe in the cervical cord, it is life threatening due to loss of the ability for the respiratory system to function on its own.

It is generally accepted that the mechanism of injury is important in determining the type of injury.

# SPINAL CORD AND SPINAL COLUMN INJURY

The mechanism of injury, extent, location, and other factors determine the damage to the patient. Primary injury is followed by secondary injury.

## Spinal Shock

When there is total damage to the spinal cord, all sensory and motor function below that level stops. Spinal, or neurogenic, shock generally occurs with injuries above the T-6 level, causing disruption of the sympathetic nervous system. Because the sympathetic system cannot respond, the body is unable to accelerate the heart, constrict the blood vessels and raise the blood pressure. Hypotension occurs. The skin is cool because the blood vessels cannot constrict and become so large that there is not enough blood volume to fill the large vessels. As a result, blood pools in the extremities, creating hypothermia due to the heat loss from the dilated vessels. The skin is pink due to the pooling blood and cool from the loss of heat. (Neurogenic shock is discussed in further detail Chapter 4, Shock/Cardiac Arrest.)

Other consequences of spinal shock are flaccid paralysis and loss of sphincter tone. When spinal shock occurs, there is the possibility of other types of shock, particularly if there are other injuries with blood loss.

## Autonomic Dysreflexia

This is a life-threatening complication of spinal cord injury above the T-6 level after spinal shock has been resolved.

The response is triggered by multiple stimuli below the point of injury. For instance, a full bladder, full rectum, or decubitus ulcer can be a trigger. Since there is lack of control below the injury from the higher nerve centers, the sympathetic system reacts without being regulated. The patient develops headache, hypertension, sweating, cardiac dysrhythmia (tachycardia or bradycardia), flushing above the level of the injury and coolness below the level of injury. The patient may have nasal congestion and become anxious.

Treatment is related to the specific trigger that caused the response, usually medication such as ganglionic blockers. The patient must be closely monitored after the medication has been given to observe for sudden blood pressure drop.

## Cervical Injury

Complete spinal cord trauma at the level C-3 most often severs the respiratory mechanism, causing the patient to die before he can be helped. Other cervical injuries will result in respiratory distress or the need for artificial ventilation as long as the patient lives. About one quarter of the patients with cervical injuries also have associated head injuries.

## Thoracic Injury

The thoracic spine receives additional stability from the ribs. Therefore, it is not injured as often as other parts of the spine. However, if thoracic injury is suspected, the neck must also be stabilized. Spinal shock often occurs with thoracic injury, affecting heart rate, blood pressure, vasodilation, paralysis, and sphincter tone. Respiratory mechanisms can also be impaired.

## Lumbar Injury

The lumbar and thoracic vertebrae join as a flexible joint, which makes it subject to injury. The T-12–L-1 area is the second most common site for injury in the spine. Spinal cord damage to the lumbar region can paralyze the legs.

## Incomplete Spinal Cord Injury

There are several types of incomplete spinal cord injuries (Newberry, 1998). They are identified by the findings of the evaluation of sensory and motor functions, as defined by the American Spinal Injury Association.

### Central Cord Syndrome

This syndrome is caused most often by hyperextension, especially by the elderly in a fall. Loss of function is in the upper extremities but not in the lower extremities. Bladder and bowel function is not affected.

### Anterior Cord Syndrome

Usually, when the anterior spinal artery is occluded, a disk is ruptured, or a transection of the anterior part of the cord occurs, the patient experiences hyperesthesia, hypoalgesia, and partial or complete paralysis. With the posterior part of the spinal column still intact, the patient is able to feel vibrations and has proprioception.

### Brown-Séquard Syndrome

Hemisection of the cord in the anteroposterior plane is most frequently caused by a penetrating injury such as a gunshot or missile fragment. Characteristics of this syndrome are ipsilateral (same side) paresis or hemiplegia; on the same side and below the level of the lesion and contralateral, (opposite side) loss of pain and temperature sensitivity. The patient has proprioception and movement on one side of the body but not the other, and has a loss of pulse and temperature sensation on the opposite side of the paralysis.

### Nerve Root Injuries

Nerve roots are often injured during spinal cord trauma. Indicators are hypoalgesia (loss of pain sensitivity), pain or referred pain.

## Penetrating Injury

The nature of penetrating injury is that there are open wounds into the spinal cord. If cerebrospinal fluid is evident, the spinal cord has been perforated, and infection is likely along with the injury.

## Impalement

An object can lodge in the spinal column, or the patient can become impaled upon an object. In any situation of impalement, it is essential to stabilize the object in order to prevent further injury to the spine.

## Injury Without Radiographic Abnormality

Children's anatomy allows for more physical flexibility than that of the adult. As a result, spinal cord injury is less likely. However, a condition known as spinal cord injury without radiographic abnormality can occur, where the child shows signs of injury without radiographic evidence. It is thought that a young child's immaturely developed spinal column can accept more flexion and extension without demonstrable vertebral damage (Soud & Rogers, 1998). Consequently, when damage occurs, it may not be immediately obvious but may progress over hours or days. The injury is more likely to occur at the cervical or thoracic levels of the cord and show neurologic deficits without evidence of bony injury. A magnetic resonance imaging (MRI) is required to detect the specific point of injury.

# ASSESSMENT

The emergency nurse should first conduct primary and secondary assessments and initiate critical interventions that are required *(see Figure 8-4)*.

As previously discussed, all patients who are unconscious, have multisystem injury or significant mechanisms of injury, should be assumed to have a spinal injury. They should arrive at the emergency department fully immobilized and kept that way until cleared by the physician. The patient should have a hard cervical collar and lateral head support. Remember not to rely too much on the collar; it does not fully immobilize the patient. The patient should be placed on a backboard with straps across the chest, abdomen and knees.

Once the critical needs have been met, a more focused assessment related to the spinal injury can be conducted.

## Signs (Observable Physical Findings)

**Unconsciousness:** The accepted rule is that an unconscious patient is assumed to have a spinal injury until proven otherwise and cleared by the physician.

**Deformity:** Although deformity is an obvious indicator of injury, most spinal cord and spinal fractures do not have obvious deformity. Only when there is severe injury with marked displacement of bony fragments is deformity obvious. Absence of deformity does not indicate lack of a fracture or displacement. When present, a deformity is most often seen in the cervical spine with the head twisted to one side.

**Tenderness:** Point tenderness over any part of the spine indicates injury. The spinous processes of all the cervical, thoracic, and lumbar vertebrae can (are able to) be palpated; with C7 being especially prominent.

**Lacerations or contusions:** Cuts and bruises often occur with strong force. A cervical spine injury usually results from a blow to the head. If the head or face is marked with lacerations or contusions, it is a reliable indication that there is spinal injury. Patients with serious lacerations or contusions over areas of the back, shoulders or abdomen are likely to have injuries to the spine.

**Paralysis or Anesthesia:** Weakness or loss of sensation identified during assessment by touching the fingers, toes, arms and legs is a sign of spinal injury. Upper extremity muscle strength is tested by judging the grip when the patient is asked to squeeze the nurse's hand. Lower extremity muscle strength is tested by asking the patient to move his feet up and down.

## FIGURE 8-4

## Summary of Observations and Possible Conclusions in Assessment of a Conscious Patient with Suspected Spinal Cord Injury

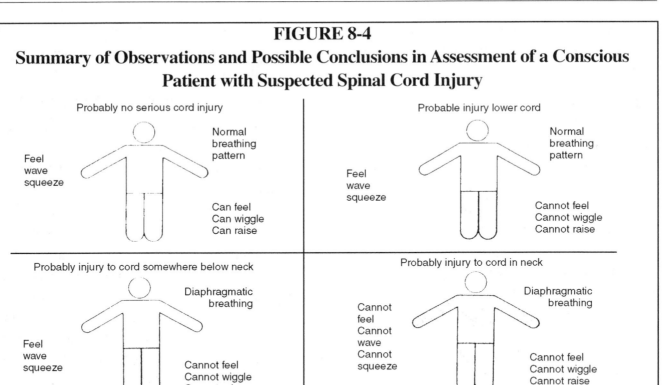

Warning: If the patient is unconscious or the mechanism of injury indicates possible spinal injury, assume that spinal injury is present.

*Reprinted with permission from* Grant, H. D., Murray, R. H., Jr. & Bergeron, J. D. (Eds.). (1990). *Brady emergency care* (5th ed.). Englewood Cliffs, NJ: Prentice-Hall.

**Respiratory Difficulty:** Difficulty breathing or inability to breathe may indicate cervical or thoracic damage.

**Priapism:** Priapism indicates loss of sympathetic nervous system control and parasympathetic stimulation.

### Symptoms (Patient Complaints)

**Pain:** Pain due to spinal injury is an important indicator. The nurse should document where the pain is, the quality of pain, and if it increases with movement, should the patient try to move. The nurse should not ask the patient to move.

**Numbness or Tingling:** Damage to the spine probably has occurred if the patient complains of numbness, tingling, loss of feeling, or weakness.

### History

If the patient is conscious when he arrives at the emergency department, it is important to verify the mechanism of injury and history that has been recorded by the rescue crew. With a suspected spine injury, signs and symptoms should be evaluated for any changes or increase in complaints. If the patient is unconscious, prehospital history is what the nurse has to rely on, along with report from the rescuers.

Information should include:

- History of significant trauma, such as a motor vehicle or motorcycle crash or a fall from a height greater than three times the patient's height, especially if there is a fracture of the heels

- Unrestrained driver or passenger

- Facial trauma

- Loss of consciousness at the site of the injury

- Altered mental status from intoxication or drugs

- Any seizure activity since the injury

- Neck pain or altered sensation in the upper extremities

- Neck tenderness

- Injury above the clavicle

- Chest or intraabdominal injuries

- A complaint of the sensation of electric shock or hot water running down the back.

Find out if the patient has been incontinent before arrival at the emergency department or, if a male, is experiencing priapism (Newberry, 1998).

### Inspection

- Look for obvious signs of injury.

- Look for abnormal shape of the spine and cervical edema.

- Identify entrance or exit wounds in the neck, chest, or abdomen.

- Identify the patient's breathing pattern, and document difficulties. Injury above C-6 disrupts ventilation. Abdominal breathing can indicate damage from C-3 to C-5.

- Document if the patient can move extremities and perceive pain.

- Priapism is associated with loss of sympathetic system control, indicated in cervical injury.

- Note any CSF leak from the nose or ears.

### Palpation

- If the cervical collar is removed in order to palpate the spine, manual immobilization must be carried out (*see Figure 8-5*).

- Feel the skin. If it is cool and looks pink, the patient may have neurogenic shock.

- Perform a quick motor evaluation, assessing the strength and equality of movement for all four extremities, feet, toes, hands and fingers.

- Briefly assess sensory status to identify if the patient can distinguish between sharp and dull and identify where there is loss of feeling.

# NURSING STRATEGIES FOR THE PATIENT WITH SPINAL CORD AND COLUMN INJURIES

The purpose of spine trauma management is the same as with any fracture: support and immobilize. The principle of immobilization is in-line position and immobilization of the joint above and below the fracture. For immobilization of any spinal injury, the anatomy of the spine dictates that the joint above means the head and the joint below means the torso and pelvis.

Since the extent of spinal injuries cannot be completely observed and since they may become progressively worse, spinal injuries should always be considered serious and potentially totally disabling or life threatening.

Administer oxygen to all patients with a suspected or known spinal injury to increase the oxygen supply to the spinal cord.

It is essential that the patient is stabilized and properly immobilized.

### Stabilization

- Spine trauma patient stabilization begins with identification and treatment of airway and vascular compromise. While the ABCs are conducted, the cervical spine must be well immobilized, as is necessary if an airway has to be established and ventilation maintained.

- The only acceptable method to open the airway of a patient with a cervical injury is the **jaw thrust** maneuver.

- Cervical spine trauma puts the patient at risk for hypoxia, respiratory arrest and aspiration.

- Post injury edema should be minimized.

**FIGURE 8-5**
**Manual Stabilization of the Head**

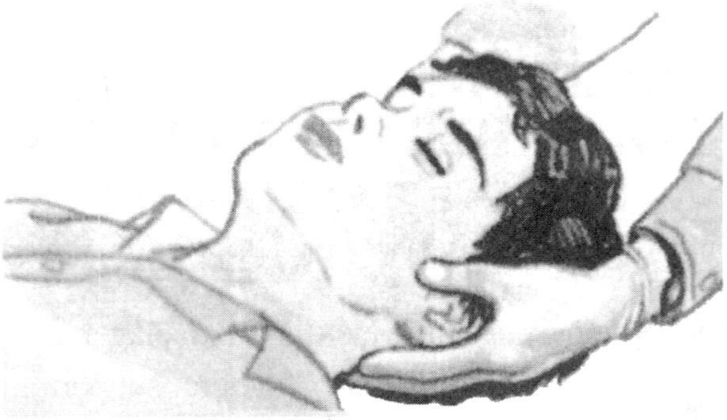

*Reprinted with permission from:* Campbell, J. E. (Ed.) (2000). *Basic trauma life support for paramedics and other advanced providers* (4th ed.). Upper Saddle River, NJ: Brady/Prentice-Hall Health.

- The airway is at risk for several problems: compromised respiratory muscles, localized edema causing obstruction of the airway and penetration of the airway.

- Advanced airway measures may have to be taken, requiring special care to immobilize the neck.

- If the patient does not have a facial or cranial injury, the airway of choice is nasal intubation because it can be done with minimal spine manipulation.

## Immobilization

The nurse must ensure the patient is correctly immobilized:

- If the patient should arrive without immobilization, a rigid collar must be immediately applied. Use a rigid cervical collar, lateral head immobilizer and backboard. The size must be correct; a collar that is too large will cause hyperextension. Someone should help apply the collar to ensure in-line stabilization of the spine.

- Care should be taken that the collar does not block the mouth.

- Too much reliance should not be placed on cervical collars; they do not hold the head

absolutely still and permit some side-to-side movement.

- The patient must be checked to see that his head is not hyperextended when he arrives at the emergency department. Padding the head will help solve that problem.

- Too much padding under the neck, along with a tie across the forehead will also cause hyperextension.

- In the concern for the spine injury immobilization, be sure that other injuries are not aggravated when immobilizing devices are applied.

- Do not remove a helmet unless it is essential for accessing the airway, sustain respirations or control hemorrhage.

## Circulation

Spinal shock/sympathetic system dysfunction will cause fluctuations in circulation, cardiac rhythm, and blood pressure. If hypotension occurs, carefully verify that it is not caused by another problem, such as hypovolemia, tension pneumothorax, or intraabdominal bleeding.

## Full Evaluation/Other Measures

- The patient should be fully evaluated after he is stabilized and immobilized.

- Remember the patient may be unable to perceive pain from other injuries. The nurse needs to be observant because the patient may not be able to relate all necessary information, due to interruption in the sensory system.

- If the patient has spinal cord damage, he may not be able to feel the sensation of a full bladder. After it is confirmed there is no urethral damage, catheterization may be necessary.

- The patient should be kept NPO until fully evaluated by the physician in case surgical intervention is necessary.

## Pharmacological Management

If the patient arrives at the emergency department within 8 hours of the injury, high-dose methylprednisolone is usually administered to manage the severity of the trauma and bring about neurological improvement. Although this is considered the current standard of care, recent research indicates high doses may put the patient at greater risk for pneumonia, decubitus ulcer development and urinary tract infections. There is also a question as to whether early administration actually improves the functional status.

# EXAMPLES OF NURSING DIAGNOSES RELATED TO SPINAL CORD AND SPINAL COLUMN TRAUMA

- Ineffective respiratory efforts related to spinal cord injury

- Ineffective airway clearance related to penetrating damage to the throat

- Potential for aspiration or pneumonia related to spinal cord injury

- Hypotension related to spinal shock

- Dysreflexia related to spinal cord trauma

- Incontinence related to sensory or neuromuscular impairment

- Inability to feel pain related to spinal cord injury

- Anxiety related to the patient's inability to breathe on his own

- Anxiety related to spinal cord injury

- Loss of skin integrity related to paralysis

- Potential for suffocation related to anterior hematoma in cervical injury

# SUMMARY

Spinal cord and spinal column injury can be devastating. The advancement of emergency medical services systems and rehabilitation have improved the patient's chances of survival and expanded the potential for recovery. Nevertheless, spinal cord trauma can affect all areas of the body.

The nervous system is complex and confusing. Basically, every function and movement in the body is directed by the brain and central nervous system, just as though they are a computer.

It is necessary to identify the cause and extent of an injury to the spinal cord or spine. Additionally, the patient must be carefully immobilized in order to prevent further damage.

The prime indications of spine injury are specific mechanisms of injury, observable signs and the symptoms the patient relates to the evaluator. However, trauma to the vertebrae may not cause immediate damage to the spinal cord or show evidence of the damage. Severe damage to the spine is possible, even though paralysis has not yet developed. A patient who presents without signs or symptoms can still have a spine so unstable that even minor movement can bring about permanent damage. The patient's ability to move his extremities or the absence of tingling and numbness only means the cord is intact at that moment.

The future of the patient's ability to recover in the best manner possible depends upon prehospital and hospital staff who understand the principles of spinal cord and column injury and can appropriately manage the care of the patient.

# EXAM QUESTIONS

## CHAPTER 8
**Questions 36–40**

36. All messages that the brain sends for the body to function are sent through the

    a. brain and spinal cord.

    b. sensory and functional nervous systems.

    c. sympathetic and parasympathetic nervous systems.

    d. vertebral ganglia.

37. Which of the following statements is true?

    a. Injury to the spinal cord always includes paralysis.

    b. Complete spinal cord trauma causes paralysis above the point of injury.

    c. Injury can occur to the spinal cord, column or both at the same time.

    d. The slight displacement of a fractured vertebra will not damage the spinal cord.

38. All patients who are unconscious and have multiple trauma should be assumed to have

    a. a spinal cord injury.

    b. an airway obstruction.

    c. neurogenic shock.

    d. paralysis.

39. A patient who develops headache, hypertension, sweating, cardiac dysrhythmia (tachycardia or bradycardia), flushing above the level of injury and coolness below the level of injury is likely to have

    a. autonomic dysreflexia.

    b. injury to the high thoracic spine.

    c. central cord syndrome.

    d. an incomplete spinal cord injury.

40. A construction worker fell from a 3-story scaffolding but managed to land on his feet, sustaining what kind of spinal cord injury?

    a. Distraction

    b. Hyperextension with loading

    c. Overrotation with compression

    d. Axial loading with compression

# CHAPTER 9

# THORACIC TRAUMA

## CHAPTER OBJECTIVE

Upon completion of this chapter, the reader will be able to indicate the major nursing strategies for managing thoracic trauma.

## LEARNING OBJECTIVES

Upon completion of this chapter, the reader should be able to:

1. Identify thoracic organs, structures and their functions.

2. Describe common mechanisms of injury to the chest.

3. Identify signs and symptoms of chest injuries.

4. Recognize complications that accompany chest injuries.

5. Describe the general principles of care and basic nursing strategies for chest injuries.

6. Indicate examples of nursing diagnoses for patients with thoracic trauma.

## INTRODUCTION

The thoracic cavity, or chest, contains organs, structures and vessels of the pulmonary, cardiovascular and gastrointestinal systems. These systems, structures and vessels are vital to life, and because of that, any damage to the chest is potentially serious. Since the body is unable to store oxygen, a chest injury interfering with normal respiration or the functioning of any of these three systems is emergent. The extent of injury depends on the force, direction, duration and physical area to which traumatic energy is applied. For example, stab versus gunshot penetrating injury and localized damage versus high velocity damage cause different types of injuries.

Chest injuries are estimated to be the cause of 25% of all trauma deaths and are a contributing factor to another 25% of the trauma fatalities. They are the second leading cause of death in trauma victims preceded only by injuries to the brain and spinal cord (Newberry, 1998).

Thoracic injuries are caused by a wide variety of mechanisms: car crashes, falls, sports injuries, crush injuries, gunshot wounds and stabbing. About 70% of the thoracic injuries are the result of auto crashes. Half of the multiple trauma victims have chest injuries. Patients with penetrating injuries below the nipple line anteriorly or inferior to the scapula posteriorly, most likely also have abdominal damage.

Today, about 85% of the trauma cases can be managed nonoperatively with analgesia, good pulmonary toilet (coughing and deep breathing), chest roentgenography, selective endotracheal intubation and tube thoracostomy. Only 10% to 15% of the victims of blunt or penetrating chest trauma will need a thoracotomy or sternotomy (Peitzman et al., 1998).

Although chest injuries have been documented for centuries, it was not until after World War II that treatment such as chest tubes connected to underwater seal drainage became standard interventions for many cases of thoracic trauma. In the past 50 years, improvements in ventilation, antibiotics, blood gas analysis and advanced emergency medical services in prehospital and emergency department areas have greatly increased the survival rates. However, despite improved diagnostics and treatment for many previously fatal chest injuries, thoracic trauma patients still require immediate systematic assessment, diagnosis and swift treatment measures.

# ANATOMY AND PHYSIOLOGY

The thorax, or chest, which extends from the top of the sternum to the diaphragm, is one of two major body cavities; the other is the abdominal cavity. Boundaries are the 12 pairs of ribs that articulate with the thoracic spine posteriorly and with the sternum anteriorly. The clavicles overlie the upper boundaries in front and joins with the scapulae in the muscle tissue of the back. The superior border of the thorax is continuous with the neck. The lower boundary is the diaphragm, which separates the thoracic and abdominal cavities. *Figure 9-1* depicts the anatomy of the thoracic cavity.

Within the thorax are structures, organs and vessels of the pulmonary, cardiovascular and gastrointestinal systems. The pleural space contains the pulmonary organs, and the mediastinal space contains the cardiovascular and gastrointestinal structures.

Important structures in the thorax are the ribs, sternum, lungs, pleurae, intercostal and accessory muscles, diaphragm, trachea, esophagus, heart, and great vessels. Twelve pairs of ribs form the rib cage, which is meant to function as a chest protec-

tor. The centrally located sternum provides additional protection but can function as a weapon to the heart and lungs if it is fractured. Essential to life by providing oxygen to the body and removing waste, the lungs fill most of the chest and are covered by the visceral pleura. The trachea funnels air in and out of the lungs, subdividing into bronchi and bronchioles. The esophagus, which lies behind the trachea, is a tube for transporting food into the gastrointestinal system. Under the sternum, slightly to the left, lies the heart with important vessels entering and leaving the heart and lungs.

## Pulmonary System

One lung occupies each half of the chest cavity, or the **hemithorax.** Between the lungs is a space, the **mediastinum,** where the heart, great arteries and veins, many nerves, esophagus, trachea, and major bronchi are located.

The lungs hang freely within the chest cavity. Because they are not made up of muscle, they have no ability to expand or contract on their own.

There is a mechanism to ensure the lungs follow the motion of the chest wall, expanding and contracting with it. A thin membrane, the **parietal pleura,** lines the inner surface of the chest cavity. The same kind of serous membrane, the **visceral pleura,** also covers the surface of each lung. Between the visceral pleural surface of the lungs and the parietal pleural surface of the chest wall is the so-called **pleural space.** In reality, this space is a "potential" space, since the visceral pleura and the parietal pleura actually lie against each other, sealed tightly with a thin film of fluid. An analogy would be two panes of glass stuck together by a thin coating of water. When the chest wall expands, the lung is pulled with it and made to expand by the pulling force of the two pleural layers.

Under normal conditions, no real space exists between the pleural layers, because the fluid causes them to adhere to each other. However, if traumatized, the potential space can hold 3,000 cc or more

## FIGURE 9-1
## Chest Cavity and Related Structures
A - Anterior View, B - Cross Section

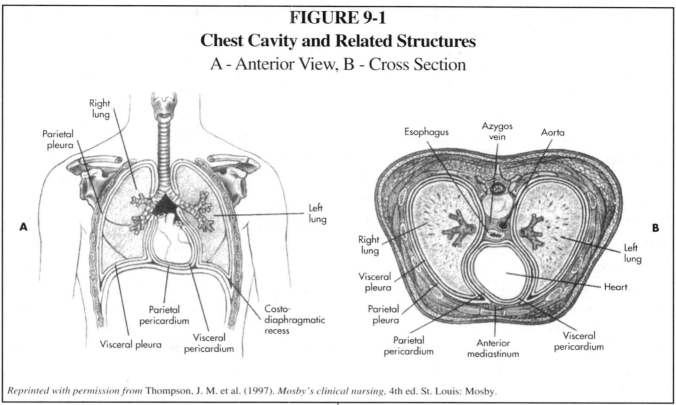

*Reprinted with permission from* Thompson, J. M. et al. (1997). *Mosby's clinical nursing,* 4th ed. St. Louis: Mosby.

in an adult. For instance, if the chest wall is lacerated, blood can separate the pleural surfaces and fill the space. A hole in the chest wall or a torn lung can cause air to enter the pleural space. In either case, the pleurae are no longer sealed together, and the means for them to expand the lungs is lost. If enough blood or air collects, the lungs can be compressed to the degree that they cannot expand at all during inspiration. At this point, there will not be enough oxygen to maintain life.

The mechanics of breathing are three dimensional. As discussed, the lungs do not contain muscle tissue and cannot expand or contract on their own. The intercostal and accessory muscles of the thorax along with the movement of the diaphragm cause expansion in three directions. The attachment of the lungs to the pleural surfaces causes them to follow the expanding motion of the chest wall, permitting air to enter the airways and the alveoli.

Although the diaphragm is skeletal or voluntary muscle, (in that one can control taking a deep breath, coughing or controling breathing patterns at will), it also performs an automatic function. Breathing occurs while asleep or awake. Conscious variations in breathing, such as holding one's breath, cannot continue indefinitely. When the balance of oxygen and carbon dioxide is disturbed enough, automatic regulation of respiration takes over.

### Negative Pressure

The chest can be thought of as a bell jar in which the lungs are suspended. The only natural opening into the chest is the trachea through which air moves in and out of the lungs. Ordinarily, the pressure in the chest cavity is slightly less than the atmospheric pressure. When the chest wall muscles and diaphragm contract during **inspiration,** the ribs expand and the diaphragm drops, so the thorax space enlarges, and the volume the chest can hold is increased.

The increased space causes the intrathoracic pressure to drop further and develop a slight vacuum. The result is that the higher outside pressure drives air through the trachea, filling the lungs. As the air moves in, the inside pressure begins to equal the pressure outside, and when it does, the air stops moving. The principle is that any gas will move from a higher pressure area to a lower pressure area until the pressure in each area is equal. In the case of respiration, when the pressures are equal, inspiration stops. At this point, **expiration** begins. The intercostal muscles and diaphragm relax, the chest contracts and becomes smaller, the pressure inside becomes higher than the pressure outside, and the air is expelled.

The key point is that the trachea is the only natural opening for air to enter the chest cavity. If there is another opening from an injury, the air cannot get to the interior of the lung through the trachea, because air or blood enters the pleural space through the injury, breaks the pleural seal, compresses the lung, and effectively stops normal chest expansion.

## Cardiovascular System

The cardiovascular system is the engine that keeps the body running, delivering oxygen and nutrients and disposing of cellular waste and carbon dioxide. Working as a closed circuit, the heart pumps the blood and makes the system go. The system is not simple. It is a complex arrangement of **systemic circulation,** the transport of blood throughout the body to exchange oxygen, nutrients, and waste products, and **pulmonary circulation,** the transport of blood through the lungs to exchange oxygen and carbon dioxide.

The heart, large vessels, trachea, esophagus, thymus and lymph nodes are situated in the **mediastinum**, a cavity between the lungs. The heart is positioned slightly on the left half of the chest, with the right ventricle lying beneath the sternum. The pericardium, a tough, layered sac that cannot expand, surrounds and protects the heart similar to the pleurae around the lungs. It is made up of an inner layer, the visceral pericardium and an outer

layer, the parietal pericardium. As with the pleural space, the pericardial cavity is a potential space between the two pericardial layers that is filled with a small amount of serous fluid. The fluid serves to prevent friction during heartbeat. The parietal pericardium attaches to the sternum, great vessels and diaphragm in order to hold the heart in place.

The right heart is a low-pressure system, receiving deoxygenated blood and pumping it to the lungs for oxygenation. Oxygenated blood returns to the left heart, a high-pressure system, to be pumped through systemic circulation. Cardiac output and function depend on contractility, heart rate, preload and afterload. Preload is the volume reached after diastolic filling of the ventricles. Afterload is the resistance the heart pumps against to push the blood out.

There are three anatomical portions of the aorta: the ascending aorta, aortic arch and the descending aorta. Just distal to the arch, the aorta is quite immobile and at risk for disruption. Over 85% of the aortic injuries caused by acceleration/deceleration forces occur to this portion of the aorta (Newberry, 1998).

# MECHANISM OF INJURY

The chest can be injured by blunt trauma, penetrating objects and compression mechanisms. The extent of injury depends upon the force, direction, duration and physical area where the traumatic energy impacts.

## Blunt Trauma

A majority of the chest injuries are caused by blunt trauma, in particular, by rapid deceleration, most often in car crashes. Energy rebounds through the thorax and may crush soft tissues against the spine, rupturing organs. Blunt trauma with force sufficient to fracture the rib cage, sternum or costal cartilages can result in heart or lung contusion.

Rapid vertical deceleration can shear the aorta and great vessels from the heart.

## Penetrating Object

Any sharp object having enough force will cause a penetrating injury. Projectiles are responsible for the majority of penetrating chest injuries, causing localized or widespread damage, depending on the extent and source of injury. Penetration can be caused by bullets, knives, shards of metal or glass and a variety of other objects that can pierce the chest. Gunshot wounds are increasing in the United States.

Penetrating injuries can lacerate, impale, puncture, or rupture an organ, structure or vessel. Stab wounds may not appear damaging but can have significant morbidity and mortality from deep penetration into the chest and its contents. Bullet wounds usually have a clear point of entry and exit, with the line of damage being obvious, but the bullet may ricochet in the chest off the ribs or sternum, causing additional injury.

## Compression

In a severe form of blunt trauma, the chest is rapidly and forcefully compressed, as by a steering wheel in a car crash or when something extremely heavy falls on the chest. The process is a sudden, severe compression of the chest, producing a rapid increase in intrathoracic pressure. Multiple fractures and flail chest can result. The increased intrathoracic pressure can cause the upper body to become swollen and cyanotic, the neck veins to distend, and the eyes appear to bulge.

## Injury to the Back of the Chest

Direct blows to the back of the chest can cause contusions or rib fracture, along with spine and airway injury. Rarely, the scapula, which is protected by large muscles, receives a blow severe enough to fracture. When this happens, there may also be damage to the underlying chest wall and lung. Direct back blows to the lower rib cage in the area of the 10th through 12th ribs can injure the kidneys.

## Categories of Chest Trauma

### Open Chest Injury

When the skin is broken or the chest wall is penetrated, it is considered to be an open chest wound. However, the term is usually taken to mean the injury has opened the chest cavity. The wound can come from the inside or the outside. An object can pass through the wall from the outside, or a fractured rib can penetrate the chest wall from within. It is not always easy to determine by looking at the wound if the chest cavity has been penetrated. The wound should not be spread apart to determine its depth. Specific signs and symptoms will aid in determining the degree of damage.

### Closed Chest Injury

With a closed chest injury, the skin is not broken and the mechanism of injury is usually blunt. Because there is no immediate obvious damage, the injury can be deceptive in not appearing serious. Even when the external injury is caused by blunt trauma, lacerations of the internal organs or structures can be caused by fractured ribs, sternum or when vital structures are torn from their attachments to the chest cavity.

# THORACIC INJURIES AND INTERVENTIONS

Thoracic injuries may involve the chest wall, pulmonary system, cardiovascular system and the esophagus. The degree of severity is based on the injury's effect on ventilation and circulation.

## Chest Wall Injury

### Rib Fracture

Frequently seen, rib fractures are most often caused by direct blunt, compression or crush injury. Car crashes and falls by the elderly are common mechanisms of injury. The fractures may be single or multiple.

It should be assumed that injury to the clavicle or above involves closed-head and neck injury and facial fractures. The upper four ribs are strong, protected by the shoulder girdle and not as likely to be fractured. A fracture to the upper three ribs indicates a powerful blow and possible accompanying serious head and neck injury. In addition, suspect trauma to the subclavian vein or aorta.

The 5th through 10th ribs are the most likely to fracture. There may or may not be deformity and contusion or laceration at the injured site. Deep breathing and movement is usually painful, so the patient will take shallow breaths and lean toward the side of the injury.

Respiratory rate and patterns should be assessed to evaluate the injury's impact on ventilation. Single fractures do not require splinting. For multiple fractures, immobilization of the chest wall provides comfort and makes breathing easier. Pain management is important and may require intercostal nerve blocks. Good pulmonary toilet of coughing and deep breathing is essential to prevent pneumonia or atelectasis.

Occasionally, the end of a fractured rib punctures or tears a lung or the chest wall, causing a hemothorax or pneumothorax.

### Flail Chest

When three or more adjacent ribs are broken, each in two places, the part of the chest wall lying between the fractures becomes a loose or *flail segment.* The injury can also be a bilateral detachment of the sternum from the costal cartilage. Both types of injuries are most often the result of a massive crush injury or a high-speed motor crash. The loose segment collapses and does not expand with the chest wall during inhalation; it moves inward. During exhalation, the loose segment protrudes slightly while the rest of the chest wall contracts. Movement of the loose segment opposite to the

normal movement of the chest wall is called **paradoxical movement** and looks uncoordinated with respiration actions.

Flail chest is serious. It takes great force to cause a series of ribs to fracture in several places and produce flail chest. The lung under the segment does not expand properly during inhalation, which decreases the efficiency of ventilation. Contusion of the lung almost always occurs simultaneously, causing immediate bleeding and swelling into the lung tissue. The contusion worsens the injury due to loss of compliance, increased airway resistance, and decreased gas exchange. Pulmonary contusion can lead to adult respiratory distress syndrome (ARDS), in which case intubation and mechanical ventilation may be necessary. Hypoventilation of both lungs can be followed by atelectasis, hypoxia, and cyanosis.

Diagnosis of flail chest can be made through visual observation or palpation of the chest wall. Palpation indicates crepitus and abnormal motion. The patient will complain of difficulty breathing. Vital signs should be monitored carefully, and the patient should have aggressive respiratory support to provide an adequate supply of oxygen.

Severe pain may be eased when the patient is positioned with the flail segment against firm external support. Pain relief with intercostal nerve blocks should be provided.

### Sternal Fracture

Enormous anterior chest impact is necessary to fracture the sternum, such as occurs with a steering wheel. There is a significant possibility for myocardial contusion or pericardial tamponade. In many emergency departments, thoracic CT scans and EKGs are routinely performed with all steering-wheel injuries to detect cardiac contusions.

Pain is severe, along with the patient having dyspnea. In order to relieve pain by minimizing chest wall movement, the patient may hypoventi-

**FIGURE 9-2**
**Conditions Produced by Chest Injuries**

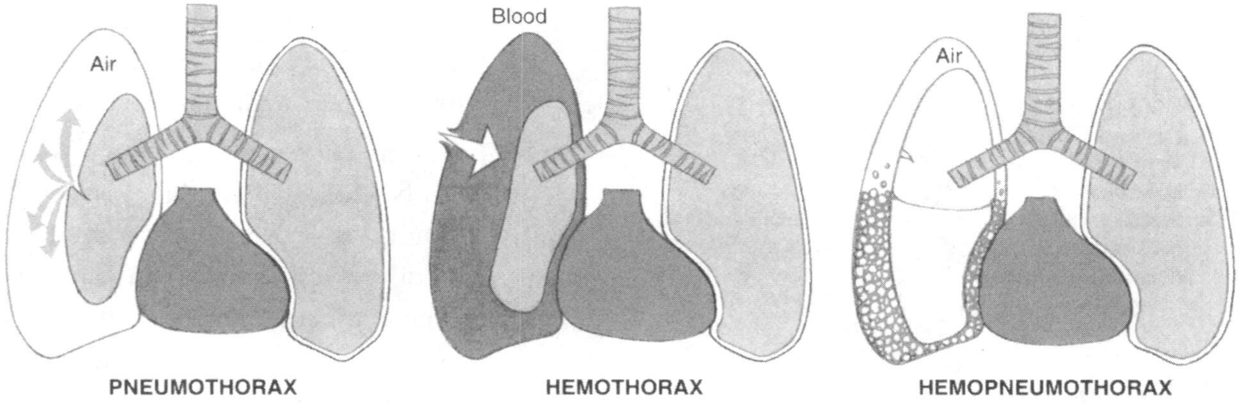

PNEUMOTHORAX     HEMOTHORAX     HEMOPNEUMOTHORAX

Reprinted with permission from O'Keefe, M. F., Limmer, D., Grant, H. D., Murray, R. H. & Bergeron, J. D. (1998.). *Brady emergency care* (8th ed.). Upper Saddle River, NJ: Brady/Prentice-Hall.

late. Chest wall ecchymosis and sternal deformity may be seen, and crepitus may be heard.

Pain relief and serial examination monitoring for hypoxia, hypotension, arrhythmias, and indications of additional thoracic trauma are required. If the fracture is displaced, surgical reduction may be necessary.

## Pulmonary Injury

### Esophageal Injury

Esophageal injuries are infrequent and deadly. Most often penetration is the cause of injury, but a severe blow to the lower abdomen can disrupt the esophagus. Other causes are accidental damage from an instrument during a procedure, caustic ingestion, crush injury and blast injury.

These injuries cause mediastinitis from contamination by saliva and gastric contents. A patient may show evidence of severe shock disproportionate to the apparent severity of the chest injury, develop pneumothorax or hemothorax without fractured ribs. Urgent surgical repair is required.

### Laryngeal Injury

Rare and life threatening, a severe blow to the anterior neck can crush the larynx. Frequent mechanisms of injury are impact by a steering wheel or

dashboard, a karate blow, and "clothesline" trauma where, for instance, a bicyclist or motorcycle rider runs into a clothesline, tree limb or other object across the throat.

Laryngeal injury is identified with a descriptive history. The neck may be marked, and the patient hoarse, have subcutaneous emphysema and crepitus. Diagnosis is confirmed with a CT of the neck. Intubation is necessary for acute respiratory distress or complete obstruction. If the injury does not permit intubation, cricothyrotomy can be done in the emergency department, followed by surgical tracheostomy in the operating room.

Penetrating injury is immediately obvious and requires immediate surgical intervention. There may also be injury to the carotid artery, jugular vein or cervical spine.

### Tracheal Injury

Trauma to the larynx can also include the trachea or the injury can be directly to the trachea. Injury is blunt or penetrating. There may be massive crepitus from the nipples up, frothy or bloody sputum in the airway and noisy breathing. Complete obstruction may take place. In the case of severe injury to the neck, bleeding may be profuse.

## FIGURE 9-3
## Paradoxical Motion in Flail Chest

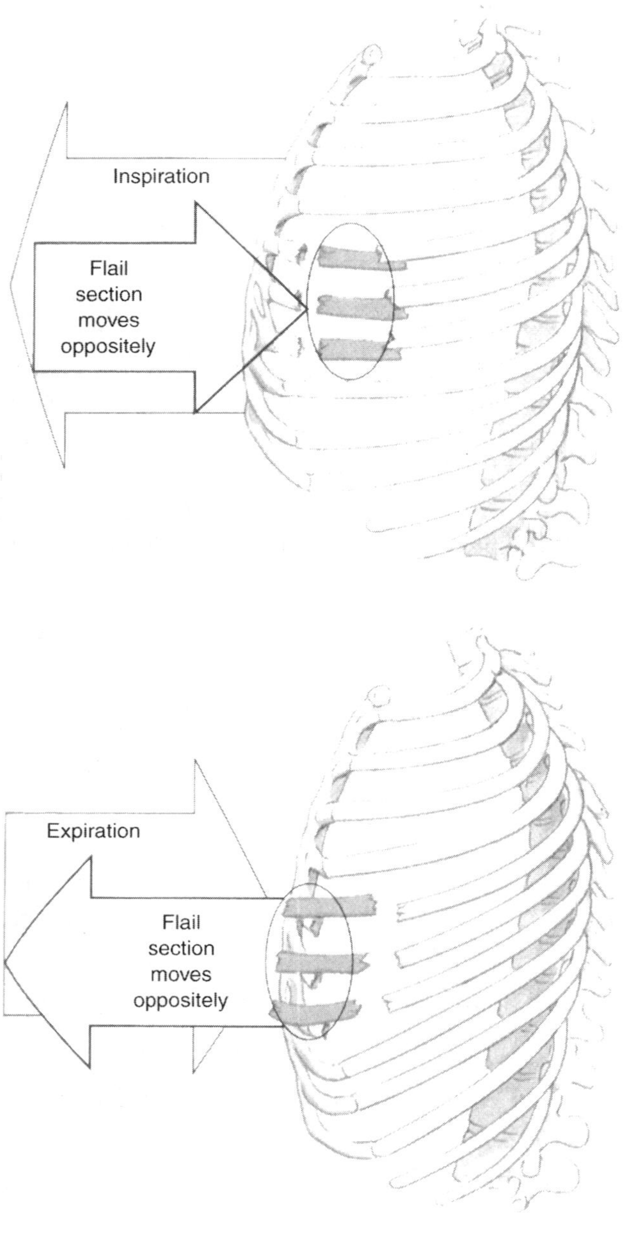

*Inspiration*

*Flail section moves oppositely*

*Expiration*

*Flail section moves oppositely*

*Reprinted with permission from O'Keefe, M. F., Limmer, D., Grant, H. D., Murray, R. H. & Bergeron, J. D. (1998.). Brady emergency care (8th ed.). Upper Saddle River, NJ: Brady/Prentice-Hall.*

looked. As a consequence of delayed or missed diagnosis, there is a high mortality rate. Many times during surgery for another reason, the bronchial injury is discovered. The injury can be severe enough for the patient to die at the site of trauma.

Any point of the tracheobronchial tree can be damaged with blunt or penetrating trauma. Because of proximity to major blood vessels, injury can cause exsanguinating hemorrhage into the chest and mediastinum or into the airway itself, producing asphyxia. Signs are severe dyspnea, hemoptysis, subcutaneous emphysema, mediastinal crunch, or tension pneumothorax. At times when there is bronchial disruption into both pleural spaces, bilateral pneumothoraces develop. The patient may have dyspnea, tachycardia, and diminished or absent breath sounds. Airway support may be adequate until inflammation and edema resolve, but surgery is necessary if the tear is significant or healing fails to occur.

### Pulmonary Contusion

Nearly 75% of the patients with blunt chest trauma have bruising of the lung. Of this group, the mortality rate is 40%. Rib fractures, flail chest, scapular fractures and hemopneumothorax can cause pulmonary contusion.

Lung contusion is when the parenchymal (essential parts of an organ related to function, as compared to structure) tissue is damaged, usually by concussive or compressive force, causing edema and hemorrhage. Injury to lung parenchyma becomes progressively worse because of rupture and bleeding into the lung tissue, alveoli and small airways. The airways collapse and ventilation is lost, resulting in hypoxemia. As inflammatory

Diagnosis may be difficult and involve a CT scan, laryngoscopy, or bronchoscopy. Treatment ranges from intubation to tracheostomy or surgery.

### Bronchial Injury

Major injuries to the bronchi are caused by blunt trauma to the chest and are frequently over-response develops, gas exchange is impaired and the patient's condition worsens.

Dyspnea, hemoptysis, hypoxia and possible chest wall ecchymosis or abrasion are present in the clinical picture. Whenever a patient has a history of chest trauma, pulmonary contusion should be suspected and looked for. Half of the patients with pulmonary contusion do not exhibit physical findings. Chest x-ray does not indicate a contusion to the parenchyma; a CT scan is a more sensitive indicator.

The immediate priority with a pulmonary contusion is to suction and place the patient in a semi-Fowler's position which improves reexpansion of the lung. Intubation and mechanical ventilation are necessary with patients who are hypoxic, show signs of shock, have eight or more fractured ribs, are elderly or have pulmonary disease.

### Diaphragm Injury

Trauma may include the diaphragm. The liver protects the right side of the diaphragm, so most diaphragmatic injuries are on the left side. In penetrating injuries, herniation may take years to manifest. Hemothorax, pneumothorax or intra-abdominal bleeding raise a flag to look for a ruptured diaphragm. Large tears may cause herniation of abdominal contents into the thorax. Other indicators are dyspnea, decreased breath sounds on the affected side, abdominal or epigastric pain radiating to the left shoulder or bowel sounds in the lower chest.

## Cardiac and Great Vessel Injuries

### Cardiac Contusion/Concussion

Blunt trauma to the anterior chest from steering wheels, falls, assaults and other direct blows can bruise the heart.

Signs and symptoms are not specific to the injury. History of significant blunt trauma to the chest is an important indicator. However, the patient may not display an indication of chest wall injury. Chest pain, abrasions and contusions to the chest and fractures are all seen in other chest injuries. Chest pain in cardiac contusion is similar to angina, but does not clear with the use of coronary vasodilators.

Mild contusions can have a dysrhythmia and normal echocardiogram. Severe myocardial contusion can mimic an acute myocardial infarction. Considerable bruising disturbs the electrical conduction that controls the heart rate. The resulting cardiac irritability produces extra heartbeats that interrupt the normal pulse rhythm and show evidence of myocardial dysfunction on the echocardiogram. Dysrhythmias include sinus tachycardia, atrial fibrillation and premature ventricular contractions (PVCs).

The patient must be monitored continuously with serial EKGs for at least 24 hours. Echocardiograms can differentiate between cardiac dysfunction and myocardial contusion, pericardial tamponade, pericardial effusion and valve rupture. Complications of contusions and concussion are dysrhythmias, valve lesion and rupture, emboli and congestive heart failure (Newberry, 1998).

### Penetrating Injury

Penetrating injuries are associated with personal violence or car crashes in the majority of cases. The patients arrive at the emergency department in cardiac arrest or serious hypotension due to hemorrhage or cardiac tamponade. If the penetration is caused by impalement, the impaling object can serve to compress damaged vessels and reduce hemorrhage if left in place until the means of intervention is determined by the physician. Because the chest contains so many great vessels, if the impalement causes massive, rapid hemorrhage, it is likely to be fatal.

If the patient does not have a heartbeat, the ABCs must be conducted immediately. The 83% mortality rate, with only 20–25% of the patients arriving at the hospital alive, calls for immediate thoracotomy in the emergency department.

### Aortic Rupture

In severe blunt injuries, when the heart's ventricles are forcefully compressed, the systolic pressure can rise to 800 mm Hg, which can cause the heart to rupture. Traumatic aortic rupture is usually caused by a deceleration injury. The heart and aortic arch suddenly move forward causing shearing at the point of the aorta's attachment to the heart. Of these injuries, 80% result in free rupture and have complete exsanguination into the pleural space in the first hour. In a very few, the tear is small and covered over by the outer fibrous layer of the aorta. This covering over will last for only a brief time and then give away. The patient will then bleed out.

Identification of aortic rupture is difficult. History of blunt trauma to the chest is helpful, considering one-third of the patients do not have any sign of chest trauma. Unexplained shock is a warning to suspect aortic rupture.

Management of aortic rupture centers around high volume oxygen administration and maintaining fluid circulation. Surgical repair must be immediate if the patient makes it alive to the emergency department.

# COMPLICATIONS OF CHEST INJURY

Although there are various mechanisms of injury, many chest injuries have similar complications.

## Subcutaneous Emphysema

A laceration of the lung or damage to the tracheobronchial tree may allow air to escape into the soft tissues of the chest wall. Air seeps in, making small bubbles in the subcutaneous tissue, resulting in a significant loss of respiratory function. Palpation over the area makes a crackling sensation as the bubbles move around. In severe cases, the emphysema will involve the entire chest, neck and face.

Fractured ribs that lacerate the lung most commonly cause subcutaneous emphysema. Respiratory support should be provided.

## Pneumothorax

A simple pneumothorax is the presence of air in the pleural space. The source of air can be external through an open chest wound from a laceration of the lung wall, such as by a fractured rib or a ruptured lung. The air separates the parietal and visceral pleura and collects in the pleural space, causing the lung to collapse. As air pressure in the pleural space increases, the lung collapses further and may fully collapse. Air can also accumulate in the mediastinum. In the case where the chest wall defect is small, the body is sometimes able to reseal itself.

The patient will complain of shortness of breath and pain. Breath sounds are down on the affected side. Tachycardia and tachypnea are usually evident.

Placement of a chest tube connected to underwater drainage (in the fourth or fifth intercostal space) is the treatment of choice to reexpand the lung. The patient should be in a semi-Fowler's position to prevent pressure against the diaphragm from the abdominal organs. High flow oxygen is administered. The patient should be monitored constantly for the development of tension pneumothorax.

## Tension Pneumothorax

Tension pneumothorax is a minute-by-minute emergency. Prompt, correct and efficient treatment will save a life.

A pneumothorax becomes life threatening when the visceral pleura or a lung injury allows the air to enter the pleural space and cannot leave. The air leaks from the lung into the pleural space. Since the air is trapped in the pleural space, the space expands with every breath, compressing the lung to the point of complete collapse. The pressure in the affected side rises with each breath so that the collapsed lung presses against the heart and compresses the other lung.

As the pressure in the chest cavity increases, it may compress the vena cava, impairing blood return to the heart for recycling through the body. The decrease in venous return to the heart decreases the cardiac output. If the mediastinal shift is great enough, the great vessels can become kinked sufficiently to prevent venous return to the heart. Death quickly follows.

Tension pneumothorax must have an intact, well-sealed chest to occur. But, it is not limited to closed chest injuries. An open wound to the chest with a severe lung laceration can develop a tension pneumothorax after the wound has been sealed with bandages. The lung continues to leak air into a pleural space that is now sealed with the dressing; the pleural air cannot escape, causing a tension pneumothorax to develop.

The patient presents with increasing difficulty breathing and shock due to the decreased flow of blood through the heart. The signs are severe and rapidly progressive. Respiratory distress, weak pulse, falling blood pressure, bulging tissues of the chest wall between the ribs and above the clavicle, distention of the veins in the neck, and cyanosis indicate an extremely critical situation.

Management is to reduce the increasing pressure in the pleural space by removing the air. In closed chest injuries, a 14 or 16 gauge needle is inserted into the pleural space through the second intercostal space by the physician or physician's assistant. If the tension pneumothorax occurs after an open wound has been bandaged, simply removing the dressing or loosening one side of the dressing will most likely resolve the problem as the air rushes out of the wound space. High flow oxygen should be administered.

## Open Pneumothorax/Sucking Chest Wound

An open thoracic injury may develop a sucking chest wound. The severity of the open pneumothorax is related to the size of the wound opening. Stab wounds generally are self-sealing. Shotgun wounds are larger.

As previously discussed, the air pressure inside the chest cavity is slightly less than the atmospheric air pressure. Inhalation further reduces the pressure. An open chest wound causes an additional loss of intrathoracic pressure.

When the chest wall is opened traumatically, the lung on the side of the wound collapses, creating an open pneumothorax. If the hole in the chest wall is larger than the glottis, air will enter through the chest wall in preference to the trachea, seriously compromising respiratory function. Air entering through the wound remains in the pleural space. The lung does not expand. When the patient exhales, some air leaves through the wound. As the air moves in and out, the mediastinum moves with respiration, compressing the opposite lung and great veins leading to the heart. The process of air moving in and out of an open chest wound makes a sucking sound.

First priority with a sucking chest wound is to put a sterile three-sided occlusive dressing over the opening, to allow air to escape but not enter the wound and to prevent a tension pneumothorax. The dressing must be large enough not to be sucked into the wound.

The patient must be closely monitored to ensure that a tension pneumothorax does not develop.

## Hemothorax

The presence of blood in the pleural space may occur in open or closed chest trauma and may be accompanied by pneumothorax. The pleural space can hold 3,000 cc of blood or more. Blood comes from lacerated or torn vessels in the chest wall, bronchi, major vessels in the chest cavity, or a laceration of the lung. The most common cause is trauma to the intercostal arteries that bleed into the pleural space. Severe bleeding into the chest cavity causes hypovolemic shock. The principle of hemothorax is the same as pneumothorax: something other than the lungs fills the chest cavity; normal lung expansion cannot be carried out due to compression; less air is inhaled; and, most likely, less blood is available to circulate oxygen.

Signs and symptoms of hemothorax are similar to those of pneumothorax. Additionally, hypovolemic shock may result from loss of circulating blood. Blood loss is not obvious, since it flows into the chest cavity.

High flow ventilation support is required. Circulatory support with electrolytes is also needed. Chest tube drainage should be carefully monitored to assess the need for autotransfusion. Observe the patient for developing tension pneumothorax.

## Traumatic Asphyxia

Although the term asphyxia is used, it is an inaccurate description. Severe blunt and crushing injuries cause a marked increase in intrathoracic pressure. The pressure forces the blood backward out of the right side of the heart into the veins of the upper chest and neck. The pressure is transmitted to the capillaries of the neck, head and brain, causing distention and the blood to pool.

Deoxygenation takes place and the blood becomes dark, making the head, neck and shoulders appear blue or purple. The face and neck are cyanotic, and the skin below is pink. Neck veins are distended. Subconjunctival hemorrhage and edema may be present.

Most likely, there are additional injuries because of the great force involved in this type of trauma. Management of the other injuries and respiratory support are required.

## Cardiac Tamponade

Tamponade means pathologic compression. Pericardial tamponade is a rapidly progressive and life threatening compression. The pericardium is a tough, fibrous, flexible but inelastic membrane surrounding the heart. As with the pleural space, there is a potential space with a small amount of fluid between the pericardium and the heart.

When the heart's blood vessels are damaged or if the myocardium is torn, blood enters the pericardial space. In the case of blunt trauma, there is no hole in the pericardium for the blood to empty from the space. With a gunshot wound, the hole in the pericardium may or may not be large enough for the blood to drain from the pericardial space.

As the blood fills and cannot empty from the pericardial space, it rapidly begins to compress the heart because of the inelastic pericardium. The ventricles are squeezed, making it more difficult for the heart to refill. Thus, less blood is pumped out of the heart, and there is decreased cardiac output. Less and less blood gets pumped out with each contraction of the heart.

Initially, there may not be any symptoms other than those related to the chest injury. An adult's pericardial space can hold about 300 cc of blood before tamponade occurs. The blood accumulates in the pericardial space, the pulse increases and pulse pressure narrows. Because the compressed ventricles cannot expand normally to accommodate the blood entering the heart, venous pooling occurs in the head and neck. Consequently, jugular vein distention (JVD) occurs. Heart sounds may be distant and muffled because the blood in the pericardium insulates the sound. Hypotension is secondary to the myocardial compression and decreased cardiac output. Shock progressively develops. Beck's Triad: hypotension, muffled heart tones and distended neck veins are the classic signs of pericardial/cardiac tamponade. Associated injuries and problems such as hypovolemia may mask the triad of symptoms.

As tamponade progresses, the patient develops air hunger, becomes agitated and his level of consciousness decreases.

The blood must be removed from the pericardial space and the source of bleeding stopped. Needle pericardiocentesis, the insertion of a needle into the pericardium to drain the blood, is potentially lifesaving. The procedure can improve cardiac function while the patient waits for surgery. Intravenous infusion increases venous pressure and helps to resolve the obstructive, or flow, shock (see Chapter 4, "Shock").

# ASSESSMENT

The effectiveness of thoracic trauma care is directly related to the patient's ability to breathe. Initial assessment is directed to the airway and respiration, the standard ABC plan. Assume head and neck injury until the patient is cleared. The upper airway must be cleared and maintained. Ventilation support and oxygen should be given if the patient has respiratory distress and before further assessment is conducted.

Thoracic trauma often includes multiple injuries. Patient history and knowledge of the mechanism of injury are important in determining the full scope of damage to the patient. Knowing the object causing the trauma, the speed of the force and the physical site of initial injury is essential information. If you are in the prehospital setting, gather information from the scene, the patient and bystanders. If you are in the emergency department, be sure to get a full report and documentation from the rescue squad transporting the patient and the patient (if possible).

Patients with obvious or suspected chest injuries must be immediately and quickly assessed in an organized and thorough manner, followed by rapid essential interventions. Speed in assessment is essential.

Basically remember there are six thoracic injuries that are thought of as lethal and should be looked for during the primary survey: airway obstruction, tension pheumothorax, cardiac tamponade, open pneumothorax, massive hemothorax and flail chest. The secondary survey should look for any of the "hidden six" injuries: thoracic aortic disruption, tracheobronchial injuries, myocardial contusion, diaphragmatic tear, esophageal injury and pulmonary contusion.

## Signs and Symptoms

- Impaled object in chest
- Open wound into the chest
- Signs of tension pneumothorax after a dressing is applied
- Obvious deformity of the chest wall, rib cage or neck, trachea displaced from the midline
- Unequal chest expansion
- Signs of flail chest
- Stressful breathing rate, depth and effort. Does the patient have dyspnea?
- Decreased breath sounds on the affected side
- Sucking respiratory sounds
- Hemoptysis, signs of hemorrhagic shock
- Hypoventilation and splinting of the injured side
- Rapidly progressing respiratory distress
- Air hunger, agitation and decreased level of consciousness
- Hypoxia
- Rapid pulse
- Hypotension, muffled heart sounds, and distended neck veins
- Weak pulse with falling blood pressure

## FIGURE 9-4
### Signs of Traumatic Asphyxia

- Distended neck veins.
- Head, neck and shoulders appear dark blue or purple.
- Eyes may be blood-shot and bulging.
- Tongue and lips may appear swollen and cyanotic.
- Chest deformity may be present.

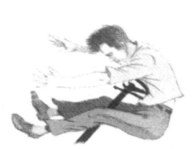
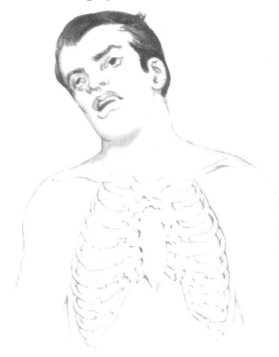

*Reprinted with permission from* Grant, H. D., Murray, R. H., Jr. & Bergeron, J. D. (Eds.). (1990). *Brady emergency care* (5th ed.). Englewood Cliffs, NJ: Prentice-Hall.

- Bulging of the tissues of the chest wall between the ribs and above the clavicle

- Cyanosis of the face and neck

- Sucking pneumothorax

- Identify subcutaneous emphysema by feeling for a crackling in the subcutaneous tissue

- Bulging eyes

## NURSING STRATEGIES FOR THE PATIENT WITH THORACIC INJURY

Although there are many types of chest injuries, the same principles of care apply to all of them:

- Rapidly conduct the ABCs, open and maintain the airway and stabilize breathing and circulation.

- Stabilize the head and neck until the patient is cleared.

- Assess the patient's breathing rate, depth, and effort after the airway is open and maintained.

- Use supplemental oxygen; provide respiratory support when necessary.

- If the patient is seriously injured, expect multiple trauma. Do not pull off clothing; it may cause more damage. Ensure patient privacy and cut off all clothing to fully inspect the patient.

- Keep the patient warm.

- Inspect the back for signs of trauma.

- *Note:* indications for emergency thoracotomy:

    — Penetrating stab wounds to the heart: entrance wound over the heart region; cardiac tamponade

    — Massive or progressive hemothorax

    — Esophageal injury: odynophagia; mediastinal or cervical emphysema

    — Major tracheal or bronchial injury: refrac-

> **TABLE 9-1**
> **Thoracic Trauma Assessment**
>
> | The following injuries must be detected and treated during the BTLS Primary Survey | Life-threatening injuries that are more likely to be detected during the detailed Exam or during hospital evaluation |
> |---|---|
> | • Airway obstruction | • Traumatic aortic rupture |
> | • Open pneumothorax | • Tracheal or bronchial tree injury |
> | • Tension pneumothorax | • Myocardial contusion |
> | • Massive hemothorax | • Diaphragmatic tears |
> | • Flail chest | • Esophageal injury |
> | • Cardiac tamponade | • Pulmonary contusion |

tory pneumothorax, massive air leak

• Be prepared for life threatening hypovolemic shock. Two large-bore intravenous catheters should be immediately inserted for fluid resuscitation, and high-flow oxygen should be administered.

• Observe and palpate neck veins for distention, which can indicate compression or obstruction of return blood flow to the heart. Check the head and neck for cyanosis. Note the turgor of the neck veins, as they may collapse if there is significant bleeding into the chest cavity.

• Promptly apply three-sided dressings to open wounds, making sure not to seal off the wound completely, which keeps air from entering the wound on inspiration, but allowing air to escape during expiration. Be sure the dressing is large enough so it is not sucked into the wound. **Do not** open the wound to assess its depth.

• Monitor for tension pneumothorax.

• If the patient shows signs of tension pneumothorax, relieve pressure by loosening one side of the dressing on the wound. If it is a closed chest injury, assist with the placement of a large-bore needle into the pleural space.

• Placing one hand on each side of the chest will allow you to compare if there is even movement, structural deformities, crepitus, subcuta-

neous emphysema, painful areas not observed by the eye and rib fractures.

• Observe, monitor and record vital signs serially; check for bilateral and equal breath sounds. Compare the findings of the vital signs measurements with the appearance of the patient's condition to see if they appear consistent.

• Monitor electrocardiogram, look for arrhythmias.

• If the patient has flail chest, splint in the inward position with bulky towels; watch for progression to respiratory failure, hypoxia and shock. After the patient has been cleared for spinal injury, he may lie on the affected side to limit movement and discomfort. Assist with positive pressure bag-mask ventilation.

• Control bleeding from the chest wall with direct pressure.

• An impaled object should be left in place and stabilized to minimize movement. Never remove or move an impaled object.

• If a rib fracture is suspected, keep the patient quiet and still so that movement does not further damage the lungs, chest wall or heart. Splint fractured ribs with external support to make the patient more comfortable.

• Keep the patient NPO until the physician clears the need for surgery and states what the patient may have by mouth.

# EXAM QUESTIONS

## CHAPTER 9
### Questions 41–45

41. The degree of severity with thoracic trauma is based upon

    a. whether it is an open or closed injury.

    b. whether the cause is blunt or penetrating.

    c. respiratory rate and patterns.

    d. the injury's effect on ventilation and circulation.

42. Complications accompanying chest injuries

    a. vary with each type of injury.

    b. may be life threatening.

    c. require surgical intervention.

    d. are noneventful.

43. Which injury is characterized by Beck's triad of hypotension, muffled heart sounds, and distended neck veins?

    a. Pericardial tamponade

    b. Tension pneumothorax

    c. Hemopneumothorax

    d. Sucking chest wound

44. An open chest wound should

    a. be opened further to evaluate if it has perforated the pleura.

    b. have a three-sided dressing applied.

    c. be tightly sealed with a petroleum dressing.

    d. be treated with chest tube drainage.

45. There are many types of chest injuries. Basic principles of care

    a. are specific for each type of injury.

    b. are the same for all types of chest trauma.

    c. require advanced life support staff to care for the patient.

    d. require surgery in 85% of the injuries.

# CHAPTER 10

# ABDOMINAL TRAUMA

## CHAPTER OBJECTIVE

Upon completion of this chapter, the reader will be able to describe the key components of managing abdominal trauma.

## LEARNING OBJECTIVES

Upon completion of this chapter, the reader should be able to:

1. Identify abdominal organs, structures and their functions.

2. Describe common mechanisms of injury to the abdomen.

3. Identify signs and symptoms of abdominal injuries.

4. Recognize complications that accompany abdominal injuries.

5. Describe general principles of care and basic nursing strategies for abdominal injuries.

6. Indicate examples of nursing diagnoses for patients with abdominal trauma.

## INTRODUCTION

Abdominal trauma is probably one of the most frequently overlooked or missed groups of injuries. Life-threatening abdominal injuries may not have any outward sign of trauma. When the injuries are undetected, they have a high potential for causing death.

Motor vehicle crashes cause approximately 75% of the blunt abdominal injuries. Falls; other types of vehicular crashes, such as bicycles or motorcycles; sports; and assaults account for most of the other mechanisms of abdominal trauma.

Patients involved in high-energy blunt injury have multiple problems that are particularly difficult to assess. They are often intoxicated, have closed head injuries and tend to have multisystem trauma (Peitzman et al., 1998).

Incidence and mechanism of injury are usually related to where the injury took place. Urban areas are often the site of penetrating abdominal injuries, although as violence escalates across the country, the suburbs are catching up. The magnitude of injury is difficult to determine outside of the hospital setting. Diagnostic methods beyond physical examination are usually necessary to identify the full extent of injuries to the patient.

## ANATOMY AND PHYSIOLOGY

The **abdominal cavity** is one of two body cavities, the thoracic cavity being the other. Beginning below the diaphragm, the cavity extends down to the pubic area. It is bounded by the spine in the back and the ribs and abdominal muscle wall in the front. When referring to descriptive geographic areas of the abdomen, it is thought of as being divided into quadrants: left and right upper quadrants and left and right lower quadrants.

The **diaphragm** is a musculomembranous wall separating the thoracic and abdominal cavities, and is attached to the ribs, sternum, and spine. It has an upward convexity that contracts and flattens downward with inhalation, returning to its original position during exhalation. The lower surface is in proximity to the kidneys, liver, spleen and the cardiac (upper) end of the stomach.

Within the abdomen there are two spaces: the **peritoneal** space and **retroperitoneal** space. They contain the major organs of the digestive, endocrine and urogenital systems, along with major blood vessels. In the peritoneal space are the stomach, bowel, liver, gallbladder, spleen, and pancreas. The retroperitoneum contains the kidneys, ureters, bladder, reproductive organs, inferior vena cava and abdominal aorta.

As in the thoracic cavity, the abdominal cavity is lined by a serous membrane, the **parietal peritoneum.** The **visceral peritoneum** covers the organs. There is also a potential space, the **peritoneal cavity**, between the parietal and visceral peritoneum. The space is closed in men and open to the exterior in women through the vagina, uterus, and fallopian tubes.

The **mesentery**, also called greater and lesser **omentum**, is formed from the peritoneum to carry blood vessels and nerves to the abdominal organs. It is a fold forming a sheet of fragile tissue that surrounds organs and suspends them from the body wall. The structure of the omentum allows the organs to hang freely, permitting movement within the abdominal cavity.

The abdominal organs are considered to be hollow, solid, or vascular.

**Hollow organs** are tubes that conduct or store material, such as food being stored in and moved

through the stomach or urine being stored in the bladder. Hollow organs include the stomach, duodenum, small and large intestine, appendix, rectum, gallbladder, bile ducts, urinary bladder, ureters, and uterus *(see Figure 10-1).*

**Solid organs** are masses of tissue where most of the body's chemical work takes place. They include the liver, spleen, pancreas, kidneys, ovaries and adrenal glands *(see Figure 10-1).*

**Vascular organs** are masses of tissue rich in blood vessels such as the liver, kidneys and spleen.

Solid organs fracture when injured; hollow organs rupture or collapse. Solid and vascular structures bleed, while hollow organs empty their contents. The consequences can be intra-abdominal bleeding, peritonitis and sepsis.

Major **vascular structures** supplying the abdomen are the abdominal aorta that bifurcates into the iliac arteries (to supply the lower extremities), the celiac trunk and the inferior and superior mesentery arteries, that supply the abdomen.

The inferior vena cava is formed by the union of two common iliac veins and is the major vein in the abdomen.

# ORGANS

## Peritoneal Space

### Stomach

Placed in the left upper quadrant and protected by the lower left ribs, the stomach is a hollow organ with the basic purpose of digestion. Having a limited ability to absorb, it receives, stores and regulates the movement of food to the rest of the digestive system. The stomach secretes gastric juice; converts proteins into peptones; destroys many microbes present in foods and aids in acid-base equilibrium in the body. It receives chemical and nervous stimulation for secretion and movement in the lower parts of the

**FIGURE 10-1**
**Major Body Organs**

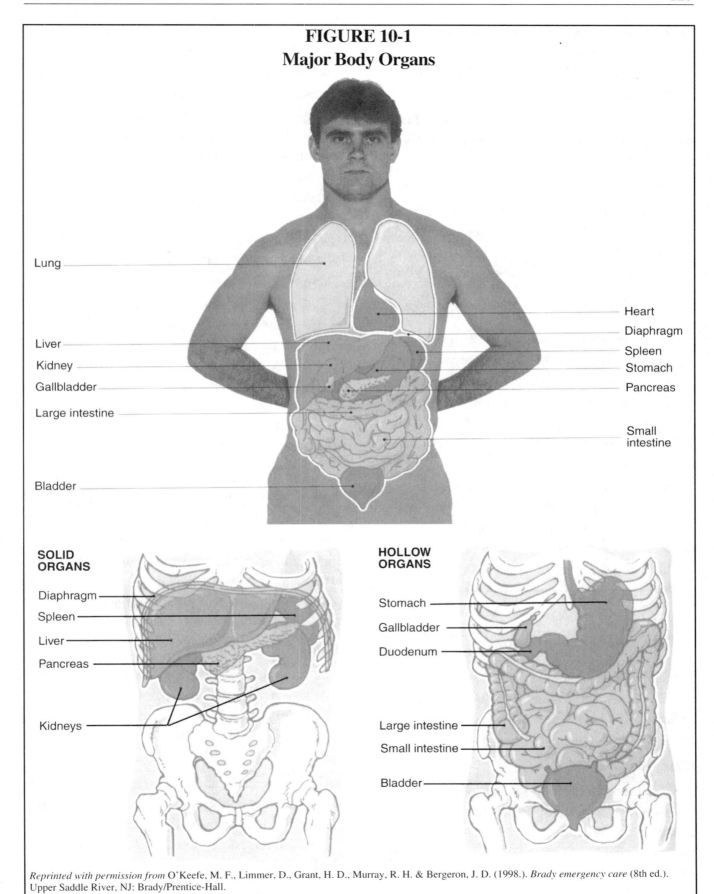

Lung

Heart
Diaphragm
Spleen
Stomach
Pancreas

Liver
Kidney
Gallbladder

Large intestine

Small
intestine

Bladder

**SOLID**
**ORGANS**

Diaphragm
Spleen
Liver
Pancreas

Kidneys

**HOLLOW**
**ORGANS**

Stomach
Gallbladder
Duodenum

Large intestine
Small intestine

Bladder

gastrointestinal tract; excretes some parenterally administered medications into gastric juices, and contains a gastric juice factor effective in the prevention of pernicious anemia.

Stomach size changes with the amount of contents, and when empty, is more able to compress and absorb energy during trauma.

### Bowel

**Small Intestine:** The pyloric sphincter in the stomach controls the emptying of contents into the small intestine and is attached to it. The small intestine is the largest hollow organ and has three sections: the duodenum, jejunum, and ileum.

Hanging from its mesentery, the small bowel lies entirely free within the abdomen. This part of the mesentery contains arteries branching from the aorta and veins that carry blood to the liver. The greatest part of digestion is continued by mucous and enzymes generated here, along with absorption.

**Large Intestine:** Also a major hollow organ, the large intestine interfaces with the small intestine proximally and ends at the rectum. About 5 feet long, the large intestine lies around the border of the small bowel. It has three sections called the cecum, colon and rectum. The primary function is to absorb the remaining 5–10 percent of the fluid from the contents and form stool. The rectum stores the stool until it is expelled.

The **appendix** is a small tube opening into the cecum in the lower right quadrant of the abdomen. It has no known function.

### Liver

A gland is an organ or structure that manufactures secretions discharged and used in another part of the body. The liver is the largest gland in the body, weighing almost 3% of the total body weight and is located in the upper right quadrant of the abdomen. Involved in more than 500 metabolic functions, the liver secretes bile to assist in the metabolism of fat; detoxifies poisons; metabolizes carbohydrates, proteins and fats; helps to maintain blood glucose and energy level; stores glycogen for energy reserve; stores copper, iron, vitamins A, B12, D, and E. It also inactivates and excretes aldosterone, glucocorticoids, estrogen, progesterone, and testosterone; forms factors necessary for blood clotting and for the production of plasma; produces many of the factors involved in the regulation of immune responses and performs many other functions.

The liver is extremely vascular, essentially being a large, dense mass of blood vessels and cells. All of the blood pumped to the gastrointestinal tract is pumped through the liver before returning to the heart. It takes only 10–20% of the liver to sustain life, but if the liver is completely destroyed, death will occur within 12 hours.

### Gallbladder

The liver's connection to the intestine is the bile duct. The gallbladder is an outpouching of the bile duct and a reservoir for bile. When food is in the duodenum, it triggers the gallbladder to send bile into the duodenum via the common bile duct. Bile is a digestive juice that, in conjunction with other juices, emulsifies fats and also stimulates peristalsis.

### Spleen

The primary function of the spleen is the production and destruction of blood cells, but it is not necessary to sustain life. If removed, the spleen's functions are taken over by the liver and bone marrow.

The spleen, located in the left upper quadrant, just beneath the diaphragm and in front of the lower ribs, is a major solid organ, smaller than the liver. The largest mass of lymphatic tissue in the body, the spleen is vascular and enclosed in a capsule supported by three ligaments. Although the ribs protect the spleen, the ligaments can be torn from the spleen in blunt injury, causing severe hemorrhage.

### Pancreas

The pancreas is a flat, solid, firmly fixed organ, lying deep in the abdomen behind the stomach, below the liver, and in front of the first and second lumbar vertebrae. Its head is attached to the duodenum and the tail reaches to the spleen. Functions are both endocrine and exocrine. Endocrine cells produce insulin, glucagon and somatostatin. Exocrine production includes lipase, amylase, trypsin and other digestive enzymes. Pancreatic ducts channel pancreatic juices directly into the duodenum.

## Retroperitoneal Space

Behind the peritoneum and outside the peritoneal cavity is the retroperitoneal space. It contains the kidneys, bladder, ureters, reproductive organs, inferior vena cava and abdominal aorta.

The organs and structures contained in the retroperitoneal space, with the exception of the major blood vessels, will be discussed in Chapter 11, "Genitourinary Trauma."

# MECHANISM OF INJURY

As with other trauma, mechanisms of abdominal injury, blunt or penetrating, may be closed or open.

## Closed/Blunt Injury

When the abdomen receives a severe blow, usually from deceleration or compression, as with a steering wheel, sports injury or assault, it is considered a closed blunt injury.

Remember that blunt abdominal injury is deceptive because damage can be severe, even life threatening, without immediate outward signs. Vital functions must be watched closely for changes in the patient's condition as indicators of unseen problems. If there is massive hemorrhage into the abdomen, there may be a blue-gray discoloration around the umbilicus, however, most often there is little visible evidence.

In **compression** incidents, the organs are crushed between solid objects, for instance, the steering wheel and spinal column. Along with direct damage, the organs are often pushed out of place, resulting in additional injuries such as herniation of the diaphragm.

**Deceleration** events may rupture solid organs or vessels in the abdominal cavity because of tearing forces exerted against stabilizing ligaments and the vessels. When hollow organs are ruptured or lacerated, their contents will spill into the peritoneal cavity, causing an inflammatory reaction. Solid organs have a large blood supply subject to hemorrhage, which is also seen in the rupture of major vessels.

Pelvic fractures causing bladder and urethral injuries may lead to hemorrhage and life threatening conditions. Loss of blood into the abdominal cavity can contribute to hypovolemic shock.

Blunt trauma from a motor vehicle crash is influenced by where the patient is sitting, speed of the vehicle, use and type of seatbelt, air bag deployment and whether there was ejection from the vehicle. Although seatbelt use has decreased fatalities, it has also created injuries to the colon, small bowel, stomach, liver, spleen, vascular structures, and the spinal cord.

Injuries from falls vary with the height of the fall, the landing surface, and the part of the body that hits the surface first.

## Open/Penetrating Injury

Open injuries range from a slight laceration of the abdominal wall to deep penetration through the peritoneum into the abdominal cavity. It may be difficult to determine if the wound extends into the abdominal cavity, but in the case of stab or gunshot wounds, it should be assumed the peritoneum has been penetrated.

The depth of injury may be deceptive; while appearing minimal, it can be devastating. Multiple organ damage is likely in the case of gunshot wounds. A clean little bullet hole may have a mess of torn vessels and tissue beneath. Stab wounds are often self-contained because they have less velocity.

It should also be noted that the diaphragm extends to the fourth intercostal space during exhalation, and penetrating injuries into the thorax may also involve the abdomen. Penetrating wounds into the flank or buttocks can also enter the abdominal cavity, hitting a major vessel, a segment of the bowel or a solid organ.

Most penetrating injuries are caused by projectiles and are intentionally inflicted. These wounds imply violence, especially as violence escalates in this country. Damage includes laceration, impalement, puncture and rupture.

The cause of the injury should be identified. In the case of a gunshot, the type of gun, caliber, proximity to the patient when fired, and number of shots that hit the patient are important in determining the likely extent of injury. It is necessary to identify the length, width, and composition of other penetrating objects as well. Injuries from wood are likely to cause infection since it is a biologic material.

**Evisceration** is the result of an extensive laceration of the abdominal wall that causes the organs to protrude through the wound (*see Figure 10-2*). The organs should not be pushed back into the abdomen but covered with a moist, sterile dressing. It is essential that the organs are kept warm and moist. Dressings should not be a material that clings or loses substance when wet, such as tissue-like paper.

**Impalement** injuries vary with the type of object lodged in the abdomen and the structures that

are damaged. The impaled object often compresses and tamponades affected organs and vessels, which acts to hold back hemorrhaging. Therefore, the impaled object should not be removed but secured in place until medical management determines the mode of treatment.

# ABDOMINAL INJURIES AND INTERVENTIONS

## Diaphragm

Ninety percent of diaphragmatic injuries are associated with high-speed motor vehicle crashes. Sixty to 80% are related to intra-abdominal injuries. Diaphragm injury may accompany, and should always be suspected, in thoracic or abdominal blunt and penetrating trauma. The injury can be easily overlooked. Diaphragmatic rupture usually occurs on the left side because the liver protects the right side of the diaphragm.

If the diaphragm is lacerated, the abdominal contents will enter the chest cavity, causing impaired breathing due to lung compression and the loss of negative pressure. Signs include decreased breath sounds on the affected side and complaints of dyspnea and cyanosis. There may be a shift in heart sounds. Bowel sounds may be heard in the hemithorax.

Diagnosis is confirmed by chest x-ray or during surgery for another traumatic repair. A hemopneumothorax may also be evident. Immediate surgical intervention is required.

## Stomach

Blunt gastric injuries are unusual because the stomach is a hollow organ that can easily be displaced and, if empty, compressed. However, the anterior position does make it susceptible to penetrating injury. Left upper quadrant pain and tenderness are signs of trauma. The stomach has an

# FIGURE 10-2
## Dressing an Open Abdominal Wound

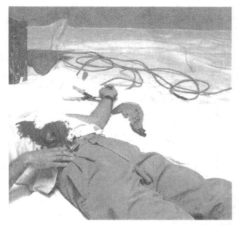

1. Open abdominal wound with evisceration.

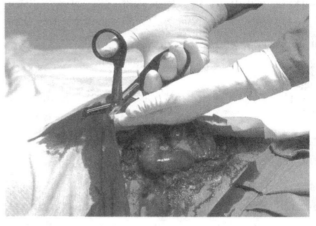

2. Cut away clothing from wound.

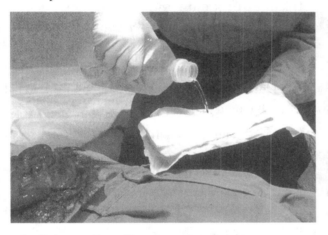

3. Pour sterile saline to soak a dressing.

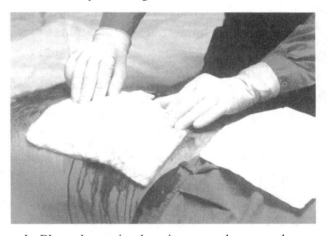

4. Place the moist dressing over the wound.

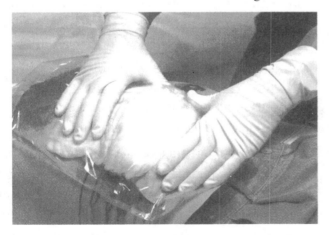

5. Apply an occlusive dressing over the moist dressing if local protocols recommend.

6. Cover the dressed wound to maintain warmth. Secure the covering with tape or cravats tied above and below the position of the exposed organ.

extensive blood supply, so that hematemesis and blood in the nasogastric aspirate are likely. Subdiaphragmatic air from blunt gastric ruptures may be seen on a chest x-ray. Surgical exploration and intervention is required.

## Bowel

The bowel is hollow, vascular, and connected to various points of the peritoneal cavity by the omentum. Anteriorly, there is little protection from injury.

The **small bowel** is the most commonly injured abdominal organ in penetrating trauma. Blunt trauma damage is not as frequent, but not unusual.

Rupture of the bowel may cause a fulminating peritonitis from the contents being spilled into the abdomen. Lap belt injuries can cause small isolated perforations. Larger perforations, complete disruption, and injuries associated with large hematomas or lacerations of the omentum are due to direct blows or shearing injuries.

Small bowel injury should be considered when there is bruising from a lap belt. There may also be a fracture of the lumbar spine. Frequently, this injury is not initially diagnosed. CT scans often show a false negative (Peitzman et al., 1998), with definitive diagnosis being made surgically.

**Colon** damage is seen in about a quarter of the gunshot and stab wounds to the abdomen. Only a small percent of colon injuries are caused by blunt mechanisms. **Rectal** injuries are a small percentage of the colon injuries, but blunt rectal perforation can be associated with pelvic fractures, concussion (explosion) injuries, devascularization from a mesentery injury or foreign objects. Gross rectal bleeding may indicate a pelvic fracture damaging the colon or rectum.

Signs include tenderness and rigidity. Contusions to the abdomen are warning signs of colon injury. If peritoneal contamination continues, fever, abdominal distention and hypoactive bowel sounds occur. Treatment is surgical.

## Liver

The location of the liver makes it vulnerable to trauma, more likely from penetrating than blunt mechanisms. Usually liver injuries are not fatal. The liver is encapsulated by a tough fibrous sheath and is vascular. Injury may only affect the capsule, or cause a contused, lacerated or fractured liver.

Physical examination in the blunt trauma victim misses an injury in nearly half of the patients. However, immediate ultrasound of the abdomen will increase the potential for correct diagnosis. Rib fractures or a blow to the right upper quadrant should raise an alert to liver damage. Most likely, there is pain and tenderness in the area of the liver, to the point of guarding, along with bruising and nausea. If the damage is severe, there will be hemodynamic instability.

More than half of the patients will not require surgery if they are hemodynamically stable.

## Spleen

Although the spleen is relatively small and not likely to be injured by penetrating trauma, it is the abdominal organ most commonly injured from blunt trauma. Blunt trauma is usually the result of compression or deceleration force seen in motor vehicle crashes, falls or direct blows to the abdomen. Like the liver, the spleen is encapsulated. A splenic injury can affect just the capsule or cause a hematoma, laceration or fracture.

Injury to the left upper quadrant and lower ribs is likely to include the spleen. There may be pain in the left upper quadrant or referred to the left shoulder. Bruising and signs of hypovolemia with tachycardia and hypotension may be apparent. Physical examination is not specific for splenic trauma. In an unstable patient, an ultrasound will provide the most rapid diagnosis of hemoperitoneum, a frequent consequence of trauma. After blunt abdominal trauma, splenic injury is the most common indication for laparotomy (Peitzman et al., 1998).

If the spleen is ruptured, or there is a penetrating wound that causes severe hemorrhage, the patient could exsanguinate rapidly without immediate surgical intervention. Management depends on the hemodynamic stability of the patient, his age, associated injuries, the degree of hemoperitoneum and the severity of the splenic injury. Surgical repair is not always necessary, but the patient must be observed carefully and have rapid access to the CT scanner, a surgeon and the operating room.

## Pancreas

The pancreas lies deep in the abdominal cavity and is well protected. Blunt trauma is relatively uncommon, with most injuries caused by penetration and usually associated with other intra-abdominal injuries. Additionally, major vascular injury of the aorta, portal vein, or inferior vena cava occurs in over half of the penetrating injuries. Organs most likely to be injured in conjunction with the pancreas are the liver, spleen, duodenum, and small intestine. Late effects from injury are infection and multiple organ dysfunction syndrome.

Diagnosis is based on the mechanism of injury and the high rate of associated intra-abdominal injury. Pancreatic injuries are rarely isolated. If the injury is confined to the pancreas, signs initially may be nonspecific. Within 24 hours of the injury, the patient will complain of mid-epigastric or back pain. Often, a laparotomy is necessary to confirm the pancreatic damage and to repair other abdominal injuries. When surgery is necessary, major efforts are made to save the pancreas because of its vital endocrine and exocrine functions.

## Pelvic Fracture

Closed fracture of the pelvis is often the result of direct compression from heavy impact that crushes the bones. The force of energy can be a fall from a height or direct impact to the pelvis. Indirect force can also cause injury. For instance, when the knee strikes the dashboard, the force is transmitted along the femur, driving the femoral head into the pelvis, causing it to fracture. Not all fractures are from violent trauma; a simple fall can cause a closed fracture, especially in the elderly.

A great deal of blood loss may occur from the large vessels in the retroperitoneal space adjacent to the pelvis. These vessels are easily torn or lacerated, with the blood draining into the retroperitoneal space. Most pelvic fractures are closed because heavy muscles surround and protect the pelvis. Once in a while, pieces of the pelvis will lacerate the rectum, vagina, or bladder. The bladder may also be ruptured. The structures that the pelvis is designed to protect, the bladder, rectum, vagina and blood vessels, are all susceptible to damage when the pelvic ring is fractured.

It should be assumed that a patient with a pelvic fracture has associated abdominal injuries until cleared by the physician.

## Vascular Structures

Any of the abdominal vascular structures are subject to blunt or penetrating injuries. Often, the identification of specific vascular damage is not made until the patient is in surgery to repair other damage. In a stable patient, diagnostic CT scan and arteriography are used to identify the extent of vascular injury.

When disrupted, the aorta, inferior vena cava, iliac arteries and hepatic veins hemorrhage severely, and death can be rapid if the damage is not repaired immediately.

Emergency department management of vascular injuries pertains to intravenous access and getting the patient to the operating room as soon as possible.

## Foreign Body

Abdominal trauma includes foreign bodies in the stomach and rectum. There are many causes, ranging from ingestion, sexual experimentation, psychiatric disorders, to assault. The patient may not initially acknowledge the problem or the presence of a foreign body. The complaint may be vague, relating only to discomfort.

Diagnosis is usually made by radiograph. Surgical intervention may be necessary.

# ASSESSMENT

As with any injured patient, the ABCs and initial stabilization are the first priority. If the patient is critically injured or unstable, the physician may elect to go directly to surgery for immediate stabilization and repair of injuries. If the patient is relatively stable, he is assessed quickly and efficiently, under controlled circumstances.

## Diagnostic Tests

Because abdominal trauma may be subtle and difficult to identify, certain tests are frequently used to more specifically identify injuries. It should be kept in mind that the most serious injuries could go undetected because the damage may only be vaguely apparent with external observation.

### Diagnostic Peritoneal Lavage

Diagnostic Peritoneal Lavage (DPL) is used to determine the presence of blood or intestinal material in the peritoneal cavity. DPL is used on a limited basis with penetrating wounds. If the patient is hemodynamically unstable, as with gunshot wounds, surgery may be required, eliminating the need for DPL. The test can be done in the emergency department.

### Computerized Tomography or CT Scan

Used in the stable patient, CT is used to evaluate peritoneal and retropertioneal injury. The test is able to identify defects and collections of fluid or air. Skeletal injuries can also be identified. Solid organ injuries are identified more easily than hollow organ injuries.

Unstable patients may not be able to tolerate the scanning process. All patients sent for the scan should be closely monitored for a change in condition.

Oral and IV contrast media can be used to evaluate abdominal structures. DPL should not be done before CT because the scan cannot distinguish between fluid and blood in the abdomen.

### Ultrasound

Ultrasound helps determine the need for surgery by detecting fluid in the abdominal cavity, and can identify as little as 70 ml. The advantage of ultrasound is that it is portable and can be brought to the patient in the emergency department. It can also be used in evaluating the pregnant patient.

Many trauma centers conduct ultrasound examinations as a routine diagnostic procedure on all abdominal trauma patients.

### Radiography

Fractures, free air or foreign objects can be identified by radiographs. Trauma centers usually have radiology components in the emergency department so that the patient can be conveniently x-rayed.

Although there are several diagnostic options that are now routinely used for a specific diagnosis, patient management is essentially the same: prevention of shock and prompt physician intervention. When the patient is hemodynamically unstable, has a dropping hemoglobin level, or has an enlarging abdominal mass without pelvic or vertebral fractures, surgical intervention should be immediate.

## Assessment Principles

• The patient with abdominal injury may be normotensive, hypotensive or exsanguinated.

- With penetrating injury, it is essential to determine the trajectory of the projectile, which is key to the determination of organs and structures most likely involved.

- If a patient is in shock with a penetrating injury or has a distended abdomen, it should be assumed that he has a major vascular injury until proven otherwise.

- If it is suspected that the patient has abdominal vascular injury, massive transfusions should be anticipated, including the replacement of platelets and plasma.

- Hemorrhage and hematoma will displace organs and structures.

- Bleeding should first be controlled with direct pressure. The physician may have to control hemorrhage directly through the hematoma by clamping or other means.

- Patient warmth must be maintained to prevent coagulopathy.

- If the patient is in extremis with shock and has an exsanguinating injury, a damage control approach should be taken: immediate control of hemorrhage and contamination, followed by resuscitation and then reexamination to determine patient status (Peitzman et al., 1998).

## Signs and Symptoms

- Note how the patient is positioned. Pain may cause guarding in an attempt to protect the injured area. The patient may have difficulty moving or have his knees drawn up to his chest to relieve pressure and make it easier to breathe. He may be taking rapid, shallow breaths to minimize abdominal movement.

- Whether the injuries are easy to identify, or not immediately apparent, relatively simple or severe and complex, the most common symptom is pain. The pain symptoms can be abdominal and/or referred.

- Nausea is a likely symptom with abdominal trauma.

- Vomiting may occur with the nausea.

- Tenderness, particularly if localized, is a significant sign indicating there may be internal damage.

- If the patient is developing peritonitis, he will want to lie still because any movement is painful.

- Abdominal distention or rigidity is an indicator of hemorrhage.

- If the patient has blunt injury bruises or crepitus, it is likely that there is internal bleeding. Bruising and discoloration around the umbilicus is called Cullen's sign, which may indicate intraperitoneal hemorhage.

- Bruising of the flank is Grey Turner's sign, and is associated with bleeding into the abdominal wall.

- Other signs of hemorrhage are hypotension, tachycardia and pallor; hematemesis; hematuria, blood, or semen (prostate disruption) at the meatus; and inability to urinate.

- Obvious deformity of the abdomen, evisceration of abdominal contents, or impalement may be associated with multiple abdominal injuries.

- Penetrating injuries cause wounds that are obvious on inspection, which make it somewhat easier to predict the extent of the injuries. Look for both entry and exit wounds. High velocity missiles often leave a small, harmless-looking wound at the entry point and a huge, gaping wound at the exit point. Always turn the patient over and examine him thoroughly.

- Bruising and swelling diagonally across the chest and/or abdomen indicates seat belt and shoulder harness injury from deceleration.

# NURSING STRATEGIES FOR THE PATIENT WITH ABDOMINAL TRAUMA

- As with any injury, the first priorities are the ABCs, and maintaining the airway.

- Serial vital signs, with temperature, should be monitored and recorded frequently, and changes promptly reported to the physician. Look for signs of shock.

- Delayed diagnosis and treatment is a major cause of death.

- Aortic trauma invariably puts the patient into hemorrhagic shock. Preparations for surgery should be swift and efficient.

- The golden hour (see Chapter 1) does not just apply to cardiac patients; all potentially acute trauma and medical patients fall within the immediacy of that first hour for assessment, decisions, and intervention. Priorities should be set with this in mind. For instance, listening for bowel sounds is not necessary in the initial assessment and management, identifying the extent of the injuries is essential.

- Because of the possibility of hemorrhage, two intravenous lines should be started immediately with large-bore needles. If the patient is transported to the hospital in a rescue unit, these lines should already be in place with fluids running when the patient arrives.

- The patient may be wearing an antishock garment to enhance venous return and maintain the blood pressure.

- If the patient is not wearing an antishock garment, cut the clothing off, as pulling can aggravate the injuries. Cover the patient with a sheet for privacy and warmth, exposing only the area being assessed.

- Be alert to indicators of multiple trauma and spinal injury. Abdominal trauma usually involves damage of more than one structure or organ. Look and feel for obvious deformities, tenderness, or abdominal tension.

- Ask the patient to describe the location and kind of pain he is feeling. Identify if the pain is direct and/or referred.

- Pain medication cannot be given until the patient's status is fully evaluated by the physician. Other means of pain relief, such as position, reassurance, mouth care and breathing techniques will help. The patient will be anxious and fearful.

- Observe for signs and symptoms of internal hemorrhaging: hypovolemic shock, abdominal pain and distention, and enlarging abdomen.

- If there is any indication of a fractured pelvis, immobilize the patient. There may be a urethral or bladder disruption.

- If a Foley catheter is ordered, it should be inserted with great care after other injuries are ruled out so that a urethral injury is not worsened.

- Blood should be typed and crossmatched for at least 4 units or according to hospital policy. Transfusion is likely.

- Do not remove an impaled object as it is likely to tamponade the bleeding. Stabilize the object, and reassure the patient as to why this is being done. The object will be removed in a surgical environment where repairs can be made.

- Any body parts that are protruding from a wound should not be returned to the abdominal cavity. Cover with a sterile dressing moistened with saline.

- The patient cannot drink or eat anything until he is cleared regarding surgical intervention and has no evidence of nausea or vomiting.

- The patient should be kept warm. He is likely to be hypothermic, which increases the need for oxygen, decreases perfusion, causes coagulation problems and decreases the chances of successful resuscitation. Warming the fluids and humidifying the oxygen reduces heat loss, as do head wraps and warming blankets.

- Be sure to explain to the patient the purpose for multiple tests and procedures if injuries are not evident; reassure him that tests are for thorough diagnosis and evaluation purposes.

# EXAMPLES OF NURSING DIAGNOSES RELATED TO ABDOMINAL INJURY

- Pain, direct and referred, related to abdominal trauma

- Fluid volume deficit related to hemorrhage

- Alteration in tissue perfusion related to hypovolemia

- Ineffective breathing pattern related to multiple injuries, abdominal trauma secondary to thoracic trauma, and shock

- Peritonitis related to penetrating injuries with biological materials such as wood or contaminated materials

- Anxiety related to pain, multiple injuries, and diagnostic and assessment procedures

- Altered thermoregulation related to shock and/or trauma

# SUMMARY

Abdominal injuries present many assessment challenges and represent 25% of all traumatic injuries. The extent of an abdominal injury is probably one of the most frequently missed diagnoses, and if unrecognized, is one of the major causes of death from trauma.

The degree of damage from blunt or penetrating injury is not necessarily evident by immediate observation. Blunt injuries can cause rupture or collapse of hollow organs, fracture of solid organs, and hemorrhaging of vascular organs and vessels. Penetrating injuries are likely to cause hemorrhage and infection. Seat belts and air bags save lives, but new injuries have developed because of them, too. Injuries are more likely to be multiple rather than isolated.

It is imperative to recognize life-threatening injuries and provide rapid surgical intervention, when necessary. Knowledge of the incident, mechanism of injury, force, velocity and time elapsed since the incident occurred are critical factors in the assessment of the patient's condition and probable injuries. Often certain diagnostic procedures including diagnostic peritoneal lavage, CT scan, ultrasound and radiography are required to make or confirm a diagnosis.

# EXAM QUESTIONS

## CHAPTER 10
### Questions 46–50

46. Abdominal trauma is

    a. easy to detect because of the anatomical location of the organs.

    b. influenced by the mechanism of injury, force, trajectory and speed.

    c. not affected by injuries to the thorax.

    d. most likely to be from violent penetrating mechanisms.

47. The organ most likely to be damaged from blunt abdominal trauma is the

    a. liver.

    b. pancreas.

    c. spleen.

    d. small bowel.

48. A passenger in a motor vehicle accident is brought to the emergency department with the history of being in a vehicle that struck a tree at the speed of 45 miles per hour. His knees struck the dashboard quite forcefully. The patient cannot move his legs without severe pain, he is bleeding from the rectum and the abdomen is taut. Likely diagnosis is

    a. fractured patella and contusion to the abdomen.

    b. multiple contusions to the lower extremities.

    c. fractured pelvis, laceration of the rectum, and rupture of the abdominal blood vessels.

    d. fracture of the head of the femur, with abdominal contusions.

49. When a patient is in extremis shock with an exsanguinating abdominal injury, appropriate damage control priorities are to

    a. resuscitate the patient and start two IV lines with large-bore needles.

    b. immediately conduct diagnostic peritoneal lavage and monitor vital signs every 5 minutes.

    c. immediately apply a pneumatic shock garment, start wide-open IVs, and order a CT scan.

    d. proceed with immediate control of hemorrhage and contamination, followed by resuscitation and reevaluate the patient.

50. When a patient with reported abdominal injuries arrives in the emergency department, the order of nursing priorities is to

    I. follow the ABCs and maintain the airway.

    II. listen for bowel sounds referred to the thorax.

    III. observe the abdomen for distention, bruising and tenderness.

    IV. observe for signs of hemorrhagic shock, take vital signs, and start two IV lines with large-bore needles.

    a. I, IV, III

    b. I, II, III

    c. I, II, IV

    d. I, III, IV

# CHAPTER 11

# GENITOURINARY TRAUMA

## CHAPTER OBJECTIVE

Upon completion of this chapter, the reader will be able to recognize the various types of genitourinary trauma and appropriate treatment strategies.

## LEARNING OBJECTIVES

Upon completion of this chapter, the reader should be able to:

1. Describe genitourinary organs, structures and their functions.

2. Identify the predominant kinds of injuries seen in genitourinary trauma.

3. Identify signs and symptoms of genitourinary injuries.

4. Describe complications that accompany genitourinary injuries.

5. Describe principles of care and basic nursing strategies for genitourinary trauma.

6. Indicate examples of nursing diagnoses for patients with genitourinary trauma.

## INTRODUCTION

Genitourinary trauma comprises only a small percent of the trauma cases. The anatomical location of the structures and organs make life-threatening injuries infrequent.

Genitourinary trauma occurs most often to the kidneys or bladder. Because the bladder is hollow, it is more likely to be seriously damaged when full and distended than when empty and collapsible.

As with the intra-abdominal injuries in the peritoneal cavity, organs and structures injured in the retroperitoneal space are difficult to immediately assess for damage. Injuries are usually not isolated to a particular organ but in association with multiple injuries. At least half of the patients with renal injuries also have skeletal injuries or multiple trauma. For instance, it takes such force to damage a kidney, that this injury is usually in association with a fractured rib or other intra-abdominal injuries. A patient with multiple injuries involving the lower abdomen or pelvis should always be considered to have a good probability for renal damage. Blunt injury is the most common mechanism in urologic trauma.

Both internal and external genitalia may be injured. Obviously, external genitalia, particularly of the male, is more vulnerable to injury. As with urologic injuries, genital injuries are rarely life threatening, but they are extremely painful and, naturally, cause great anxiety for the patient.

# ANATOMY AND PHYSIOLOGY

## Urinary System

The urinary system controls the elimination of specific toxic waste products filtered from the blood, along with managing the body's electrolyte and water balance. Additional functions include renin production, activation of vitamin D, insulin degradation, and stimulation of red blood cell production through the production of erythropoietin.

The kidneys are solid organs and the bladder, ureters and urethra are hollow organs. All the organs are contained in the retroperitoneal space. *Figure 11-1* depicts the anatomy of the urinary system.

### Kidneys

The kidneys lie in a fatty tissue layer on the left and right side of the posterior wall of the abdomen, just above the waist at the costovertebral angle (CVA). They are enclosed in a strong fibrous capsule. The right kidney lies below and behind the liver and posterior to the ascending colon and duodenum. It is slightly lower than the left kidney. The left kidney lies posterior to the descending colon and adjacent to the spleen and pancreas. The kidneys are well protected by the vertebrae and muscles of the back and abdominal viscera in the front. Each kidney drains into a ureter connected to the bladder.

Kidneys are very vascular; nearly 20% of the cardiac output passes through them every minute. The renal arteries branch off the aorta to bring the blood supply to the kidneys. Renal veins join the inferior vena cava as the blood returns to the heart.

Waste products and water are continuously filtered from the blood to form urine. Filtered urine is

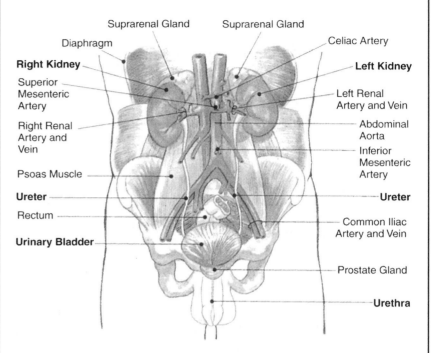

**FIGURE 11-1**
**The Urinary System**

*Reprinted with permission from* O'Keefe, M. F., Limmer, D., Grant, H. D., Murray, R. H. & Bergeron, J. D. (1998.). *Brady emergency care* (8th ed.). Upper Saddle River, NJ: Brady/Prentice-Hall.

concentrated by the reabsorption of water through specialized tubules that form a collecting area, the renal pelvis. The normal adult produces from 1.5 to 2 liters of urine a day. The renal pelvis connects the kidney with the ureter.

Kidneys are vital organs. They are essential to life, along with the heart and brain. When the body is in an extreme medical or traumatic state, the vascular system diverts blood to the vital organs to maintain perfusion and life.

A child's kidney is more likely to be injured because is it relatively larger than the adult's, has less protection from the thoracic cavity, has less fat surrounding the kidney and the muscles protecting the kidneys in the back are not as well developed.

### Ureter(s)

Small flexible muscular tubes, the ureters drain the urine from each kidney into the bladder. There are no valves or sphincters in the ureters, so it is possible for urine to reflux into the ureters from a distended bladder. Peristalsis is the action that moves the urine into the bladder. Blood is supplied to the ureters from the renal artery, aorta and iliac artery.

The ureters are so well protected, lying deep in the retroperitoneal space, that they are rarely injured from blunt trauma.

### Urinary Bladder

The urinary bladder is supported by ligaments and protected behind the symphysis pubis in the pelvic cavity. Ureters enter at the base posteriorly at each side of the bladder. Urine capacity ordinarily is about 500 ml and emptying occurs through the urethra.

The bladder has an abundant blood supply, primarily from branches of the internal iliac artery.

Until the age of 6, the bladder is in the peritoneal space, lying just beneath the anterior abdominal wall. This position makes it more susceptible to injury than in the adult. In the adult, the bladder is covered with a patch of peritoneum and is located in the retroperitoneal space.

The bladder collects, stores, and releases urine. It is formed from smooth muscle and has a specialized membrane lining. Although urination is essentially an automatic process, the muscular sphincters are voluntarily controlled.

### Urethra

In the male, the urethra is about 20-cm long and passes through the penis on the exterior of the body. It expels urine and reproductive fluids. In the female, the urethra is short, about 3.8 cm. Protected internally by the symphysis pubis, the woman's urethra opens in front of the vagina.

## Genital/Reproductive System

The male genitalia, with the exception of the prostate gland and seminal vesicles, lie outside the pelvic cavity. Female genitalia, including ovaries, fallopian tubes and uterus, are entirely within the pelvis. The only exterior female structures are the vulva, clitoris and labia. Both male and female genital systems contribute to reproduction.

### Male Reproductive System

The male reproductive system comprises the testicles, vas deferens, seminal vesicles, prostate gland, urethra, and penis. *Figure 11-2* depicts the male reproductive system.

**Testicles** are made up of cells and ducts that produce male hormones and sperm. The hormones are absorbed directly into the bloodstream. The **vas deferens** is the excretory duct of the testis; a tube for the transport of sperm from each testis up through an opening in the abdominal wall and down into the prostate gland to connect with the urethra. Two saclike **seminal vesicles** lie inferior to the bladder, adjacent to the prostate gland, and empty into the urethra. They store sperm and seminal fluid.

The **prostate gland** is small and partly muscular and partly glandular. It encircles the urethra at the point it leaves the urinary bladder. Ducts open into the prostatic portion of the urethra. Fluid made by the prostate becomes part of the seminal fluid. A neurologic mechanism allows either urine or seminal/prostate fluid to pass through the urethra, but not both at the same time.

**Penile** tissue is erectile and becomes engorged with blood in order to become firm and enter the vagina. The urethra passes through the penis as it leaves the abdominal cavity.

### Female Reproductive System

Female reproductive organs are the ovaries, fallopian tubes, uterus, and vagina. They are contained in the retroperitoneal space. *Figure 11-3* depicts the female reproductive system.

**Ovaries** produce sex hormones and reproductive cells corresponding to the testicles. As in the male, the hormones are absorbed directly into the blood. The reproductive cell, or ovum, is periodi-

## FIGURE 11-2
## Description and Care of Injuries of the Reproductive System in Males

**MALE REPRODUCTIVE SYSTEM**

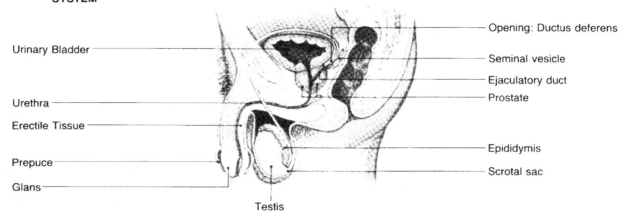

| STRUCTURE | INJURY | CARE |
|---|---|---|
| Scrotum (SKRO-tum) surrounds and protects the testes | Blunt trauma | Padded ice pack, transport. |
| | Lacerations and avulsions (rare) | Direct pressure, dressing, and triangular bandage applied like diaper. Keep avulsed parts moist, wrapped, and cool. |
| Testes (TES-tez) produce sperm cells and male hormone | Blunt trauma<br>Lacerations and avulsions (rare) | Same as scrotum<br>Same as scrotum |
| Spermatic (sper-MAT-ic) cords: suspend testes, contain blood vessels, nerves and vas deferens (vas DEF-er-en's) which transport sperm | Blunt trauma<br>Lacerations (rare) | Same as scrotum<br>Same as scrotum |
| Prostate (PROS-tat) gland: produces seminal fluids | Rare, usually gunshot wounds | Pressure dressing, treat for shock, oxygen, apply PASG when appropriate |
| Seminal vesicles: store seminal fluids | Rare, usually gunshot wounds | Same as prostate |
| Penis<br>Erectile organ containing the urethra | Blunt trauma<br>Lacerations and avulsions (also called amputation), self-mutilation | Same as scrotum<br>Same as scrotum |
| | Blunt trauma of the erect penis (known as "fracture") | Padded ice pack and transport |

## FIGURE 11-3
## Description and Care of Injuries of the Reproductive System in Females

**FEMALE REPRODUCTIVE SYSTEM**

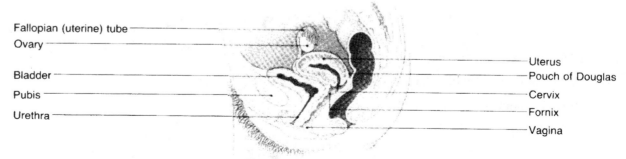

| STRUCTURE | INJURY | CARE |
|---|---|---|
| Vulva (VUL-vah); external genitalia | Blunt trauma | Padded ice pack, transport. |
| | Lacerations and avulsions | Sanitary napkin and triangular bandage applied like diaper. Keep avulsed parts moist, wrapped, and cool. |
| Vagina (birth canal) | Lacerations (seen in rape, self-mutilation cases, abortion attempts) | External application of sanitary napkin and triangular bandage. |
| Uterus (U-ter-us) womb for the developing baby (fetus) | Rupture due to extreme blunt trauma or crushing injury | Unable to tell in field that specific organ is injured. Vaginal bleeding is often profuse. Treat as internal injury with internal bleeding; apply sanitary napkin and triangular dressing over vaginal opening. This is a **true emergency.** Apply PASG garment when appropriate. |
| | Lacerations (rare), usually due to gunshot or stab wound, abortion attempts | Treat as penetrating or perforating wound. Vaginal bleeding may or may not be seen. Apply PASG when appropriate. |
| Oviducts (O-vi-dukt's) or fallopian (fah-LO-pe-an) tubes: carry egg (ovum) from the ovary to the uterus | Lacerations (rare), usually due to gunshot wound | Treat as penetrating or perforating wound. Vaginal bleeding is usually not seen. Apply PASG when appropriate. |
| Ovaries (O-vah-re's) produce female hormones and ova (O-vah) or eggs | Lacerations and puncture wounds (rare), usually due to gunshot or stab wounds | Treat as penetrating or perforating wound. Associated vaginal bleeding is not likely. Apply PASG when appropriate. |

*Reprinted with permission from* Grant, H. D., Murray, R. H., Jr. & Bergeron, J. D. (Eds.). (1990). *Brady emergency care* (5th ed.). Englewood Cliffs, NJ: Prentice-Hall.

cally produced during the female's reproductive years. The mature ovum is released and passes from the ovary through the **fallopian tubes** to the uterus.

The **uterus** is a hollow pear-shaped muscular organ. Its purpose is to contain and nourish the embryo and fetus from the time the ovum is fertilized and implanted to the time of birth.

The **vagina** connects the uterus with the vulva (external female genitalia). Vaginal functions are to channel the menstrual flow from the uterus, receive the penis during intercourse, and serve as the birthing canal.

# MECHANISM OF INJURY

Blunt and penetrating trauma are the injury mechanisms. Blunt mechanisms are the most common of all urologic injuries, accounting for 70–80% of the trauma. Examples of blunt mechanisms are motor vehicle deceleration impact, a fall, an object such as a bat or fist striking the flank or external genitalia, blunt force strong enough to fracture the pelvis and cause damage to the bladder and urethra, rape.

Blunt trauma to the back or flank related to kidney damage is most often a simple self-healing renal contusion. In cases of severe lower abdominal injury or pelvic fracture, urologic damage should always be considered. If the trauma is severe, the kidney will fracture.

Most penetrating genitourinary trauma is caused by projectiles. Impalement, laceration and puncture wounds result from knives in stab wounds, missiles such as bullets from gunshot wounds and objects of impalement. The ureters are damaged more often from penetrating trauma than blunt trauma. Genitalia may be injured in industrial accidents from machinery or burns.

All patients with penetrating injuries to the abdomen, chest or flank should be observed for evidence of urogenital injury.

# GENITOURINARY INJURIES AND INTERVENTIONS

## Urinary Injury

### Kidneys

Blunt injuries account for 70–80% of the renal trauma, but renal injuries are infrequent, and severe renal injuries are even less frequent.

There are three means of blunt injury to the kidney: a direct blow to the flank, laceration from a blunt injury fracturing a rib or vertebrae and sudden deceleration causing shearing that results in renal damage. To seriously damage a kidney, a blow must be powerful, most likely powerful enough to cause other intra-abdominal injuries. Even though rare, a fractured or severely lacerated kidney or renal pelvis can hemorrhage enough to be life threatening.

Penetrating injuries are most often caused by gunshot or stab wounds. The nature of damage from a gunshot is more complex than a stab wound. Other penetrating wounds may be fragments from blasts, impalement, and shards of material. These injuries require surgical repair.

History of a direct blow; evidence of abrasion; laceration; ecchymosis; or a penetrating wound in the lower rib cage, flank or upper abdomen should immediately suggest kidney damage. Other external signs of possible renal injury are bruising of the body wall, flank mass and flank tenderness. Fractures of the lower rib cage, lower thoracic or upper lumbar vertebrae are likely to have an associated kidney injury. With significant blood loss, there may be signs of shock. Hematuria is an indicator of injury, but the amount of blood in the urine does not always correspond with the severity of damage. Further, there may be injury without hematuria in a small number of cases.

Renal injuries are classified by the Organ Injury Scaling Committee of the American Association for the Surgery of Trauma. Classifications range from Grade I, minor, to Grade V, the most severe. A more practical system of staging divides renal injuries into contusions, minor lacerations confined to the renal cortex, major lacerations that involve the collecting system and vascular injuries (Newberry, 1998).

Because kidney injuries are so difficult to identify and confirm by external observation of the patient, additional diagnostic tools are used.

**Ultrasound** is good for patients who do not appear to have a severe injury or to confirm the absence of injury. Ultrasound cannot differentiate between a hematoma, laceration or urine.

**Radiographic evaluation** of the kidneys, ureters and bladder (KUB) is used to identify the path and appearance of the projectile in penetrating trauma.

**Intravenous pyelogram (IVP)** is used for patients with penetrating injuries, who are unstable and need immediate surgery. It can give information about the condition and function of the kidney, ureter and bladder. Blockage can be detected. The IVP is limited in identifying intra-abdominal injuries and staging renal injuries and should not be used as the initial study in blunt trauma patients who are stable.

**Computerized tomography (CT scan)** is the most accurate diagnostic tool for staging renal injuries because it can identify renal pedicle injuries, identify the size and degree of a retroperitoneal hematoma and identify related intra-abdominal injuries.

**Magnetic resonance imaging (MRI)** is a companion diagnostic tool to the CT scan for the patient with a severe renal injury, preexisting

abnormality, indefinite CT findings, or a repeat radiographic follow-up.

**Angiography** is invasive, sensitive and used for ruling out vascular injuries. It is used only on high-risk patients who have an inconclusive CT scan. The test cannot evaluate other abdominal injuries.

**Radionucleotide** renal scans are particularly good at identifying large arterial injuries but minor arterial injuries and lacerations may be missed.

Blunt or penetrating injuries may not require surgical intervention. Criteria used for surgical intervention is not universally agreed upon. Unstable patients having pedicle or ureteral injuries, expanding retroperitoneal hematoma, falling hemoglobin levels, extensive extravasation and other serious problems may require immediate surgery. Bed rest, serial urinalysis and close follow-up monitoring may be the treatment of choice in hemodynamically stable patients with severe renal injury.

Renal complications occurring soon after a traumatic incident include delayed onset of bleeding, renal insufficiency, urinary extravasation, urinoma (cyst containing urine), abscess formation, and fistula formation. Late complications are arteriovenous fistulas, hydronephrosis, stone formation, chronic pyelonephritis and pain. Renal artery or compression injuries may result in hypertension within a half an hour after the injury or be delayed up to 10 years.

Long-term monitoring after a renal injury should be done to see if hypertension, perinephric cysts, arteriovenous fistulas and stones develop.

### Bladder

Major trauma to the urinary bladder is uncommon, but when it occurs, it is usually not an isolated injury. The mechanism of injury varies, as well as the patient population, amount of bladder contents at the time of injury, and type and location

**FIGURE 11-4**
**Bladder Rupture Caused by Blunt Trauma**

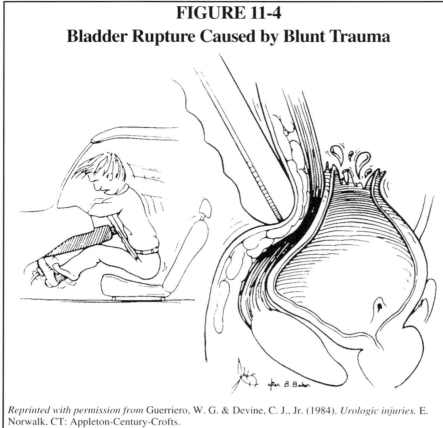

*Reprinted with permission from* Guerriero, W. G. & Devine, C. J., Jr. (1984). *Urologic injuries.* E. Norwalk, CT: Appleton-Century-Crofts.

trauma to the lower abdomen, pelvis or perineum, blood at the urethral meatus, or associated leg fractures are indicators of likely urinary bladder trauma.

Most patients with bladder perforation are unable to urinate and have suprapubic pain. Gross hematuria and pelvic fractures are present in 90% of all bladder ruptures. Whether the urine appears bloody or not, it should be sent for analysis. If there is a large amount of blood loss into the pelvis, the patient will become hemodynamically unstable. Late signs of injury are abdominal distention, an acute abdomen, and increased blood urea nitrogen (BUN) and creatinine levels.

Diagnostic evaluation includes retrograde urethrogram and cystogram studies in all male patients having a pelvic fracture, gross hematuria, inability to urinate, blood at the urethral meatus, perineal swelling or a prostate that cannot be palpated. A cystogram is the most accurate method of diagnosis. Plain films are done before the cystography. CT scans can detect a bladder rupture but are not as good a diagnostic tool as cystography.

Intraperitoneal ruptures do not heal spontaneously. Most extraperitoneal ruptures are the result of bony injuries or other intra-abdominal trauma. Both injuries usually require surgical exploration and repair. In situations with minimal bleeding and no infection, conservative treatment of maintaining adequate drainage with a catheter, antibiotics and close observation is most likely the treatment used.

of injury in the bladder. The mortality rate is low and is usually caused by severe associated injuries.

Bladder injuries are classified as contusions, extraperitoneal ruptures and intraperitoneal ruptures. Most of the injuries are nonpenetrating.

Blunt or penetrating trauma to the urinary bladder usually causes a rupture with the urine leaking into the surrounding area. Urine that is able to pass through the urethra most likely will be bloody. Lower abdominal or pelvis blunt injuries frequently result in an explosive rupture of the bladder, especially if it is full. An empty bladder lies low in the pelvis and can collapse and be more flexible with blunt force than a full, distended bladder.

Sharp, bony fragments from a fractured pelvis can tear into the bladder. Mid or lower abdominal and perineal penetration may have associated bladder involvement. In the male, sudden deceleration can shear the bladder from the urethra. A history of

## FIGURE 11-5
## Mechanisms of Extraperitoneal Bladder Rupture

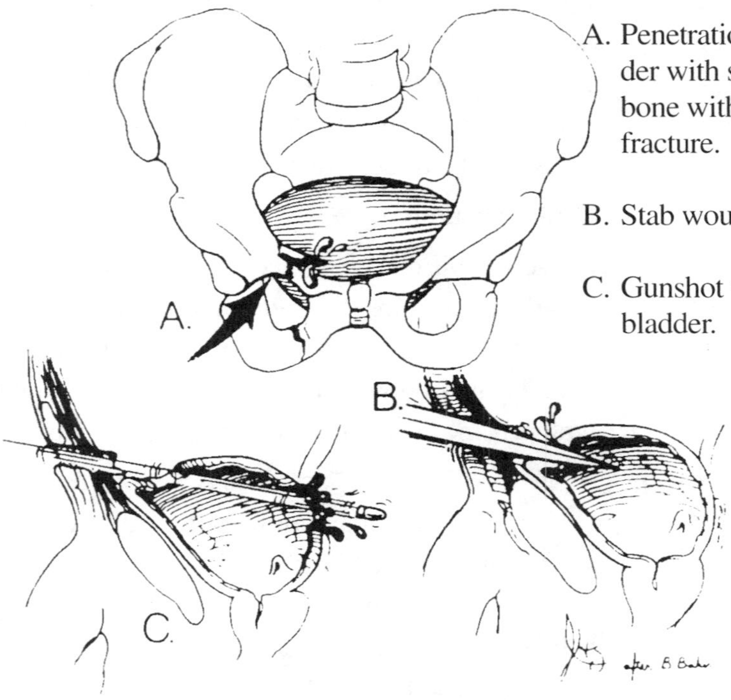

A. Penetration of bladder with spicule of bone with pelvic fracture.

B. Stab wound.

C. Gunshot wound to bladder.

*Reprinted with permission from* Guerriero, W. G. & Devine, C. J., Jr. (1984). *Urologic injuries.* E. Norwalk, CT: Appleton-Century-Crofts.

Consequences of bladder injuries can be urinary ascites, abscesses, and the formation of urinary fistulas.

### Ureters

Injuries to the ureters are unusual and almost always from penetrating trauma of the abdominal cavity. Injury may cause partial or complete ureteral transection. Penetrating lower abdominal injuries require careful examination for indications of ureteral damage.

Blunt injuries with major hyperextension of the upper lumbar and lower thoracic areas can avulse the ureteropelvic junction. Ureteral avulsions at the ureteropelvic junction can occur after falls from heights.

Signs of ureteral injury may not be evident on initial examination. Findings are usually related to other intra-abdominal injury. The only sign specific for ureteral injury is when obstruction causes classic pain radiating to the groin. Microscopic hematuria is present in most instances.

Diagnosis is made with IVP and retrograde uteropyelography. Surgery for other abdominal injuries will confirm any ureteral injury. Surgical repair includes pyeloplasty with ureteral stenting and a nephrostomy tube. If untreated, injury can lead to urinoma, abscess or stricture.

### Urethra

Any patient with a pelvic or perineal injury should be assessed for urethral damage. These injuries are rare in females. When damage does occur, obstetric injury, pelvic fracture and anterior vaginal lacerations are the mechanisms of injury.

A small percent of males have urethral injuries, and because of the anatomical position of the urethra, males are more likely than females to have this type of damage. Proximal urethral injuries occur almost solely in men. A few males have the posterior urethra damaged when they suffer a pelvic fracture. Injuries are more frequently caused from shearing than direct laceration.

Signs of urethral injury in the male range from blood at the meatus, inability to urinate and a distended bladder to being able to void and absence of bleeding, depending upon the extent of the urethral tear. There can also be pain when urinating, perineal/scrotal/penile swelling, hematuria, and displacement of the prostate. A classic sign of posterior urethral injury is the inability to palpate the prostate. All patients should have a digital rectal exam to exclude associated rectal damage.

A retrograde urethrogram is used as a diagnostic procedure. If injury is suspected, urinary catheterization should not be attempted, as it can change a partial urethral disruption to a complete one and may cause contamination, infection and increased hemorrhage. If the prostate is palpable on digital exam and there is no blood at the meatus, it is probably safe to insert a catheter. If any resistance is felt while attempting to pass a urinary catheter, the procedure should immediately be stopped.

Minimal disruption of the urethra may only require placement of a soft Foley catheter. Complete urethral disruption requires prompt suprapubic cystostomy drainage.

The most severe complications of posterior urethral disruption are impotence, stricture and incontinence. Complications of injuries to the anterior urethra are strictures and occasionally, impotence and incontinence.

## Genital Injury

Trauma may occur to the internal and external reproductive organs. External organs are called external genitalia and they are more susceptible to injury than internal reproductive organs.

### Male Genitalia

Injuries to the male genitalia are uncommon, are soft tissue injuries, and are mostly from blunt trauma. Rarely are these injuries life threatening, but they are extremely painful and cause a great deal of anxiety.

### Testicular Trauma

The scrotal skin protects the testicles. It may be lacerated with or without damage to the internal structures. Avulsion injuries can cause all or part of the scrotal skin to be lost. Total skin loss leaves the testicles unprotected. Skin grafting should be immediate, and if there is a delay, the testicles should be placed in thigh pouches. Penetrating injuries to the testicle should be explored and repaired.

Large scrotal hematomas make examination difficult, so sonography should be used. Blunt injury may rupture the testicle or cause an accumulation of blood. Pain is acute and the patient will experience syncope, nausea, vomiting, and urinary retention. Rupture of a testicle should be repaired immediately. Reconstruction is possible.

### Penile Trauma

**Avulsion** of the penile skin, especially if the patient is not circumcised, occurs most often in industrial accidents. Every effort should be made to save the avulsed skin. The denuded penis should be wrapped in a soft sterile dressing that is wet with saline.

Partial or complete **amputation** of the penile shaft causes severe blood loss. The bleeding is controlled by direct pressure with a sterile dressing. When a complete amputation occurs, every effort must be made to find the amputated part. As with any amputated part, it should be wrapped in a sterile, wet dressing. It can be reattached and reconstructed with microsurgery. If the amputation is an act of self-mutilation, the patient should be observed carefully and treated for both the medical and psychological problems.

Acute **angulation, or "fracture"** of the penis, occurs while it is erect. During sexual activity the patient will hear a snap or cracking sound, followed by intense pain and collapse of the erection. Rupture of the supporting erectile tissues causes a hematoma and swelling in the shaft. The urethra can also be lacerated. A hematoma and edema can cause external compression of the urethra and subsequent urinary retention. Management is debated as to the best approach. Early surgical repair usually has a lower risk of persistent penile angulation, more rapid return to functioning and a shorter period of recovery. If the hematoma is minimal, sedation, elevation of the penis and ice packs are the conservative treatments.

**Laceration** of the skin at the penile head is usually caused by an accident that occurs when the penis is erect. Severe bleeding occurs. Direct pressure with a sterile dressing will control the bleeding. The **foreskin** is sometimes caught in the zipper of trousers, especially by children. Cut the zipper away from the rest of the fabric to release tension on the skin.

## Female Genitalia

### Internal Genitalia

The ovaries, fallopian tubes and uterus are internal female genitalia that can be injured the same as any other internal organ. However, they are small, protected by the pelvis, and not likely to be injured. Because these organs are not adjacent to the pelvis as the bladder is, they are not usually injured when the pelvis is fractured.

### External Genitalia

The major and minor labia, vulva and clitoris are the external female genitalia. The urethra opens at the anterior vagina. The external genitalia do not contain structures such as the testicles.

Injuries to external genitalia consist of soft tissue damage: contusions, abrasions, lacerations, and avulsions. Rich innervation to the external genitalia is the reason for extreme pain when these areas are injured. Treatment is direct pressure and iced compresses. A diaper-type dressing will hold compresses in place. Dressings and packs should never be inserted into the vagina.

### Straddle Injury

Straddle injuries occur when a patient falls, and has trauma directly to the perineum. Mostly occurring in children, the mechanisms of injury usually are falls from bicycles, fences and motorcycles.

In females, a vulvovaginal laceration with extensive ecchymosis of the perineum may be seen. Vulvar hematomas may extend into the retroperitoneal space. Urethral damage and rectal tears can also occur.

Treatment includes repair of the laceration and evacuation and drainage of the hematomas. Complications are infection and sexual dysfunction.

### Foreign Bodies

A myriad of foreign bodies have been documented to be found in the vagina, urethra and bladder. Anything small and firm can be passed into the vagina and urethra. Children insert foreign bodies because of orifice curiosity. Adults insert foreign bodies into children as a perversion. Adults use the foreign bodies as erotic stimulation, sometimes under the influence of drugs, or because of psychiatric disorders.

Patients are often embarrassed to seek help for removal of a foreign object and only do so when a complication or symptom evolves. Dysuria, suprapubic or urethral pain, urethral discharge, difficulty urinating, swelling and abscess formation are the usual complications.

A history of chronic urinary tract infections is a tip-off to investigate for foreign bodies. Radiographs are useful in locating radiopaque objects. Xeroradiography detects nonmetallic foreign objects traumatically or deliberately placed into the body. If the object is below the urogenital diaphragm, it can be palpated and removed endoscopically. If the object is above the urogenital diaphragm, greater endoscopic manipulation, perineal urethrostomy or suprapubic cystotomy will be necessary.

### Sexual Assault and Rape

Sexual assault and rape occur frequently, to males and females, to all ages and in any demographic area. It is a very sensitive issue psychologically, medically and legally, especially with children.

Examination requires a chaperone to be present. The victim should not be washed, urinate or defecate until the physician has completed the entire examination. Sometimes, the patient does not want to be questioned or examined, particularly if well-known in the community. An adult has the right to make the choice of refusing an examination. Children's services should be called for pediatric cases. Confidentiality is of great importance to both the patient and the hospital facility.

# ASSESSMENT

Genitourinary trauma seldom occurs as a singular injury and most often is associated with other abdominal injuries. Further, the injuries are almost never life threatening. Consequently, rapid assessment and treatment of genitourinary injuries is difficult and usually secondary to other abdominal injuries.

The first priority, as in every assessment of trauma, is to conduct the ABC protocol, followed by identification of any injuries that threaten life or limb. Once these areas have been managed and maintained, the genitourinary evaluation may be started. The top priority is to aggressively look for and diagnose genitourinary injuries, considering they are not obvious on initial inspection. The absence of external signs of trauma does not eliminate the presence of injury. A fractured kidney or ruptured bladder can cause substantial blood loss into the abdomen.

- History: It is important to get information about how, when and where the incident happened. Certain mechanisms of injury carry a greater incidence of genitourinary trauma, such as being struck by a vehicle, rapid deceleration or penetrating trauma.

- Previous genitourinary injury, illness, surgery, defects, abnormalities and anomalies, should be documented. Are there chronic infections or adhesions? Does the patient have renal failure or insufficiency? Does the patient have renal artery stenosis? Find out if there are other medical problems. All of this information has a great bearing on the initial assessment, treat-

ment and long-term care. Be sure to document allergies and current medications.

- Look for any external injuries or deformities. Look for bruising or lacerations in the flank area. Several patterns of contusion and bruising are specific for genitoruinary trauma. Grey Turner's sign of bruising over the flank and lower back is the result of retroperitoneal hematoma, and often present in pelvic fractures. A swollen and contused scrotum may be from a straddle injury, pelvic fracture or dissecting retroperitoneal hematoma. A late sign of a fracture of the pelvic rami or symphysis pubis is perineal bruising.

- Palpate the abdomen, looking for rigidity and tenderness. If there is urine in the abdominal cavity, gentle palpation of the abdomen will have rebound tenderness. Listen for bowel sounds; their absence may indicate intraperitoneal urine extravasation or renal injuries.

- Pain: Where is the pain and what kind of pain is it? Pain may be very severe, especially if external genitalia are involved. Is the pain directly identifiable, such as in the flank, pelvic or suprapubic area, or is it referred? There may be abdominal pain due to other abdominal injury.

- Shock: Kidney damage may cause severe blood loss and shock.

- Hematuria: The patient may or may not have hematuria. All urine should be sent to the lab for testing. The absence of hematuria does not rule out damage to the kidney.

- Inability to urinate: Is the patient able to void, and when was the last time he urinated?

- Has he been incontinent since the injury?

- Inspect the external genitalia for soft tissue injury or lacerations.

- Check for blood at the urinary meatus. Is the blood dried or fresh? In the male, check for signs of semen at the meatus, which may be due to prostate damage from a pelvic fracture.

## NURSING STRATEGIES FOR THE PATIENT WITH GENITOURINARY TRAUMA

- Follow the ABC protocol and maintain the airway.

- Due to the possibility of accompanying abdominal injuries, serial vital signs should be monitored and recorded frequently, and changes should be promptly reported to the physician. Look for signs of shock.

- Assess and manage injuries that threaten life or limb, which most likely would be abdominal or other injuries rather than genitourinary injuries.

- Management of GU trauma is aimed at maintaining the structure, function and sexual integrity of the patient.

- Protect the patient's privacy by working efficiently, covering the genital area as much as possible during assessment and treatment and having a professional manner.

- Follow through with diagnostic orders for radiographic and laboratory procedures, reporting abnormal results to the physician.

- Send urine for lab analysis, even if hematuria is not apparent. Do not catheterize until the patient has been cleared by the physician for genitourinary damage.

- Do not let rape victims void or defecate until the physician has completed an examination or ordered otherwise.

- Lacerations and abrasions of the genital area should be covered with moist, sterile dressings.

- Apply padded ice packs to external genitalia to reduce swelling. Periodically recheck for temperature and change in status. If there are moist, sterile dressings in place, apply the ice packs over the dressings.

- Keep the patient NPO until it has been determined immediate surgical intervention has been ruled out by the physician.

- Keep the patient warm and warm IV fluids and blood products.

## EXAMPLES OF NURSING DIAGNOSES RELATED TO GENITOURINARY TRAUMA

- Pain, direct and referred, related to genitourinary injury

- Fluid volume deficit related to trauma

- Altered tissue perfusion related to injury

- Altered patterns of urinary elimination related to trauma

- High risk for infection related to trauma or the use of a urinary catheter

- High risk for injury related to the insertion of a urinary catheter

- High risk for sexual dysfunction related to complications from trauma

- High risk for body image alteration related to trauma

- Complex medical, legal, psychological and social issues related to rape

- Anxiety related to alteration of body image

## SUMMARY

The structures and organs of the genitourinary system are located in the abdominal retropertioneum, and well protected by other abdominal structures. As a result, injuries to the genitourinary system are rarely singular and usually associated with skeletal and other intra-abdominal injuries. It is unusual for these injuries to be life threatening, but they are very painful and can have image-altering complications.

Genitourinary injuries are difficult to detect with visual inspection. Any patient with blunt or penetrating trauma to the abdomen, a pelvic fracture or who suffers a severe blow to the back in the costovertebral angle should be evaluated for GU damage. Confirmation is often through radiographic or surgical procedures. The kidneys and bladder are the most frequently injured organs and result from blunt or penetrating trauma.

## CHAPTER 11
### Questions 51–55

51. Which of the following is true about genitourinary trauma?

    I.   GU trauma occurs frequently because of the location of the organs and structures in the abdomen.

    II.  It takes such force to damage a kidney that other structures are usually also injured.

    III. The kidney can be fractured.

    IV.  The urinary bladder is more likely to rupture when it is full.

        a. I, II, III

        b. II, III, IV

        c. I, III, IV

         I, II, IV

52. A mechanism of blunt injury to the kidney is

    a. severe compression to the mid-thoracic area.

    b. laceration from a blunt injury fracturing a rib.

    c. severe anterior abdominal contusion.

    d. stage III contusion to the back.

53. Grey Turner's sign indicates

    a. bruising over the flank and lower back, resulting from a retroperitoneal hematoma.

    b. contused scrotum from a straddle injury.

    c. a fracture of the pelvic rami.

    d. a syndrome of renal anomalies.

54. General principles of care include

    a. sending urine samples to the lab, even if hematuria is not obvious.

    b. conducting GU assessment secondary to abdominal assessment.

    c. GU injuries are not obvious to visual observation and other diagnostic tools are often necessary to confirm injury.

    d. All of the above

55. Complications occurring after a traumatic incident to the kidney are

    a. urinoma, abscess or renal insufficiency.

    b. rupture with urine leaking into the abdominal cavity.

    c. abdominal distention.

    d. inability to urinate.

# CHAPTER 12

# OBSTETRIC AND GYNECOLOGIC TRAUMA

## CHAPTER OBJECTIVE

Upon completion of this chapter, the reader will be able to describe the principles of treating gynecologic and obstetric trauma.

## LEARNING OBJECTIVES

Upon completion of this chapter, the reader should be able to:

1.  Recognize normal changes in anatomy and physiology during pregnancy.

2.  Identify frequent causes of obstetric and gynecologic trauma.

3.  Identify frequent injuries seen in obstetric and gynecologic trauma.

4.  Describe complications that accompany obstetric and gynecologic trauma.

5.  Describe general principles of care and appropriate basic nursing strategies for obstetric and gynecologic trauma.

## INTRODUCTION

Obstetric trauma involves the safety and lives of the mother and child or children she is carrying. Specific data on the incidence of obstetric trauma is vague, but it is estimated to occur in only about 6% to 7% of pregnant women.

Most injuries are not serious. Blunt injuries are secondary to auto crashes, falls and assaults. Falls are the most common cause of injury. Penetrating injuries are predominantly gunshot and stab wounds. Physical abuse during pregnancy is increasing in severity and frequency. Head injury and hemorrhagic shock account for most of the maternal deaths from trauma.

Fetal death is usually the result of maternal death but can also occur after relatively minor injury of the mother.

Gynecologic trauma is often the result of violent sexual assault, although there are other sources of injury. Rarely, males are sexually assaulted. However, since this chapter discusses gynecological trauma, with sexual assault being the primary cause, only female assault will be discussed. Other trauma is caused by falls, straddle injuries and motor vehicle crashes.

## CHANGES IN ANATOMY AND PHYSIOLOGY DURING PREGNANCY

### Terminology

**Amniotic Sac:** A thin, transparent sac, which is the part of the fetal membrane in the uterus that holds the fetus and the fluid in which the fetus is suspended. At the end of the third month of pregnancy, the amnion fuses with the chorion to form the amniochorionic sac. Another term is the "bag of waters."

**Amniotic Fluid:** The fluid, also known as the liquor amnii, is in the amniotic sac that surrounds the fetus. Transparent, the liquid protects the fetus from injury, maintains an even temperature and prevents the formation of adhesions between the amnion and the skin of the fetus.

**Embryo:** The stage in prenatal development between being an ovum and a fetus, from the 2nd to the 8th weeks of gestation.

**Fetus:** The developing child in utero from the 3rd month to birth.

**Gestation:** The period of time from conception to birth. The length of pregnancy is normally 38–40 weeks. Fetuses have survived as early as 24–26 weeks of gestation.

**Gravid:** Pregnant

**Ovum:** The female germ cell capable of developing into a new organism after being fertilized. The egg.

**Placenta:** A spongy structure in the uterus through which the fetus is nourished. The amnion encloses the embryo and is attached to the margin of the placenta. The umbilical cord is attached at the center of the concave side. Two arteries and one vein comprise the umbilical vessels that pass through the cord. At birth, the cord can be 50 cm in length. After the birth, the placenta is expelled and is called the afterbirth. Maternal blood enters the placenta through branches of the uterine arteries. Nourishment, oxygen and antibodies from the mother pass into the fetal blood; metabolic waste products pass from fetal blood into the mother's blood. There is no direct mixture of the fetal and maternal blood. The placenta also functions as an endocrine organ, producing gonadotropins (which, if present in urine, is one way to determine pregnancy), estrogen and progesterone.

**Parturient:** The woman in childbirth

**Umbilical Cord:** The cord connects the fetus with the placenta and contains two arteries and one vein and is surrounded by a jelly-like substance, Wharton's jelly. After the child is born and after the umbilical vessels have stopped pulsating, the umbilical cord is severed. When the stump of the cord dries and falls off, it leaves a depression in the abdomen called the navel or umbilicus.

## Structures, Organs and Systems

### Uterus

The uterus is shaped like a pear and expands as the fetus grows. During the **first trimester,** the uterus is small, self-contained and protected within the pelvis. As the uterus grows, the walls become thinner as it expands outward and upward, pushing on the peritoneal cavity and confining the intestines to the upper abdomen.

In the **second trimester,** the uterus becomes more susceptible to abdominal injury. The fetus still remains small and well cushioned by the amniotic fluid.

The uterus is large and thin walled by the **third trimester.** In the last 2 weeks of gestation, the fetus descends and the head becomes "engaged," or fixed in the pelvis, preparing for birth.

Blood flow in the uterus increases from 60 ml/min to 600 ml/min during the third trimester. Total maternal blood volume circulates through the uterus approximately every 8 to 11 minutes. Uterine blood flow is not automatically regulated, *and depends completely on the perfusion pressure of the mother.* By the third trimester, the uterus and placenta have reached the maximum ability for vasodilation and cannot increase blood flow any further in response to decreased perfusion. Uterine trauma may be a cause of major blood loss.

If there is maternal stress or injury, the sympathetic nervous system releases catecholamines that

# FIGURE 12-1
## The Structure of Pregnancy

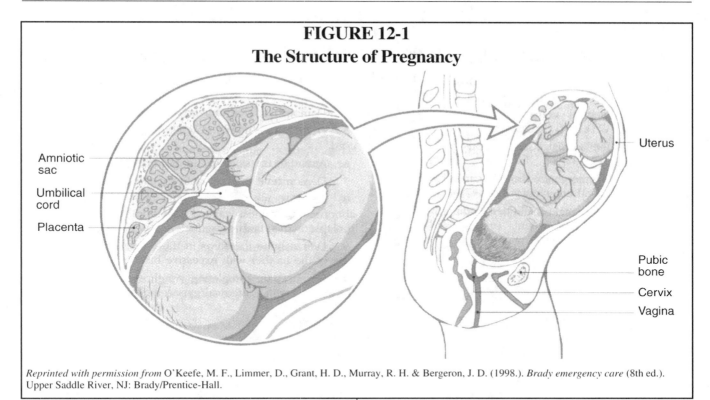

Amniotic sac

Umbilical cord

Placenta

Uterus

Pubic bone

Cervix

Vagina

*Reprinted with permission from* O'Keefe, M. F., Limmer, D., Grant, H. D., Murray, R. H. & Bergeron, J. D. (1998.). *Brady emergency care* (8th ed.). Upper Saddle River, NJ: Brady/Prentice-Hall.

cause uteroplacental constriction and decreased perfusion. Fetal distress is the consequence.

### Cardiovascular

The physiology of the heart changes considerably during pregnancy. The needs of the fetus and mother are very demanding. Maternal blood flow increases 40% to 50% by the 28th week. Further, during vaginal delivery, blood loss is about 500 ml, and 1 litre during a cesarean delivery.

In the first trimester, systolic and diastolic pressures decrease and then level off in the second trimester. By the last trimester, prepregnancy pressures are reached again. The resting heart rate increases until the second trimester and stays elevated 10 to 20 beats. Complications of pregnancy, such as preeclampsia, will cause a rise in the blood pressure, which may become critical.

The uterus pushes up the diaphragm so that it elevates the heart and rotates it forward. The shift in position can cause cardiac electrical changes, which are expected in pregnancy.

After 20 weeks' gestation, when the mother is lying down, the fetus may compress the aorta and vena cava, decreasing cardiac output. The occurrence is called **inferior vena cava syndrome** or **supine hypotensive syndrome.** By 20 weeks, the uterus has grown to the level of the inferior vena cava. Compression of the vena cava may decrease the cardiac output by as much as 28% and the systolic blood pressure by 30 mm Hg. Because blood flow in the uterus is controlled by the maternal perfusion pressure, the changes can decrease perfusion in the uterus. At a time when uterine vasodilation is expanded to the maximum point, the vessels are unable to respond any further to the demand for increased blood flow. If the mother lies in the left lateral decubitus position, the aortocaval compression is relieved.

Hemodynamic measures change during pregnancy. Usual indicators of shock, hypotension and tachycardia are often just normal changes. On the other hand, "normal" findings may be masking underlying shock. For instance, gestational hypovolemia allows the mother to tolerate greater

**FIGURE 12-2**

**Effects of the Pregnant Uterus on the Inferior Vena Cava (I.V.C.) and the Aorta in the Supine (A) and Lateral (B) Positions**

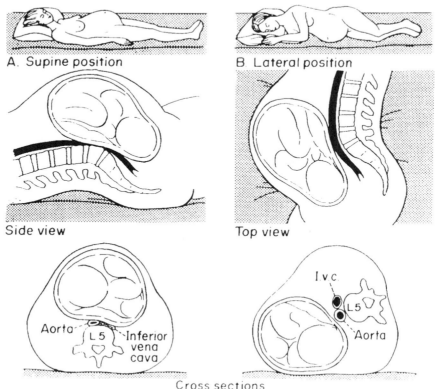

*Reprinted with permission from* Bonica, J. J. (Ed.). (1980). *Obstetric analgesia and anesthesia* (2nd ed. rev.). Amsterdam: World Federation of Societies of Anesthesiologists.

blood loss, acute or gradual, without a change in vital signs. Pregnant women in shock do not always have the physical indicators of cool, clammy skin, due to vasodilation in the first two trimesters. Vasoconstriction response to stress is seen in the third trimester.

The central venous pressure (CVP) may remain normal. Serial readings should be made to get a good picture of response to fluid resuscitation. Fluid delivery to restore maternal and uteroplacental perfusion should be adequate and appropriate. Lactated Ringers is recommended.

Blood transfusions should be with Rh-compatible blood. In cases of impending shock, *only* O negative or type-specific blood is acceptable (Newberry, 1998).

*Pulmonary*

Significant changes in the pulmonary system occur during pregnancy.

As the uterus enlarges, it pushes the diaphragm up as far as 4 cm. There is also a flaring of the ribs. If chest tubes are inserted in the third trimester, it should be in the third or fourth intercostal space to avoid damaging the diaphragm.

Elevation of the diaphragm reduces the mother's pulmonary functional reserve capacity. The capacity is also reduced because of increased maternal oxygen consumption. The diminished functional oxygen reserve in the mother makes the uterus susceptible to hypoxia, which affects fetal oxygenation. When fetal respiratory compromise occurs, the first sign is often a change in the fetal heart rate. In the case of maternal trauma, blood gas levels should be monitored to determine if hypoxia and acidosis have occurred. Supplemental oxygen at 100% is required.

Pregnancy causes the capillaries of the mucosal lining of the respiratory tract to become engorged and swollen, which may cause nosebleeds and airway obstruction. Therefore, placement of a nasal airway should be cautious.

### Neurologic

The nervous system does not normally have physiological changes during gestation. Changes in the central nervous system (CNS) during pregnancy only indicate abnormal circumstances.

Pregnancy-induced hypertension (PIH), also known as toxemia, includes preeclampsia and eclampsia. It is a syndrome occurring between the 20th week and the end of the first week postpartum, and usually is seen in primigravida women younger than 20 years or over 35 years. Indications of preeclampsia are hypertension, headaches, proteinuria, decreased urinary output, and edema of the lower extremities. If left untreated, CNS irritability can lead to eclampsia, which magnifies and worsens preeclamptic symptoms and leads to seizure activity. Seizures can cause hypoxia, placing the mother and fetus at risk. Coma may also occur, and pulmonary edema may develop. The condition is an immediate threat to mother and fetus and a leading cause of maternal morbidity and mortality.

Head injury can cause altered mental status, seizures and hypertension. Careful neurologic assessment is essential in the pregnant trauma patient.

### Endocrine

The pituitary gland will double in size and weight and need an increased blood supply by the end of the pregnancy. Low perfusion will bring about ischemia and may lead to pituitary necrosis.

Sheehan's syndrome is necrosis of the anterior pituitary and has long-term complications related to decreased hormone levels.

Shock from hypoperfusion should have rapid and aggressive treatment to prevent ischemia and necrosis. Reperfusion can bring about intrapituitary hemorrhage; carefully monitor the patient.

### Gastrointestinal

Several anatomic and physiologic changes occur during gestation. The small bowel is pushed into the upper abdomen by the uterus. The large bowel moves posteriorly. Bowel sounds may be diminished as a normal condition or may be a sign of intraperitoneal injury. Progesterone affects the gastrointestinal tract by reducing motility and tone while relaxing the gastric sphincter. Gastroesophageal reflux is a frequent occurrence because of delayed gastric emptying and increases the possibility of aspiration.

It should be assumed that all pregnant trauma patients have a full stomach and require a nasogastric (NG) tube to minimize the risk of aspiration. Remember that the mucosal lining of the respiratory tract is engorged and susceptible to nosebleeds. Extra care should be taken while the NG tube is being inserted.

As the abdominal wall stretches, it becomes less sensitive to peritoneal irritation, making muscle guarding, rigidity or rebound tenderness dulled or absent.

### Genitourinary

By the end of the first trimester, the bladder moves from a pelvic position to an intra-abdominal position, making it more vulnerable to injury.

The uterus compresses the bladder by the third trimester, causing urinary frequency. Urinary stasis may occur from dilation of the ureters, due to compression by the ovarian plexus.

The filtration rate of the kidneys increases by about 30%.

### *Musculoskeletal*

As the pelvis prepares for pregnancy, it becomes more flexible. Hormonal changes loosen the ligaments of the symphysis pubis and sacroiliac joints. By the seventh month, the pelvis has widened. The "waddle" and unsteady gait characteristic of the late term mother is caused by pelvic widening and a heavy abdomen. In this condition, the mother is more likely to fall.

### *Hematology*

The increase in plasma volume is much greater than the increase in erythrocyte volume, which causes dilutional anemia. Hematocrit and hemoglobin levels drop because of the red blood cell dilution in the plasma volume. These changes are referred to as physiological anemia of pregnancy.

Platelet levels may stay the same or decrease slightly. By term the white count and sedimentation rate have elevated. Fibrinogen levels rise, causing an increased tendency to clot and a risk of deep vein thrombosis or pulmonary embolism. Inactivity aggravates the risk.

# MECHANISM OF INJURY

Obviously, trauma can affect both the mother and child. Risks vary according to the stage of gestation and the changing vulnerability of the uterus.

In the first trimester, the fetus has little chance of direct injury because the uterus is still small and protected by the pelvis. However, if the mother is injured, the fetus may suffer consequences from her injuries, such as hypoxia and decreased perfusion. By the last trimester, the uterus and fetus are more likely to be injured from direct trauma because of the expanded anatomical position.

The most common causes of abdominal trauma are motor vehicle crashes, falls and assaults. Other sources of injury are penetration, domestic violence, burns and smoke inhalation.

As in any case of blunt trauma, the severity of injury ranges from minor to life threatening to the mother and fetus. Blunt abdominal trauma from rapid forward deceleration such as car crashes, directs the energy through the abdomen, compressing the organs and structures against the spine. In the third trimester, when the uterus is high in the abdomen, the transferred energy can be a deadly force. The uterus may rupture or the placenta may separate from the wall of the uterus. Massive hemorrhage and death of the mother and fetus can result. If the force is great enough to fracture the pelvis of the mother, the fetal skull may also be fractured.

Choosing not to wear a seat belt based on the erroneous idea it might injure the fetus only contributes to the possibility of injury. Ejection from the vehicle is more likely to occur when a shoulder harness and/or lap restraints are not used. The mother is apt to have head trauma when ejected and fetal fatality is more apt to happen. Seat belts can cause serious injury, but the risks to mother and fetus are greater without them.

The potential for a fall increases because hormonal changes soften joints and relax the pelvic ligaments. As a result, the mother has unstable balance and gait, a protruding abdomen and she is easily tired. All of these factors make her more susceptible to a fall. Most falls happen during the third trimester.

Gunshots and stab wounds are the predominant cause of penetrating trauma. The probability of fetal injury is related to the point of contact of the penetrating mechanism, the stage of pregnancy, and fetal position. Uterine growth displacing the stomach and small intestines provides some protection for the mother against penetrating trauma. Although multiple organ injury to the mother is less likely to occur, the fetus is often wounded. Fetal mortality rate in penetrating trauma is 70%.

### FIGURE 12-3
### Abruptio Placentae with Large Blood Clot Between Placenta and Uterine Wall

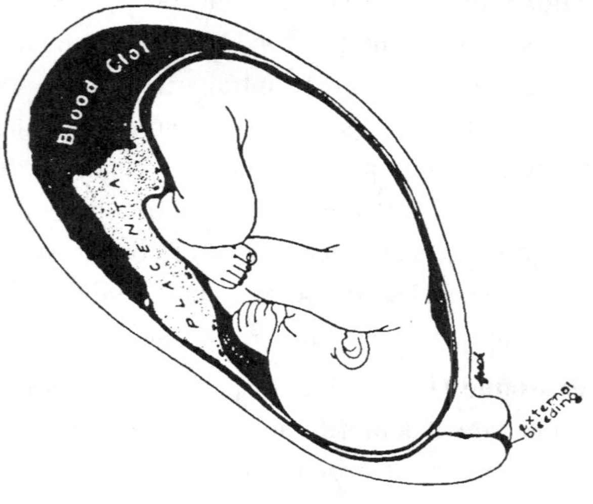

*Reprinted with permission from* Reeder, S., Mastroianni, L., Jr., Martin, L. L. & Fitzpatrick, E. (1976). *Maternity nursing* (13th ed.). Philadelphia: Lippincott.

Physical abuse is increasing, and is more frequent in teens than adult women. However, adult women are likely to sustain more severe emotional and physical abuse. Domestic violence also has a potential for repeat attacks.

# OBSTETRIC INJURY, COMPLICATIONS, AND INTERVENTIONS

## Blunt Trauma

### Premature Uterine Contractions

The most frequent obstetric trauma complication is the onset of premature uterine contractions.

Damaged cells release prostaglandin, a chemical that begins contractions. Basically, the degree of uterine damage, fetal age, and amount of prostaglandin released determine the progression of the contractions and labor. Generally, the contractions are self-limiting, and medical suppression is not necessary. If the contractions proceed, it may indicate other uterine complications such as abrup-

tio placentae. Tocolysis, pharmacological suppression of contractions, may be effective in abating the contractions. Appropriate fluid replacement and positioning the mother in the left lateral tilt position will minimize the uterine irritability.

### Abruptio Placentae

Most of the fetal deaths from blunt maternal injury are due to separation of the placenta from the uterus. Rarely, minor injury will cause abruption. Abruptio placentae is premature separation, and in blunt trauma, is partial or complete shearing of the placenta from the wall of the uterus. Since all gas exchange between the mother and the fetus is across the placenta, the oxygen to the fetus decreases in abruptio while the carbon dioxide increases in the fetal circulation. Fetal insult or death may occur and is related to the time between the separation of the placenta and delivery of the infant.

Signs and symptoms may be vague or absent. They range from vaginal bleeding (due to the collection of blood between the placenta and uterine wall), uterine tenderness and abdominal pain to uterine contractions, maternal shock, increasing fundal height and fetal distress. Vaginal bleeding is not always present.

Fetal distress may be the first sign of uteroplacental injury and abruption. Fetal monitoring should continue until the obstetrician states otherwise. Fetal distress requires immediate surgery. It is possible for the fetus to survive a small abruption.

### Uterine Rupture

Blunt trauma directly to the abdomen occasionally causes a rupture of the uterus. When rupture does happen, the injury is disastrous and occurs in mid to late pregnancy. Previous cesarean section is vulnerable at the suture line, making it a predisposing factor. The unscarred uterus usually ruptures at the posterior aspect and is likely to also involve bladder injury. Because the maternal blood volume and perfusion are increased, risk is high for maternal hypovolemic shock with uterine rupture. Maternal death generally is associated with additional injuries and happens in less than 10% of the injuries. Fetal death is close to 100%. The uterus cannot be repaired and a hysterectomy is indicated.

### *Pelvic Fracture/Direct Fetal Injury*

When blunt trauma fractures the mother's pelvis, direct fetal injury of the skull or other bones may also be involved. Fetal skull fractures with intracranial hemorrhages are most commonly seen. If the injury is late in the pregnancy when the fetal head is engaged, it may become trapped and injured by the fractured pelvis. A restraining seat belt or striking object may trap the fetal skull against the mother's spine. Other fractures seen in the fetus are the clavicle and the long bones.

## Penetrating Injury

Gunshot wounds to the abdomen are more common than stab wounds. The degree of injury is relative to the type, caliber and range of the weapon. Nearly a quarter of the gunshot wounds also involve visceral injuries. Upper abdominal wounds can include perforation of the bowel or retroperitoneal injuries. Lower abdominal wounds can cause direct injury or fatality of the fetus.

The mother and fetus fare better with stab wounds than gunshots because the visceral organs may slide away from the penetrating object.

Upper abdominal trauma from either gunshot or stab injuries may require exploratory surgery. Lower abdominal injury can be treated more conservatively if the mother is stable, the bullet can be identified and positioned radiographically and there is no evidence of gastrointestinal or genitourinary damage. Although there are several diagnostic options, the exploratory laparotomy is still the most accurate means to identify and treat penetrating injuries.

# ASSESSMENT

## Diagnostic Tests

**Diagnostic Peritoneal Lavage (DPL)** has been safely and accurately conducted in the pregnant woman to determine intraperitoneal hemorrhage, but it does not assess retroperitoneal or intrauterine injury. Indications for the procedure are blunt trauma with abdominal signs and symptoms, altered level of consciousness, unexplained shock, severe thoracic injuries and multiple or severe orthopedic injuries.

**Ultrasound (US)** is able to specifically determine the intra-abdominal injury and fetal status. It is a good tool for determining the need for a laparotomy.

**Cardiotocography** for fetal monitoring should begin as soon as possible but not interfere with maternal resuscitation and stabilization. Doppler is good for hearing the initial fetal tones, but this form of continuous electronic monitoring is also necessary to keep track of fetal heart tones, patterns and uterine contractions.

**Radiographics** are necessary for trauma evaluation of the gravid patient. Radiation exposure risks should be limited as much as possible to decrease potential fetal injury. Radiation has the greatest effect on the fetus during the first week after conception. After the embryo is successfully implanted, the potential for ill effects on the well-protected fetus is low.

## Assessment Principles

Changes to the mother's body during pregnancy can alter her response to trauma. The mother's compensatory mechanisms will protect her vital functions at the expense of the fetus.

To survive, the fetus must have adequate uterine perfusion and gas exchange. These needs require rapid and efficient assessment and appropriate intervention.

*Primary Assessment*

- Immobilize the spine if a neck injury is suspected or the patient is unconscious, and proceed with the standard ABC evaluation and maintenance. Tilt the head of the spine board or gurney up 15 degrees to maintain immobilization and prevent compression of the inferior vena cava. If an airway is used, oral or nasal should be used. Be careful to prevent bleeding from engorged mucous membranes.

- All gestational trauma patients should have 100% supplemental oxygen to handle the pulmonary changes typical of a pregnant woman, such as decreased functional pulmonary reserve and increased maternal oxygen consumption. Oxygen is also critical to the fetus to prevent hypoxia, which it cannot tolerate. Remember that as a rule, fetal death during trauma is the result of maternal death.

- The next priority is to determine if there is internal or external hemorrhage. External bleeding can be controlled with direct pressure. It is possible for the mother to lose up to 1,500 ml of blood internally without signs of shock. Undetected hemorrhage can be retroperitoneal or uteroplacental. Determine if the patient has hypovolemic shock.

  Fluid volume replacement should be aggressive to maintain maternal blood volume and delivery of oxygen to the mother and fetus. An arterial line and/or central venous line will provide the means for accurate monitoring of circulation and the patient's response to treatment.

  When blood is given, it should be Rh-compatible. If the mother is more than 20 weeks' pregnant, aortocaval compression may be relieved and cardiac output increased by 20% by displacing the uterus to the left. Optimizing position is helpful in making the mother more comfortable and improving perfusion.

- When assessing neurologic problems, be sure to consider the possibility of eclampsia.

*Secondary Assessment*

- Obtain the history and identify other injuries and their severity. A complete obstetric and trauma history should be documented. Identify the last menstrual period; expected due date; any medical problems the mother has had during the pregnancy, such as gestational diabetes; and the number of previous pregnancies and live births she has had. Additionally, identify medical diseases or disorders the mother has, such as a seizure disorder, diabetes, or hypertension.

- Abdominal assessment: As with other abdominal trauma, determination of specific injuries or intraperitoneal irritation may be difficult to assess. Intra-abdominal hemorrhage may not give signs of impending shock. There may be liver or splenic injury, which occurs in nearly a quarter of the serious motor vehicle crashes. The most common cause of intraperitoneal hemorrhage in gestational trauma is splenic rupture (Newberry, 1998).

  Inspect the abdomen for abrasions, contusions and ecchymosis. When the contour of the abdomen is irregular or deformed, it may be a sign of uterine rupture. Palpate the abdomen for masses and tenderness. Don't forget that abdominal rigidity, rebound tenderness and guarding may be blunted by the stretched abdominal wall.

- Fetus and uterus: Abdominal pain, uterine tenderness and contractions may be indicators of uteroplacental injury and maternal-fetal compromise.

  Knowing the gestational age, which is obtained by a detailed maternal history, affects the evaluation and interventions of fetal problems. If the patient is unsure of being pregnant, testing is necessary. The fundus is usually able to be palpated by 12 to 14 weeks' gestation, and it reaches the umbilicus by 20 weeks. When the fundus is just below the xiphoid, the fetus is full term.

Unless the fundus is filled with blood and firm, it will feel relatively soft. Determine if the mother is having contractions.

Check the perineum for blood or amniotic fluid. Blood may point to separation of the placenta from the uterine wall, or penetration or rupture of the uterus. Nitrazine paper can differentiate vaginal fluid from amniotic fluid. A general pelvic exam will determine crowning, fetal presentation, blood and fluids. The trauma physician will determine if a speculum exam by an obstetrician is necessary.

Determine fetal movement. Ultrasound will detect fetal cardiac activity, movement, location, approximate age and the amount of amniotic fluid. Fetal death can also be determined. The fetal heart sounds are ordinarily heard with a special fetal stethoscope, but without one, a standard stethoscope can sometimes detect fetal heartbeats. Fetal heart tones are audible by Doppler at the end of the first trimester. The fetal heart rate normally ranges from 120–160 beats/min. Bradycardia is considered to be less than 110 beats/min. If the fetus has tachycardia sustained at greater than 160 beats/min, it indicates fetal distress.

# NURSING STRATEGIES FOR THE PATIENT WITH OBSTETRIC TRAUMA

As with any trauma patient, the first priority for the obstetric patient is ABC evaluation and maintenance. In the case of pregnancy, the oxygenation and perfusion of the mother will affect both her survival and the survival of her fetus.

Patient management should be within the parameters of professional training, legal limitations and hospital policy. While conducting assessments and interventions, protect the patient's privacy and be sure to tell her what is being done and why.

- Provide oxygen to the mother at a high concentration to cope with maternal and fetal increased needs.

- Remember that the airway of the pregnant woman is engorged and swollen. Consequently, intubation may be more difficult than usual. It may be necessary to perform a tracheostomy if intubation is too difficult or traumatic to the airways. Be prepared for the potential of airway bleeding.

- If the injury is penetrating, do not remove any object embedded in the abdomen and stabilize the object as discussed in Chapter 10, "Abdominal Trauma." If there is no impalement, bleeding can be controlled with direct pressure. Fluid replacement should be started immediately.

- Conduct serial uterine muscle tone evaluations with fundal palpation in order to identify the onset of contractions or firmness indicating intrauterine bleeding.

- Periodically check for vaginal bleeding or leaking of amniotic fluid. After the fluid has been tested to determine if it is amniotic, a sterile pad can be placed against the perineum and changed as necessary if there is vaginal bleeding. Do not throw the pads away; the obstetrician may want to examine them for the amount of bleeding and the presence of tissue.

- Never insert anything into the patient's vagina. Pelvic examination should only be conducted by a professional with special training and skills in order to prevent introducing infection or causing injury.

- Begin fluids as ordered to meet the increased needs of maternal blood volume and oxygen carrying capacity. Remember that the blood pressure is slightly lower in the first trimester and heart rate is slightly higher in the gravid woman, making detection of hypovolemic shock more difficult than in the non-gravid woman.

- Position the patient to avoid aortocaval compression: elevate the spine board or gurney by 15 degrees, and place the patient on her left side to displace the uterus. The uterus can also be displaced manually by pushing it toward the patient's left side.

- Mark the height of the fundus on the abdomen with a pen in order to identify any changes that may be due to intrauterine hemorrhage.

- Do not allow anything by mouth until the patient is cleared by the physician. She may need an exploratory laparotomy. Note the last time the patient ate or drank any fluids.

- If the fetus should die as a direct or indirect result of the trauma, spontaneous vaginal delivery ordinarily begins within hours. If the uterus has also been injured, every attempt will be made to save it.

- Ask the patient if she would like anyone to be notified or to be with her. Ensure privacy.

# EXAMPLES OF NURSING DIAGNOSES RELATED TO OBSTETRIC TRAUMA

- Impairment in gas exchange related to increased oxygen demands of the gravid patient along with altered oxygen circulation

- Fluid volume deficit related to internal or external bleeding

- Altered perfusion to the fetus related to maternal volume and perfusion pressure loss

- Respiratory complications of suffocation and aspiration related to increased risk of bleeding in the respiratory tract due to engorgement and swelling

- Decrease in cardiac output related to aortocaval compression

- Risk of infection related to organisms being introduced into the retroperitoneum or the vagina

- Anxiety and fear related to the potential death of the fetus

- Anxiety and fear related to the potential loss of ability to have other children

# GYNECOLOGIC TRAUMA

Most gynecologic injuries are not severe. Internal and/or external reproductive organs may be damaged.

Blunt mechanisms are the predominant form of injury in gynecologic trauma. Injuries are mostly the result of motor vehicle crashes, falls and assaults. Falls are the most common reason for straddle injuries, hematomas and lacerations. Chapter 11 on genitourinary trauma discusses straddle injuries, foreign bodies, sexual assault, and rape.

Sexual assault in the female is seen more often than in the male and includes all ages, from the very young to the old. It is accepted that sexual assault is an act of violence. The rape-trauma syndrome is the physical and emotional consequence of sexual assault. Emotional reactions of anger, fear, embarrassment, shame, humiliation and self-blame are to be expected. Physical signs and symptoms of genitourinary discomfort, gastrointestinal upset and sleep disturbances may continue after initial treatment.

Data show that a woman is raped every 6 minutes, with 10,000 female victims being less than 18 years old and nearly 4,000 of those victims being less than 12 years old (Vachss, 1993; Thomas,

1994). Most of the attacks are by relatives or someone the victim knows.

For several years, special teams have provided non-physician services for sexual assault victims. Sexual assault response teams (SART) and sexual assault/abuse nurse examiners (SANE) have trained staff who are nurses, rape crisis advocates and law enforcement personnel. They provide evidentiary and support services in the emergency department.

## NURSING STRATEGIES FOR THE PATIENT WITH GYNECOLOGIC TRAUMA

- As the first priority, follow the ABCs and manage any injuries that threaten life and limb.

- Staff should be aware of their verbal and nonverbal behaviors' effect on the patient, particularly in cases of sexual assault. It is essential to communicate support and understanding.

- In as supportive manner as possible, document the history of the assault, time, place, names, witnesses and so on. In order to expedite care, you should be familiar with your hospital's policies and procedures on patients who have been sexually assaulted. By law, most cities and states require the hospital to report rape and sexual assaults to the police authorities, particularly if the patient is a child. It may also be necessary to notify children's services and other agencies. If the patient is an adult woman, she should be offered the opportunity to file police charges.

- Find out if the patient has anyone she wants contacted to come to the hospital for support. Do not leave the patient alone; she is probably very fearful.

- Many hospitals have specially trained staff and are affiliated with rape counselors or other related agencies that can begin immediate intervention aimed at dealing with emotional and physical problems. Nurses or clinicians are also able to examine the patient; gather evidence; administer treatment, including prophylaxis and specific therapy for sexually transmitted diseases; and arrange for follow up support and counseling.

- Explain to the patient the necessity for not changing clothes, brushing teeth, washing out her mouth, bathing, washing hands, eating, drinking, urinating or defecating. It is essential that all body cavities are examined and evidence is collected for testing before she is cleared by the physician to do any of these activities. Clothing will be given to the police for examination. Eating or drinking could destroy evidence or cause serious complications such as aspiration, if surgery is necessary. If the patient does not want to be examined or counseled, she cannot be made to comply.

- Do not catheterize the patient unless absolutely necessary as it may destroy evidence and aggravate injuries.

- If your emergency department uses the services of SART or SANE, follow protocol in contacting their staff.

## EXAMPLES OF NURSING DIAGNOSES RELATED TO GYNECOLOGIC TRAUMA

- Rape-trauma syndrome related to the emotional and physical consequences of sexual assault

- Anxiety related to the feeling of powerlessness from the violence of sexual assault

- Loss of self-esteem related to the demeaning feelings from sexual abuse

- Altered family dynamics related to incest

- Sexually transmitted disease related to sexual assault

# SUMMARY

Many changes in anatomy and physiology take place naturally during pregnancy. Demands on the heart for increased maternal blood flow are considerable. Uterine blood flow is not automatically regulated and is dependent upon the perfusion pressure of the mother. The nervous system does not have to alter to accommodate to gestational needs. Any neurologic change such as preeclampsia or eclampsia, is the result of a medical problem. The growth of the uterus pushes gastrointestinal and genitourinary organs out of place, causing symptoms such as reflux and urinary frequency. All the changes the mother experiences during a normal pregnancy affect her response to trauma and physical damage.

Injuries to the mother may or may not affect her gestational status. Head injuries and hemorrhagic shock account for most of the maternal deaths from trauma. Obstetric complications the mother may develop from blunt trauma include premature contractions, abruptio placentae, uterine rupture and pelvic fractures. Penetrating injuries are infrequent, most often from assault with the mechanisms being gunshot and stab wounds.

Obstetric trauma affects the fetus directly and indirectly because of its dependence on the mother's oxygenation and perfusion pressure and the fetus' vulnerability in the later trimesters. Fetal demise from trauma is most often the result of maternal death.

Most injuries are not severe and the incidence of obstetric trauma occurs in less than 10% of all pregnancies. Blunt injuries are secondary to motor vehicle crashes, falls and assaults. Falls, especially late in pregnancy, are the most common cause of injury.

Most gynecologic injuries are not generally physically critical, but considering they include sexual assault as a mechanism, the emotional damage may be severe. Sexual assault occurs to all ages and across all demographic descriptions. Assessing and caring for the victim of sexual assault requires particular training and sensitivity. Knowledge of the laws and facility policies and procedures are required in order to serve the patient appropriately and provide necessary interventions.

# EXAM QUESTIONS

## CHAPTER 12
### Questions 56–60

56. Which of the following statements is accurate?

    a. Neurologic changes during pregnancy cause preeclampsia.

    b. Cardiac demands on the mother during pregnancy are great.

    c. The pregnant woman experiences reflux because of poor diet.

    d. Perfusion in the uterus is determined by the fetal age.

57. Traumatic fetal death is most often due to

    a. direct injury.

    b. indirect injury.

    c. traumatic preeclampsia.

    d. the death of the mother.

58. The most frequent cause of obstetric trauma is

    a. falling.

    b. motor vehicle crashes.

    c. assault.

    d. gunshots and stabbings.

59. It is important to provide a high concentration of oxygen to the injured mother because

    a. it relieves her anxiety and complications of stress.

    b. administration of oxygen will prevent abruptio placentae.

    c. oxygen prevents hypotension.

    d. perfusion and oxygenation of the mother affects the fetus.

60. The rape-trauma syndrome

    a. is the physical and emotional trauma resulting from sexual assault.

    b. is the triad of external injury to the genitalia, vaginal abrasions and emotional stress resulting from sexual assault.

    c. causes injury to the fetus after sexual assault of the mother.

    d. is not a real syndrome.

# CHAPTER 13

# ORTHOPEDIC AND NEUROVASCULAR TRAUMA

## CHAPTER OBJECTIVE

Upon completion of this chapter, the reader will be able to identify the proper procedures for managing orthopedic and neuromuscular trauma.

## LEARNING OBJECTIVES

Upon completion of this chapter, the reader should be able to:

1. Describe basic structures and functions of the musculoskeletal system.

2. Identify frequent causes of orthopedic trauma.

3. Describe frequent orthopedic injuries and associated neurovascular problems.

4. Identify appropriate basic nursing strategies for orthopedic injuries and associated neurovascular problems.

5. Indicate examples of nursing diagnoses for patients with orthopedic trauma and associated neurovascular problems.

## INTRODUCTION

Musculoskeletal injuries, including fractures, dislocations and sprains, are a significant group in the emergency department population. Injuries can be the result of direct or indirect force. Most of the mechanisms of injury are motor vehicle crashes, assaults, falls, athletic injuries, and injuries that are work or home-related.

Orthopedic injuries are a significant cause of short and long-term disabilities. Although injuries usually are not critical unless accompanied by severe hemorrhage, such as traumatic amputations, they may be urgent because of potential arterial occlusion or neurovascular damage.

Quick and appropriate evaluation and intervention may prevent permanent disability.

## ANATOMY AND PHYSIOLOGY

Musculoskeletal and related neurovascular structures are bones, joints, tendons, ligaments, muscles, blood vessels, and nerves.

### Bones

Bones are the 206 skeletal structures that provide support, give solidity, strength, movement and protection to the body and its organs. They are also involved in blood cell formation and storing calcium.

Identified as long, short, flat or irregular, bones are designed for a particular function. The **axial skeleton** is the central structure of the body, made up of the skull, spine, sternum and ribs. The **appendicular skeleton** is made up of the rest of the bones in the body, including long, short and flat bones.

There are two types of bones: cancellous or spongy, found in the skull, vertebrae, pelvis, and long-bone ends, and cortical or dense bones, found in the long bones.

Bones are richly supplied by blood vessels, nerves and lymphatic vessels for nourishment and self-repair. Covering the bone is the periosteum, which provides an additional blood supply and osteoblasts for new bone formation after injury. Along with being a supporting structure for blood vessels, the periosteum is the point of attachment for muscles, tendons and ligaments and covers the entire bone except for the points of articulation.

Ligaments connect bones to other bones, and tendons connect muscle to bone.

## Joints

A joint is the point of connection between two bones, held together by fibrous connective tissue and cartilage, the joint capsule. The inner surface of the joint capsule, the **synovial membrane,** produces **synovial fluid,** which lubricates and nourishes the articular cartilage. There are two classifications of joints: **nonsynovial,** or immovable and slightly immovable, and **synovial,** or freely movable. Functions of joints are to give stability and mobility, flexion and extension, medial and lateral rotation, and abduction and adduction.

Joints are grouped according to motion: ball and socket, hinge, condyloid, pivot, gliding and saddle joint. There are four kinds of joint movements: **gliding** of one surface upon another without angular or rotary motion; **angular** is forward and backward movement to increase or decrease the angle between long bones; **rotation** around a central axis without moving away from the axis and **circumduction** in joints (having the head of a bone and an articulating cavity) with the long bone able to move in circles. Some joints have a combination of movements, such as the ball and socket hip,

which allows rotation as well as bending. Movement is aided by muscles and ligaments connected with the joint.

Because of their function and location, joints are vulnerable to stress, inflammation and trauma. Injuries are in the form of contusions, sprains, dislocations and penetration.

## Muscle

Muscle facilitates movement. The body's 600 muscles basically are divided into three types: skeletal, smooth and cardiac.

**Skeletal or voluntary** muscle forms the major muscle mass of the body and attaches to the skeletal bones. These muscles are under the direct control of the nervous system's commands to the brain, contracting or relaxing at will and related to all body movement. Specific nerves pass directly from the brain to the spinal cord, where they connect with other nerves leaving the spinal cord and then with each skeletal muscle. In most circumstances, a specific movement is the result of several muscles working together contracting and relaxing.

All skeletal muscles must have adequate perfusion in order to function. When nutrients are inadequate or acidic waste products accumulate, muscles will cramp.

Smooth muscle does much of the automatic or involuntary work in the body. Examples are the gastrointestinal tract, blood vessels, urinary system and bronchi. These muscles are found in the walls of most of the body's visceral organs and tubular structures. Contraction and relaxation moves the contents through the system, as seen in peristalsis. Involuntary responses are to primitive stimuli such as heat or the need to eliminate waste.

Cardiac muscle is a special adaptation of involuntary muscle, with its own regulatory system. It requires a continuous supply of oxygen and glucose or it cannot function.

## Ligaments

Ligaments are sheets or bands of strong fibrous connective tissue that connect bone to bone at points of articulation. Their purpose is to align the bones and allow or limit motion.

The bone ends of a joint are held together by a fibrous joint capsule. At points around the joint, the capsule is thin to provide the means for motion. At other points, the fibrous tissue is a band, thick, tough, and resistant to stretching or bending, which is the ligament. Some joints, such as the sacroiliac, are essentially surrounded by tough ligamentous tissue and allow little motion. On the other hand, the shoulder has few ligaments, which allows for free movement in almost any direction, and also makes it more prone to dislocation.

Freedom of joint motion is determined by the limitations the ligaments place on holding the bone ends together and by the configuration of the bone ends.

## Tendons

Cords of fibrous tissue that attach most skeletal muscle to bone are tendons. The cords are a continuation of the fascia covering all skeletal muscles, similar to the way skin covers a sausage. At each end of the muscle, the fascia continues beyond the muscle to attach to the bone, crossing the joint as the musculotendinous unit. It is this muscle-tendon unit that moves the joint.

When a muscle contracts, the line of force between the origin and insertion of the muscle pulls these points together at the joint between the two bones.

## Cartilage

Cartilage is a specialized type of dense connective tissue and has a limited vascular supply. It is found between the ribs, in the nasal septum, ear, larynx, trachea, bronchi, between the vertebrae, and articulating surfaces between bones. In joints where motion occurs, the ends of bones that articu-late are covered with articular cartilage. The inside of some joints, such as the knee, cushions of cartilage called the meniscus, fill the space between the bones and aid in the gliding motion of the joint. When the meniscus is torn, it can result in locking or catching in the joint.

**Nerves and blood vessels** lie close to bones and muscle groups. Arterioles run throughout the periosteum, providing nutrients and removing toxins. Nerves activate sensation and movement. In traumatic situations, these structures are at risk for damage, along with the adjacent muscles and bones.

# MECHANISM OF INJURY

Musculoskeletal injuries account for a large percent of the emergency department trauma patients. Because there are so many of these injuries, a solid basic knowledge of the anatomy and physiology, mechanisms of injury, types of injuries and interventions is essential.

Blunt and penetrating, direct and indirect, twisting or high-energy trauma is involved in orthopedic and related neurovascular injuries. When there is trauma to the musculoskeletal system, damage also occurs to the surrounding tissues such as the nerves and vessels. Additionally, other areas of the body may have sustained injury. Therefore, it is important not to focus on the assessment of a musculoskeletal injury to the exclusion of other possible injuries.

Considerable force is involved in fractures and dislocations. Direct blows can fracture. Indirect forces also cause fractures when energy strikes one part of a limb, and the fracture occurs some distance from the point of impact. Twisting is often the cause of the tibial fractures and knee and ankle ligament injuries seen in athletic trauma. In cases of severe trauma, when the bones are broken and torn or sheared from the surrounding tissues, amputation occurs. Other times, when the bone does not break, tendons, ligaments and muscles may be strained, sprained or torn by the force of the trauma.

High-energy injury from auto crashes, falls from heights, gunshot wounds or other extreme forces result in severe skeletal, surrounding soft tissue and adjacent vital organ damage. Multiple injuries generally are associated with high-energy trauma.

Penetrating injuries from gunshot wounds and knives may cause shattering of bones and lacerations of the muscles, tendons and ligaments. When a projectile passes through bone, the bone fragments along with the foreign object cause additional tissue and structural damage. The ends of the broken bone may also protrude through the skin, inviting bacteria and infection along with bringing about additional tissue damage.

Age is a factor in the results of a musculoskeletal injury. With the same mechanism of injury, the older person may incur a fracture, while a younger person will have a dislocation. Twisting and rotational forces can fracture a bone along with rupturing ligaments and tendons and often are a hallmark of abuse in young children. Biceps tears may happen with relatively little effort in middle-aged or older adults.

# ORTHOPEDIC TRAUMA AND ASSOCIATED NEUROVASCULAR PROBLEMS

## Types of Orthopedic Injuries

### Soft Tissue Injuries

Most orthopedic trauma involves soft-tissue injuries of the skin, muscles, tendons, ligaments, cartilage, vessels, and nerves that may compromise circulation and function.

Injury to the skin includes abrasions, avulsions, contusions, hematomas, lacerations and puncture wounds. Open wounds stand the chance of hemorrhage and contamination. Radiographs are used to rule out foreign bodies and fractures.

### Strain

A strain is sometimes referred to as a muscle pull and is the stretching or tearing of a muscle. Damage includes only the muscle, not the joint or ligament. The muscle fibers are weakened, overstretched or partially pulled apart at the point of attachment to the tendon, causing pain and possible swelling and ecchymosis of the soft tissues around the muscle damage.

Strains occur from many mechanisms of injury that overstretch, twist, wrench or cause violent muscle contraction.

Therapeutic interventions include cold packs, light or no weight-bearing and if the injury is moderate or severe, compression bandage and elevation. Analgesics ease the pain. A complete rupture may require surgical repair.

### Sprain

A sprain may have the same mechanism of injury as a strain, but generally, a more traumatic force is involved. In a sprain, the joint exceeds its normal limits and some of the supporting capsule and ligaments are stretched or torn. Injuries are commonly in the knee, ankle or shoulder. The joint may be partially dislocated. After the injury, when the force of injury is released, the joint falls back into place without continuing displacement.

The degree of injury varies from mild to severe, depending on the amount of damage to the supporting ligaments. Severe sprains may have as much damage to the joint capsule and ligaments as a complete dislocation. In children, epiphyseal disruption is common.

Signs of a sprain are tenderness over the damaged ligaments, swelling and ecchymosis from the tearing of blood vessels at the point of ligament injury, and inability to use the related extremity because of pain.

Mild sprains cause slight pain and swelling. Intervention includes compression bandage, elevation, cold pack for 12 hours and light weight-bearing. A moderate sprain results in pain, point tenderness, swelling and being unable to use the injured limb for more than a short period of time. Intervention is the same as for mild sprains, except that the cold pack should be used for 24 hours and light weight-bearing is aided with the use of crutches. If the sprain is severe, the ligaments are torn and there is a longer period of time that the joint cannot be used. Along with point tenderness and pain, there is swelling and discoloration. A splint or cast is used, along with a cold pack for 48 hours and light to no weight-bearing with the use of crutches.

### Peripheral Nerve and Artery Injury

Joints are well supplied with nerves and vessels. Causes of peripheral nerve and vessel damage are dislocations, fractures, lacerations and penetrating wounds. Neurovascular damage is likely with a joint injury.

High impact and rapid deceleration mechanisms are the major causes of arterial injuries. Pulse quality, capillary refill, skin color and temperature, bleeding, hematomas and bruits are indicators of arterial ischemia. Doppler pulses may be absent. Subjective symptoms of neurovascular damage are aching pain, weakness or paralysis, paresthesias, pallor and pulselessness.

Arterial injuries are sometimes difficult to identify because distal pulses may be detectable. A Doppler should be used when pulses are questionable. If collateral circulation is sufficient to prevent ischemia, surgical repair may not be necessary. Undiagnosed arterial disruption complications include thrombosis, arteriovenous fistula,

aneurysm, false aneurysm and tissue ischemia with limb dysfunction.

### Tendon and Muscle Rupture

Traumatic tendon and muscle ruptures are ordinarily seen in sports or recreation injuries. Runners experience quadriceps tears. Achilles tendon ruptures are seen in start-and-stop sports, where there is an abrupt step-off on the forefoot with the knee in forced extension. Sharp pain extends from the heel into the back of the leg. There is a sudden inability to use the foot and obvious deformity.

For an incomplete tear, rest and ice for 24 to 48 hours followed by heat is the usual treatment. A compression bandage may be applied. In complete tears, surgical repair is necessary.

### Knee Injuries

One of the most common forms of soft tissue injuries, most knee injuries are rotational or extraflexion that strain or tear the medial meniscus, collateral ligament, or cruciate ligament. Swelling, ecchymosis, effusion, tenderness and pain accompany the injury.

Interventions include compression bandage, knee immobilizer or cylinder cast, elevation, intermittent cold pack application over 24 hours and nonweight-bearing with the use of crutches. In the case of a ligament tear, surgical repair is necessary.

### Compartment Syndrome

Soft tissue injuries, fractures, casts or antishock garments can compress soft tissue. Other causes are prolonged pressure on a limb, frostbite or snakebite. When swelling and/or compression causes pressure in the muscle compartment to rise to the point that microvascular circulation is compromised, it is known as compartment syndrome. The result is tissue ischemia, which threatens the limb.

This syndrome is most often seen in compartments of the lower leg and forearm, with symptoms developing within 6 to 8 hours but possibly delayed up to 96 hours.

Signs and symptoms are deep throbbing pain much greater than the pain caused by the original injury and without relief from narcotics; pain with passive flexion; decreased mobility of digits; paresthesia; coolness; pallor and tight overlying skin. Pulses may or may not be absent.

Within 4 to 6 hours, irreversible tissue damage will occur from the inadequate perfusion. This is an urgent situation and should be identified and reported to the physician as soon as possible.

Position the limb on the same level as the heart. Frequent neurovascular checks are necessary. Changes should be reported immediately to the physician.

**Fingertip Injuries**

Fingertip injuries ordinarily are the result of crushing, secondary to an object falling on the distal phalanx or a finger being slammed in a door. High-pressure paint or grease guns are also a source of these injuries. These guns release a stream of paint or grease into the finger or hand, leaving a small pinhole, and potentially are limb-threatening. Debridement of the paint or grease is an immediate priority.

A subungual hematoma is a likely consequence of the injury, which is painful, and can be relieved by evacuation.

Fractures may also be caused by the force of the injury.

**Crush Injuries**

Crush injuries range from a fingertip to a large body area. Mechanisms of injury are common in an industrial environment: conveyor belts, grinders, wringers and machine presses, for example.

Complications depend upon the specific mechanism of injury and the extent of damage. When there is significant tissue necrosis, systemic crush syndrome may occur, marked by extracellular fluid loss, myoglobinuria (myoglobin in the urine due to muscular activity, trauma or a deficiency in muscle phosphorylase), acidosis, increased potassium, shock, renal failure, and cardiac disruption may occur (Newberry, 1998).

**Impaling Injuries**

Impalements may occur secondary to falling on a piercing object, be sustained from machinery or pneumatic tools (nails from nail gun), or by an impaling object, either a weapon or other instrument. The wound will vary in size and the depth is difficult to determine. Sometimes, the object will still be embedded in the patient when he arrives at the emergency room.

Impaled objects should not be removed immediately. There may be damage to muscles, tendons, bones, organs, and vessels. Surgical intervention may be necessary for removal of the object. A potential complication is infection from organisms and foreign bodies introduced by the impaling object.

*Dislocations*

Defined as a complete loss of articular contact between two bones in a joint, dislocation causes direct injury to ligaments and capsule tissues. The joint exceeds its normal range of motion, so the surfaces are no longer intact. The injury within the joint capsule and to the surrounding ligaments can cause nerve, vein, and artery damage. Diagnosis is confirmed by radiograph.

Signs and symptoms are pain, point tenderness, swelling, loss of motion, joint deformity, shortening of the extremity, and possible related nerve and vascular damage. There is a likelihood of nerve damage and vascular compromise, resulting in permanent disability or the loss of a limb. If the dislocation self-reduces, it still should be evaluated by an orthopedic physician.

## FIGURE 13-1
## The Dislocated Shoulder Loses its Full Lateral Contour and Appears Indented Under the Point of the Shoulder

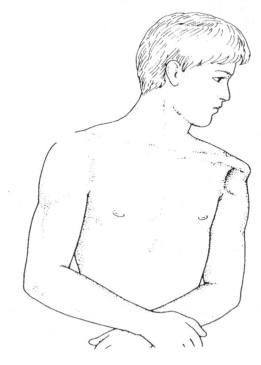

*Reprinted with permission from* Kitt, S., Selfridge-Thomas, J., Proehl, J. A. & Kaiser, J. (1995). *Emergency nursing: A physiologic and clinical perspective* (2nd ed.). Philadelphia: Saunders.

It is essential to assess the pulse carefully and serially. Palpate and splint the joint in the position as it presents and until the physician manages the injury. If reduction is necessary, it will be conducted with analgesia and sedation, and the patient is carefully monitored.

### Acromioclavicular Dislocation

The acromioclavicular (ACL) joint is between the acromion (the lateral projection of the scapula that forms the point of the shoulder and articulates with the clavicle) and the acromial end of the clavicle. Separations, commonly seen in athletes, are secondary to a fall or a force on the point of the shoulder.

The patient is unable to raise the arm or bring it across the chest. Pain is severe. Deformity, point tenderness, swelling and hematoma over the injury are characteristic.

The separation will be reduced. The arm and shoulder is immobilized with a sling and swath. Pain may be severe, even after reduction. The patient may need surgery to reduce and wire the joint if the injury is severe.

### Shoulder Dislocation

Probably the most commonly dislocated joint in children and athletes; there are two areas affected:

**Anterior:** Generally seen in athletic injuries when there is a fall on an extended arm that is abducted and externally rotated. The force pushes the humeral head in front of the shoulder joint.

**Posterior:** Not frequently seen, these dislocations can occur in seizure patients when the arm is abducted and internally rotated. Deformity is not always readily apparent.

Either type of dislocation has severe pain, deformity and inability to move the arm. More than half of the shoulder dislocations seen in the emergency department are recurrent.

After the arm is placed in the position of most comfort, distal pulses, skin temperature and moisture, and neurologic status should be evaluated. Unless there is neurovascular compromise, radiographs should be taken before and after reduction is done. After reduction, the shoulder is immobilized with a sling and swath bandage or shoulder immobilizer. Referral should be made to an orthopedic surgeon.

Complications can be neurovascular compromise to the brachial plexus and axillary artery and there may be associated fractures.

### Elbow Dislocation

Although a common athletic injury, elbow dislocations are seen most often in children, teenagers, and young adults. In athletes, the injury is usually caused by a fall on an externally rotated arm. Children's dislocations are usually from being jerked or lifted by one arm hard enough to cause a dislocation or "nursemaids' elbow." With nursemaid's elbow, the parent will bring the child to the hospital with the complaint that the child refuses to use his arm but does not seem to be in pain.

The patient's elbow may feel "locked." He complains of pain in the joint, especially with movement. Swelling, displacement, and deformity are evident.

The arm should be immobilized in the position of greatest comfort while waiting to be reduced. Radiographs are obtained after the reduction and the elbow immobilized again. If the dislocation is easily reduced with good return of mobility, follow-up radiographs may not be necessary.

Complications are neurovascular damage to the median nerve or the brachial artery.

### Hand or Finger Dislocation

Hand and finger dislocations are generally seen in athletes who fall on an outstretched hand or finger or who have direct trauma to the finger, such as when catching a ball.

Pain and inability to move a deformed joint are the patient's complaints.

The hand or finger should be splinted in the most comfortable position, and an ice pack applied. Once radiographs are obtained, reduction can be carried out, followed by splinting for immobilization.

### Hip Dislocation

Dislocation of a hip is a serious injury and is considered an orthopedic emergency. The dislocation may be anterior or posterior and is seen in all age groups.

Mechanism of injury may be secondary to major trauma. For example, in head-on auto crashes when the leg is extended with the foot on the break pedal or when the knee is jammed into the dashboard at the time of impact, and the result-

ing force dislocates the hip. Dislocation of the hip can also be caused by a fall or crush injury.

The complaint is of pain in the hip. Signs are that the patient's hip is flexed, adducted and internally rotated with posterior dislocation; or flexed, abducted and externally rotated with anterior dislocation. The patient cannot move his leg and his hip feels locked.

The patient's hip should be splinted in the position of greatest comfort or as it presents. There may be other injuries, which should be identified and assessed.

After reduction, the patient should be on bed rest with traction. Children are treated with a spica cast.

Posterior hip dislocation can cause sciatic nerve injury and permanent disability. Other complications are femoral artery and nerve damage. Blood supply to the femoral head may be impaired and cause necrosis if the dislocation is not reduced within 6 hours. In this situation, a hip replacement will become necessary.

### Knee Dislocation

Generally the result of major trauma, knee dislocations are seen in all age groups. Types are anterior, posterior, medial, lateral or rotary.

The patient has severe knee pain, swelling, deformity and cannot move the leg. Immediately splint the limb in the presenting position or the position of the most comfort. Knee dislocations urgently need reduction and immobilization. Treatment is a splint or hinged brace. The patient should be on bed rest after reduction, with the leg elevated and intermittent cold packs applied for about a week.

Arterial assessment is a high priority. Injury to the popliteal artery occurs in about one quarter of the cases because the artery can become caught between the adductor hiatus proximally and the interosseous membrane distally. Arteriography or immediate operation is necessary if there is unequal neurovascular evaluation. There is a risk of undetected arterial injury with late occlusion in knee dislocations. Therefore, even though there may not be any signs of arterial damage, arteriography should be considered.

Tibial, popliteal and peroneal nerve injuries are common in knee dislocations, as are fractures of the tibia.

**Patellar Dislocation**

Trauma to the lateral aspect of the knee or rapid rotation on a planted foot can cause patellar dislocations.

The patient experiences severe pain, holds his knee in a flexed position and is unable to use the knee. There is significant swelling and tenderness.

Splint the knee in the presenting position, and apply a cold pack. Reduction is carried out after radiographs are reviewed. After reduction, the knee is placed in a compression bandage and knee immobilizer or compression cast. Sometimes the patella will spontaneously reduce with extension of the leg.

*Subluxation*

Partial loss of articular contact, as compared to complete loss in dislocations, is referred to as subluxation. Sufficient ligament and capsular structure is intact to prevent a complete dislocation. There is less damage than in a dislocation. A dislocation that has partially self-reduced may be mistaken for subluxation.

*Fractures*

A broken bone is a fracture. Or, to be technical, a structural break in bone continuity is a fracture. The break may be caused by trauma or certain diseases, such as osteoporosis, osteomalacia, osteomyelitis, malignancies or syphilis that cause a spontaneous or pathologic fracture.

In the case of trauma, the fracture may be **direct,** occurring at the point of impact, or **indi-rect,** occurring at a distance from where the force is applied. An example of indirect fracture is when a person falls on an outstretched arm and the fracture is in the clavicle. In other situations, a sudden, violent contraction of a muscle may fracture the associated bone.

Severity of a fracture ranges from a simple crack to severe shattering that produces many fragments. The break may happen anywhere on the surface of the bone, including the articular surface.

Fractures have several potential complications. Bones can puncture or lacerate vessels, nerves, organs and structures causing hemorrhage or neurovascular compromise. Open fractures have the potential for infection from bacteria and foreign bodies, leading to serious limb dysfunction or loss.

Fat embolism is unusual but life-threatening when it occurs. It becomes apparent 24 to 48 hours after bone injury. This complication is seen most often with pelvic, femoral or tibia fractures. When a fracture occurs, it causes the release of fat particles into the blood. These particles may embolize to the lungs, signaled by sudden tachycardia, tachypnea, shortness of breath, cyanosis, cough, temperature elevation, altered level of consciousness, and pulmonary edema leading to adult respiratory distress syndrome (ARDS).

Long-term complications are non-union, deformity, disability, chronic pain, avascular necrosis from decreased blood supply, and Volkmann's contracture (ischemia, contracture fibrosis and atrophy of a muscle due to injury of the blood supply) secondary to untreated compartment syndrome.

Complications of pediatric fractures are addressed in Chapter 15, "Pediatric Trauma and Child Maltreatment," and elderly fractures in Chapter 16, "Elder Trauma, Abuse and Neglect."

*Classifications of Fractures*

Fractures are classified with respect to the following (Peitzman et al., 1998):

## TABLE 13-1
## Estimated Blood Loss in Fractures

| Fracture of | Blood Loss (L) |
| --- | --- |
| Humerus | 1.0–2.0 |
| Elbow | 0.5–1.5 |
| Forearm | 0.5–1.0 |
| Pelvis | 1.5–4.5 |
| Hip | 1.5–2.5 |
| Femur | 1.0–2.0 |
| Knee | 1.0–1.5 |
| Tibia | 0.5–1.5 |
| Ankle | 0.5–1.5 |

*Reprinted with permission from* Kitt, S., Selfridge-Thomas, J., Proehl, J. A. & Kaiser, J. (1995). *Emergency nursing: A physiologic and clinical perspective* (2nd ed.). Philadelphia: Saunders.

- **Integrity of the skin:** Open or closed

- **Pattern:** Transverse, oblique, spiral, greenstick, impacted, compression, depressed, avulsion

- **Morphology:** Simple (two parts) and comminuted (three or more parts)

- **Location:** Proximal, middle or distal; extra-articular or intra-articular

- **Radiographic parameters:** Displacement, angulation, rotation, shortening, apposition

The most important factor in the assessment of a fracture is the integrity of the skin over the break and the surrounding soft tissues. The degree of soft tissue damage in closed or open fractures is important. Extensive soft tissue injury increases the risk of compartment syndrome.

**Open or compound** fracture is any bone break where the overlying skin is damaged. Laceration may occur when the bone ends protrude through the skin or when the skin is broken from the exterior at the time of the injury. The wound may vary in size from small to gaping with exposed bone and soft tissue. The broken bone does not have to be visible in the wound to be considered an open fracture. Open fractures are more serious than closed because of the potential for hemorrhage, shock, foreign bodies and infection. Infections can cause

long-term problems for the patient. For this reason, open fractures are considered surgically urgent.

Wound care includes sterile saline irrigation, sterile dressing, intravenous fluid replacement, antibiotics and analgesia. Wound cultures should be done before irrigation is begun.

A **closed fracture** is a bone break with no apparent open skin damage over the fracture. Closed injuries will tamponade and limit blood loss.

A **comminuted fracture** is one in which the bone is broken in more than two fragments.

**Greenstick fracture** is only seen in children and is partially bent and partially broken, causing the bone to bow.

**Epiphyseal fracture** is seen in growing children when there is an injury to the growth plate of a long bone. If not properly treated, bone growth may be slowed or stopped.

**Pathologic fracture** occurs when a bone is weak or diseased. Minimal force can cause the break. This type of fracture may be seen in the spine without the patient being aware of the fracture, and just "seems to get shorter."

The degree of displacement is another classification that should be noted. If there is no displacement, there will not be a deformity, making intervention relatively simple. In these cases, in order not to identify the injury as just a sprain or contusion, diagnosis is confirmed radiographically. However, if there is displacement, deformity will be obvious and a reduction will be necessary. Different types of displacement may occur, such as angulation or rotation of the limb. Additionally, the limb may be shortened when the fractured bone ends overlap.

### Upper Torso Fractures

The clavicle and scapula are in the upper torso and relate to the upper extremities.

**Clavicle Fracture:** Clavicle fractures are found in all age groups, particularly in children. A fall on the shoulder or when two people run into each other in direct frontal contact, as in contact sports, are common mechanisms of injury. Most fractures are in the middle third of the clavicle.

Point tenderness, pain, swelling, deformity, crepitus, inability to raise the affected arm, and tilting the head toward the side of the injury are indicators of clavicle fracture. Neurovascular status should be assessed.

The shoulder should be held in a figure-of-eight support. In the elderly, a sling or sling and swath are used. Cold packs are used intermittently for 15–24 hours. Referral should be given for orthopedic follow-up.

Complications are brachial plexus injuries and pneumothorax or hemothorax, especially in more severe frontal impact trauma.

**Scapula Fracture:** Infrequently seen, young men involved in violent, direct trauma may fracture their scapula. Severe muscle contraction may also cause these fractures. Other mechanisms are auto crashes, falls, and crush injuries.

Pain and point tenderness during movement are the patient complaints. Swelling and bone displacement may be seen.

As always in musculoskeletal injuries, neurovascular status should be checked. A cold pack is used the first 24 hours. If the fracture is not displaced, a compression bandage, sling and swath or shoulder immobilizer is placed for 1 to 2 weeks.

Injury to the underlying ribs or viscera resulting from the force of the trauma is a complication.

## Upper Extremity Fractures

**Shoulder Fracture:** The glenoid, head of the humerus or neck of the humerus are the areas of shoulder fracture. Shoulder fractures occur, especially to the elderly, after a fall on an outstretched arm or from direct trauma. The same degree of injury in younger persons usually results in a dislocation rather than a fracture.

Shoulder pain, point tenderness, immobility of the affected arm, gross swelling and discoloration are the usual presenting signs. Most fractures are impacted or nondisplaced, needing only a sling and swath or shoulder immobilizer for treatment. If the fracture is serious, reduction is ordinarily closed, but open reduction or skeletal traction may be needed. This type of fracture is tremendously inconvenient for the patient in performing activities of daily living.

Neurovascular compromise of the axillary nerve and adhesive capsulitis or frozen shoulder, may be complications.

**Humerus Fracture:** The humerus is a long, strong bone, which generally requires considerable force to fracture. Children and seniors are the most likely to fall on their arms, receive direct trauma, or experience a shoulder dislocation and fracture the shaft of the humerus. A stress fracture may happen in weight lifting.

Point tenderness, swelling, difficulty using the arm, crepitus, angulation or deformity occur.

Neurovascular checks and assessment for other injuries should be conducted. A sling and swath or sugar-tong ("Y" splint) are the usual therapeutic interventions. Additional stabilization is done by securing the arm to the chest. Fingers should be wiggled frequently for exercise and circulation.

Fracture of the middle or distal shaft of the humerus may damage the radial nerve. There may be severe blood loss if bleeding is not controlled immediately.

**Elbow Fracture:** Elbow fractures are mostly seen in young children and athletes who fall on an extended arm or flexed elbow.

Fracture of the elbow involves the distal humerus, head of the radius or head of the ulna. Supracondylar fractures of the humerus are typically extension injuries and may damage the brachial artery. Ulnar head fractures are usually comminuted and result from a direct blow.

The injury causes considerable swelling, with a high risk of neurovascular compromise. Assessment should be prompt and serially.

Splint as found, and use a sling. If there is closed reduction, the arm is casted and put in a sling. Radial head fractures may need only a sling. If the fracture is comminuted or intra-articular, open reduction will be necessary.

Associated complications are brachial artery laceration; median, radial or ulnar nerve damage, and Volkmann's contracture. Signs and symptoms of contracture are an inability to move the fingers, severe pain with manipulation, severe pain in the forearm muscles continuing after reduction, pulse deficit, swelling, coolness of the extremity, cyanosis, and decreased sensation. The cast should be removed, and an immediate orthopedic consult obtained. Without prompt attention to Volkmann's contracture, atrophy and a claw-like deformity will result.

**Forearm Fracture:** The bones of the forearm, the radius and ulna, may be fractured individually or together. A fall on an extended arm or a direct blow can result in a fracture.

Pain, point tenderness, swelling, deformity, angulation and occasionally, shortening are indications of forearm fracture.

Splint to immobilize the arm and use a sling for support. In the use of a sling, the entire arm and hand should be supported, being careful not to let the hand droop at the wrist or assume a dependent position.

Closed reduction and casting with the elbow in

90° flexion with the shoulder and fingers free is the treatment used in many situations.

There is a risk of Volkmann's contracture with these injuries.

**Wrist and Hand Fracture:** Fractures of the wrist include the distal radius, distal ulna and carpal bones of the hand. The scaphoid is the carpal bone most likely to fracture. The most common mechanism is a fall onto an extended arm and open hand, especially in the elderly. A Colles fracture (a transverse fracture of the distal end of the radius, with displacement of the hand backward and outward) may occur in a fall from a height.

Closed reduction and casting are the usual interventions. In place of a sling, for better elevation of the wrist, some physicians prefer a hanging apparatus, such as an IV pole, to suspend the hand for 2 days, which can be done at home.

Complications can include avascular necrosis or tissue death from loss of blood supply.

**Pelvic Fracture**

Pelvic fractures happen most often in middle-aged and elderly adults. Mortality occurs in about 8% to 10% of the cases; and is higher with open fractures. Open fractures into the rectum or vagina are seen in a small percent of the patients, and have a 40% to 60% risk of mortality.

More than half of the patients with pelvic fractures have additional injuries, particularly in vehicular trauma of pedestrians. Other causes are direct trauma, falls from a height, sudden contraction of a muscle against resistance and sports injuries.

Acetabular, or hip socket, fractures are complicated and can be associated with hip dislocation and injuries to the pelvic ring. These fractures are significant injuries, and can result in lifelong disabilities. Temporary skeletal traction is used to maintain the reduction and prevent soft tissue contracture. If the fracture is displaced, delayed open reduction after about 3 to 7 days, reduces the chance for bleeding complications.

Classifications of pelvic fractures are stable or unstable, depending on the condition of the pelvic ring and degree of bone and tissue damage. Neurovascular structures at risk for injury are the iliac artery, sciatic nerve and the venous plexus.

When gentle pressure applied to each side of the pelvis is painful, fracture should be suspected. Pelvic fractures tend to bleed profusely and may cause abdominal distention from internal hemorrhage, hypovolemic shock and hematuria. There may also be paraspinous muscle spasm, sacroiliac joint tenderness, paresis or hemiparesis, and pelvic ecchymosis.

Interventions include high-flow oxygen, vital signs every 5 minutes with observation for hypovolemia, establishing 2 intravenous lines for volume replacement, and immobilization of the spine and legs on a long board with the knees flexed. Blood type and crossmatch should be conducted, along with peritoneal lavage and radiographic studies. Orders may include a Foley catheter, but not when there is blood at the meatus.

External fixation is used with unstable weight-bearing fractures. Nonweight-bearing, less severe fractures are treated with bedrest and traction.

Other problems with pelvic fractures are varied and may be severe, including bladder trauma, genital trauma, lumbosacral trauma, rupture of internal organs, sepsis, shock, and death. Post-traumatic arthritis, chondrolysis and heterotopic ossification are the most common complications. Long-term problems, aside from chronic pain and loss of function, are thrombophlebitis and fat embolism.

## Hip Fracture

Hip fractures are common in elderly people, usually after a fall or minor trauma. Auto crashes and other sudden deceleration incidents also contribute to hip fractures. Hip fracture in the younger person is usually the result of major trauma and generally causes a fracture to the femoral head, femoral neck or intertrochanteric area. Femoral head fractures are infrequent, usually the result of a high-speed motor vehicle crash. A fall or minor trauma may cause a hip fracture in the elderly.

The patient feels pain in the hip, groin and leg when moved. Those with greater trochanteric fractures can ambulate. Extracapsular trochanteric fractures have pain in the lateral hip, shortening of the leg and external rotation.

The patient should arrive in the emergency department with the hip splinted to a long board or the other leg. Buck's traction or surgical repair may be necessary.

Complications are hypovolemia, shock, avascular necrosis with femoral head and neck fractures, and non-union.

### Lower Extremity Fractures

**Femoral Fracture:** It takes substantial force to fracture the femur, a serious injury, that usually occurs in conjunction with other musculoskeletal and soft tissue damage. Be sure to evaluate for other injuries, especially of the knee.

Severe pain, inability to stand on the affected leg, swelling, crepitus, deformity, external rotation or angulation indicate a femoral fracture. Shortening may develop due to severe muscle spasms.

Initially, the use of Hare traction, Sager or Thomas splints will provide traction. Long air splints with an enclosed foot or splinting to the other leg does not provide enough stability for this type of fracture. Blood loss may be severe, so the patient may arrive with a pneumatic antishock garment, in order to compress the bleeding and splint the fracture.

At least one intravenous site should be established, with frequent vital signs and circulation checks conducted. Nothing for the patient by mouth until cleared by the physician, and it is confirmed that surgical intervention is not necessary.

Shock secondary to hypovolemia is the primary complication. It is not unusual for approximately 2 liters to bleed into the thigh. Severe muscle spasms are able to move bone ends, causing further soft-tissue injury, muscle damage and pain. Neurovascular damage can include the peroneal and sciatic nerves and popliteal artery.

**Knee Fracture:** Supracondylar fracture of the femur or intra-articular fractures of the femur or tibia fall into the category of knee fractures. Occurring in all age groups, these injuries are mostly the result of vehicular or vehicle-pedestrian accidents. Inability to flex or extend the knee, pain, swelling and tenderness are signs of knee fracture.

A long-leg splint or splinting the injured knee to the other leg are the usual interventions. If the injury is severe, surgical repair may be required.

Complications include neurovascular compromise of the peroneal or tibial nerve, or popliteal artery.

**Patella Fracture:** Direct impact from a fall or contact with a dashboard; or indirect trauma, with a severe muscle pull, can cause a patella fracture. The patient has pain and the fracture may be able to be palpated. The fracture may also be open.

Cover the open wound with a sterile dressing, and use a long-leg splint. Nondisplaced fractures are usually put in a long-leg cylinder cast. Displaced fractures have closed reductions. Surgery is necessary for open reductions and pinnings. The patella is a key part of the knee, aiding in leverage and protecting the knee joint. Disruption of extension requires surgical intervention.

**Tibia and Fibula Fractures:** Direct and indirect trauma and rotational force cause tibial/fibula fractures. Many of these fractures are open. There is pain, point tenderness, swelling, deformity and crepitus. Splint as found. Open wounds should be covered with sterile dressings. Long-leg splint is applied; and reduction is closed or open. It is rare for the fibula alone to be fractured. Because the fibula is not a weight-bearing bone, a walking cast can be applied.

Complications are severe blood loss, soft tissue damage, neurovascular compromise, compartment syndrome and Volkmann's contracture.

**Ankle and Foot Fracture:** Ankle fractures include the distal tibia, distal fibula or talus breaks from direct or indirect trauma or torsion. There may be open fractures or dislocations. The patient has pain and point tenderness in the area of damage, is unable to bear weight, and has swelling and deformity. Closed reduction and casting is the treatment. If the damage is severe, open reduction and pinning may be necessary. The most frequent complication is neurovascular compromise of the peroneal nerve.

Fracture of the metatarsals and tarsals occur from vehicular crashes, sports injuries, crush injuries or direct trauma. Inversion foot injuries cause fifth metatarsal fractures. Compression dressing and soft splint is the usual intervention. If the fracture is minimal, treatment is an open-toed orthopedic shoe or cast. Severe displacement may require open reduction. Crutches assist with weight bearing or non-weight bearing.

### Traumatic Amputations

Amputation trauma has the potential of significant morbidity. Dysfunctional limbs should be treated at facilities with the capability of microvascular surgery. This trauma is life and limb threatening, is a true emergency, and treatment must be immediate.

Mechanisms of injury are most frequently industrial or recreational accidents. Lawn mowers and snowblowers also cause a large number of amputations.

The most frequently amputated parts are fingers and toes, distal half of the foot, leg, forearm, hand, ear, nose, and penis.

High-flow oxygen, two large-bore intravenous lines and control of bleeding are top priorities. Splint and support the limb in a position of anatomic function if the amputation is partial. In total amputations, the stump should be elevated, irrigated with sterile saline and sterile dressings applied. Orders will include antibiotics, tetanus booster and immune globulin. Tourniquets should not be applied unless ordered by the physician.

The amputated part should be brought with the patient to the emergency department for possible reimplantation. The amputated part should be wrapped in sterile gauze, wet with saline. Place in a water-tight plastic bag or container, which is then put in a container with iced saline. DO NOT USE DRY ICE, DISTILLED WATER, PLACE DIRECTLY ON ICE OR ALLOW TO FREEZE AS IT WILL DAMAGE THE TISSUE. Label the container with the patient's name, time and date (Peitzman et al., 1998).

Success of reimplantation is very limited. The availability of a reimplantation team, the type and degree of damage to the stump and amputated part, and the amount of time that has passed since the incident are the key factors in the success of reimplantation. Other factors are age, general physical condition, occupation and motivation.

Amputations caused by sharp cuts have a better outcome than crush injuries and avulsions. Muscles can survive 12 hours of cold ischemia; and cooled, bone, tendon and skin can survive 24 hours

(Newberry, 1998). Without cooling the amputated part, survival time is greatly diminished.

# ASSESSMENT

As discussed in the previous chapters, the ABC assessment and maintenance is always the first priority. It is important not to allow dramatic orthopedic injuries to distract from more serious trauma.

Rapid assessment follows the ABCs to identify serious injuries of the head, cervical spine, chest, and abdomen and identify the prioritization of actions. Musculoskeletal injuries are not isolated in serious traumatic incidents.

- Intervene in life-threatening injuries first, limb-threatening injuries second and then other injuries according to severity. Injured nerves and vessels have the potential for causing permanent disability.

- Obtain as accurate a history as possible while examining the patient. Ascertain any previous musculoskeletal injuries, diseases or surgeries.

- Do not pull off clothing, but cut it away, being careful not to disturb the injured area and always protecting the patient's privacy.

- Assess for open wounds and skin integrity, checking for internal as well as external bleeding.

- Compare the injured extremity with the opposite limb, checking for pain, point tenderness, swelling, discoloration, and temperature.

- Palpate injured areas gently, feeling for irregularities and signs of dislocations and fractures.

**Signs and symptoms of fractures: Deformity** or irregular position, angulated, rotated, shortened; **point tenderness** sharply localized at the injury site; **guarding** or inability or refusal to use the injured part; **swelling and ecchymosis** of tissues around the point of injury; **crepitus** or a grating feel due to raw bone ends rubbing together; **false motion,** which is motion at a point in a limb where it does not naturally occur; and **exposed fragments** in an open fracture, either protruding through the skin or seen through the wound. Determine if the patient heard a popping sound.

- If the patient is a child, look for indicators of abuse when the patient has a spiral fracture.

- Palpate for pulses distally and in both extremities; compare extremities.

- Assess neurovascular status, checking for numbness and paresthesia. Determine if the patient can wiggle his fingers or toes.

- Assess the circulatory status of extremities.

# NURSING STRATEGIES FOR THE PATIENT WITH ORTHOPEDIC TRAUMA AND ASSOCIATED NEUROVASCULAR PROBLEMS

Remember that with major trauma, there will be multiple injuries. The primary goal is to limit current damage, prevent further damage, and preserve the structure and function of the injured extremity as much as possible.

- Conduct the ABCs and immobilize the neck until cervical injury has been cleared.

- Let the patient know what you are doing and why. Be comforting.

- Maintain perfusion of the injured limb.

- If there is bleeding or signs of internal hemorrhage, start an intravenous with a large-bore needle.

- If the patient has multiple severe injuries, a long bone fracture or possible pelvic fracture, administer intravenous fluids and provide oxygen to keep the patient adequately perfused, since hypovolemic shock is likely.

- If there is an open wound, culture if ordered, gently irrigate with sterile saline and cover with a sterile dressing. Do not spread the wound apart to determine its depth.

- Do not apply a tourniquet unless ordered by the physician.

- Nothing by mouth until the physician determines surgical intervention is not necessary or if the patient is nauseated.

- Maintain warmth of patient to help prevent coagulopathy.

- Reassess the injured limb serially and after each time the limb has been moved.

- Splint the injured extremity if there is a question of an orthopedic injury. See earlier described injuries in this chapter for information regarding the best immobilization techniques for specific injuries.

- Once spinal injury has been ruled out, elevate a sprained or strained extremity and apply a cool pack to reduce swelling. Periodically assess the site under the cool pack for any change in the status of the injury. **Do not** use ice; it can impair the integrity of the tissues.

- Do not attempt to straighten a dislocated or fractured limb. If not already splinted, immobilize the limb in the most comfortable position or as the limb presents.

- Do not attempt to remove any impaled object; stabilize the object until the physician arrives for trauma management.

- Exposed bones should not be pushed back into the wound; it will aggravate the injury, increase the potential for infection and be painful.

- If there is an amputation, transport the amputated part to the emergency department with the patient. It is not advisable to suggest to the patient that reimplantation is usually successful. It is not.

- If the amputation is partial, the limb should be supported and splinted in a position of anatomic function (Newberry, 1998).

- A full amputation should have the stump gently irrigated for gross contamination, sterile dressing applied and elevated.

  The amputated part should be wrapped in sterile gauze, wet with saline. Place in a water-tight plastic bag or container, which is then put in a container with iced saline. DO NOT USE DRY ICE, DISTILLED WATER, PLACE DIRECTLY ON ICE OR ALLOW TO FREEZE AS IT WILL DAMAGE THE TISSUE. Label the container with the patient's name, the time and date (Peitzman et al., 1998).

  Amputated parts should not be soaked in any liquid, cleaned or rinsed; as it will ruin the integrity of the tissue.

# EXAMPLES OF NURSING DIAGNOSES RELATED TO ORTHOPEDIC TRAUMA AND ASSOCIATED NEUROVASCULAR PROBLEMS

- Potential alteration in tissue perfusion related to musculoskeletal injury

- Fluid volume deficit related to blood loss in musculoskeletal injury

- Potential neurovascular compromise related to orthopedic injury

- Physical mobility impairment related to damage incurred in orthopedic trauma

- Potential infection related to open wounds in musculoskeletal injury

- Impaired skin integrity related to musculoskeletal trauma

- Pain related to damage to musculoskeletal tissues and structures

- Anxiety related to severe orthopedic injuries

# SUMMARY

A large portion of the trauma patients seen in emergency departments have musculoskeletal injuries. Most of these injuries are not threatening to life or limb, although orthopedic trauma with associated neurovascular damage is a significant cause of short- and long-term disabilities. Orthopedic trauma includes soft tissue injuries, dislocations, fractures, and traumatic amputations. There may be multiple injuries in addition to the musculoskeletal trauma.

Recent progress in emergency care and treatment and surgical techniques have improved the outcome potential for patients with musculoskeletal trauma.

The primary objective for emergency care of orthopedic trauma and potential neurovascular injury is to restore or preserve the injured limb with the greatest integrity possible and prevent further injury. Quick and appropriate evaluation and intervention may prevent disability.

The caregiver must have a solid basic knowledge of the musculoskeletal and neurovascular anatomy and physiology in order to properly assess the patient and provide the best possible interventions.

# EXAM QUESTIONS

## CHAPTER 13
**Questions 61–65**

61. Musculoskeletal injuries, including sprains, dislocations and fractures

    a. are mostly seen in middle-aged patients.

    b. have little risk of neurovascular compromise.

    c. specifically relate to muscles tearing away from long bones.

    d. are a significant cause of short and long-term disabilities.

62. Most orthopedic trauma involves

    a. soft tissue injuries of the skin, muscles, tendons, ligaments, cartilage, vessels, and nerves.

    b. tendons and ligaments that are over-stretched and pulled apart.

    c. severe swelling and neurovascular compromise.

    d. compartment syndrome.

63. When assessing for musculoskeletal injury

    a. splint the injured extremity to immobilize it before carrying out any assessments.

    b. the most important factor in the evaluation of a fracture is the integrity of the skin over the point of injury and surrounding tissues.

    c. pull off clothing as fast as possible if a fracture with hemorrhage is suspected.

    d. perfusion is not a problem in these types of injuries.

64. Nursing strategies for the patient with orthopedic trauma include

    a. replacement of exposed bone back into the limb.

    b. placing an amputated part in saline and then on ice.

    c. placing a fractured elbow in a Thomas splint.

    d. establishing an intravenous infusion with a large-bore needle in patients who have a suspected long bone or pelvic fracture.

65. Complications of fractures include

    a. Volkmann's contracture.

    b. transverse avulsions.

    c. partial loss of articular contact.

    d. structural inversion.

# CHAPTER 14

# BURN INJURIES

## CHAPTER OBJECTIVE

Upon completion of this chapter, the reader will be able to describe the concepts important in the management of burn injuries.

## LEARNING OBJECTIVES

Upon completion of this chapter, the reader should be able to:

1. Identify the epidemiology and incidence of burns.

2. Describe the pathophysiology of burn injuries.

3. Identify types of burn injuries and the criteria for describing the extent and severity of burns.

4. Identify priorities in the assessment of burn patients.

5. Identify appropriate basic nursing strategies for the burn patient.

## INTRODUCTION

Burns are one of the most serious and painful injuries a person can sustain. These injuries are the fourth leading cause of death from trauma in this country. Between 2 and 2.5 million persons in this country are treated for burns each year. Residential fires are the primary cause of burn deaths.

A large part of the morbidity and mortality in burn patients is related to associated injuries. Pulmonary disorders from inhalation damage lead to many of the deaths. The more serious burns are often disfiguring and many require long-term treatment and rehabilitation.

Taking immediate action when a person is burned can have enormous effect on the rest of his life. Removing the patient from the source of the burn; the burning process, stabilizing him; and providing safe, rapid access to treatment is essential.

More than 90% of all burns are preventable. Because of recent strong public education programs and legislative mandate regarding construction codes and smoke/fire detection devices, efforts are met with increasing effectiveness in decreasing the number of burn injuries.

## EPIDEMIOLOGY

Of the 2 million plus burn injuries in this country each year, 60,000 to 100,000 victims are hospitalized, 20,000 require the expertise of a burn center and 7,500 to 10,000 die at the scene or subsequently from burns or associated injuries or complications (Newberry, 1998; Peitzman et al., 1998).

Residential fires are the main cause of burn deaths, with the predominant mechanisms being heating unit failure, kitchen accidents, incendiary devices/arson, and smoking materials.

In the home, pediatric burns most often are caused by scalding. They may be unintentional or deliberate, and it takes careful observation and history-taking to determine if the child's burn is the result of abuse.

High-risk groups for fire incidents include those who smoke, especially in bed; children; the elderly; and the disabled.

Fire is not the only source of burns. Electricity, including lightening; ultraviolet rays; superheated steam; chemicals; tar; explosions; and frostbite are also mechanisms that cause burns.

# ANATOMY AND FUNCTIONS OF SKIN

## Anatomy

Skin is the largest single organ in the body, and as a true organ, it has functions. Three major functions are to protect the body in the environment, regulate the temperature of the body, and transmit information about the environment to the brain—protect, regulate and inform.

### Layers of the Skin

**Epidermis:** Of the two main layers of skin, the epidermis is the tough outermost layer. There are several layers within the epidermis. The base epidermal layer is the germinal layer, which continuously produces new cells that rise to the surface, die and form the watertight covering. The epidermis varies in thickness in different parts of the body.

**Dermis:** A deeper layer, the dermis, is below the germinal layer and consists of collagen and elastic fibers. Within the dermis are specialized structures that give the skin its characteristic appearance: sweat glands, sebaceous glands that secrete oil to lubricate the skin, hair folli-

cles, blood vessels, and specialized nerve endings.

**Subcutaneous Tissue:** Lying below the dermis, this fatty layer varies in thickness in different parts of the body and in each person.

**Fascia:** Below the subcutaneous layer lies the deepest layer, the fascia, which covers the muscles.

## Functions

### Protection

The skin is watertight. More than 70% of the body is made up of water containing an exact balance of chemical substances in its solution. The watertight quality of the skin keeps the balance of the internal water solution stable. The body is also protected from the invasion of infectious organisms, bacteria, viruses and fungi, as they cannot pass through unbroken skin.

### Regulation

Skin is the major organ in the body for temperature regulation. The metabolic process can only function within a narrow temperature range. If the temperature is too low, reactions cannot occur, metabolism stops and the body dies. If the temperature is too high, the rate of metabolism increases, sometimes resulting in permanent tissue damage and death.

When the environment is cold, constriction of the blood vessels shunts the blood away from the skin's surface to decrease the amount of heat radiated. When the environment is hot, sweat is secreted to the skin's surface for evaporation. Evaporation of sweat uses energy, which is taken from the body as heat, causing the body temperature to fall. In other words, sweating itself does not reduce the body temperature; it is the process of evaporation pulling energy from the body in the form of heat that reduces the temperature.

### Information

Sensory nerves originating in the skin, carry information about the environment to the brain, including sensations of pressure, pleasant stimuli and pain.

# PATHOPHYSIOLOGY

The generally accepted definition of a burn is that it occurs when the skin is exposed to more energy than it can absorb. There are many causes of burns, but local and systemic responses are similar in all cases.

## Zones of Damage

When a burn occurs, it causes three zones of damage (Newberry, 1998).

### Zone 1

**Central zone of coagulation:** The contact burn area of irreversible damage.

### Zone 2

**Stasis:** The area where capillary and small vessel stasis (stagnation of the normal flow of fluids, in this case, blood) occurs and surrounds Zone 1. The outcome of the burn wound depends upon resolution or progression of this area of stasis. Edema formation and continued compromise of blood flow to this zone will cause a deeper and more extensive wound. When there is decreased perfusion to the skin, it can convert the zone of stasis to one of coagulation, causing the burn to become deeper. Because of this, determination of the depth and severity of burn wound may not be known for 3 to 5 days.

### Zone 3

**Hyperemia:** This is an area of superficial damage that heals quickly. After a burn, there is immediate hemolysis of red blood cells; the remaining red cells have their life span reduced by about one third. Platelet count and survival time

drastically fall and continue to do so for about a week, after which they begin to increase for several weeks.

Response to a burn is tissue damage, cellular impairment and fluid shifts. In a burn involving less than 20% total body surface area (TBSA), burn response is usually limited to the burn area. Beyond 20%, the response goes from local to systemic.

After a burn occurs, there is a brief decrease in blood flow to the burned area. Then there is a marked increase in arteriole vasodilation. The burned tissues release mediators that cause an inflammatory response. Release of the vasoactive substances along with the vasodilation increase capillary permeability, or the ability of the capillary

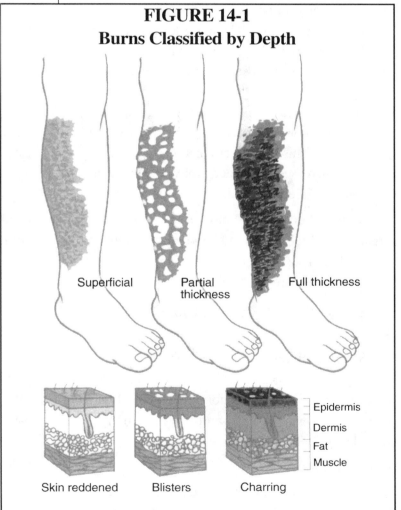

## FIGURE 14-1
## Burns Classified by Depth

Superficial    Partial thickness    Full thickness

Skin reddened    Blisters    Charring

Epidermis
Dermis
Fat
Muscle

*Reprinted with permission from* O'Keefe, M. F., Limmer, D., Grant, H. D., Murray, R. H. & Bergeron, J. D. (1998.). *Brady emergency care* (8th ed.). Upper Saddle River, NJ: Brady/Prentice-Hall.

wall to let substances in the blood move back and forth into tissue spaces or cells. As a result, there is intravascular fluid loss and wound edema.

Increased capillary permeability also causes hypoproteinemia that aggravates edema in tissue that is not burned. Insensible fluid loss increases the basal metabolic rate, that coupled with the fluid shift, causes hypovolemia.

The capillary permeability increase has the most significant changes in the first 24 to 36 hours and continues from 2 to 3 weeks.

Vascular fluid shifts into the interstitium (the small space between body parts, cells or tissues) make the blood more viscous. The decreased intravascular fluid volume, increased blood viscosity and increase in peripheral resistance causes the cardiac output to drop. Capillary leak and falling cardiac output may depress central nervous system function, shown by increasing restlessness, then lethargy and coma. The drop in cardiac output and blood volume and the nervous system sympathetic response decreases perfusion to the skin, viscera and kidneys. This drop in circulating plasma along with the increased hematocrit may lead to hemoglobinuria and renal failure.

Serious burn injury may affect all the body organs. Cerebral perfusion abnormalities, impaired cardiac blood supply, renal insufficiency and metabolic imbalance are likely consequences of burns.

## Pulmonary Response to Smoke Inhalation

Smoke inhalation causes a syndrome with three specific problems: carbon monoxide intoxication, upper airway obstruction and chemical damage to the lower airways and lung parenchyma (Newberry, 1998).

### Carbon Monoxide Intoxication

The most frequent cause of death in fire occurs in victims who have been overcome by carbon monoxide before they are burned. Carbon monoxide is a gas released during a fire, and when inhaled and absorbed, it binds with hemoglobin, displacing oxygen and blocking oxygen-binding sites.

Carbon monoxide has an affinity for hemoglobin that is 200 times greater than that of oxygen. When carbon monoxide binds to hemoglobin, it interferes with adequate amounts of oxygen getting to the tissues. Additionally, carbon monoxide combines with myoglobin in the muscle cells, causing muscle weakness. The tissue hypoxia that results in muscle weakness and mental confusion is thought to be a primary contributor to fatalities.

### Upper Airway Obstruction

Thermal injury to the upper airway is usually related to facial burns. Intrinsic or extrinsic edema may occlude the airway at the level of the vocal cords or higher. Edema progresses rapidly, causing total occlusion within minutes to hours.

Tissue damage in the posterior pharynx is usually from thermal causes. It is not likely that thermal damage occurs below the posterior pharynx because this area is an efficient system for heat exchange. When there is true thermal injury below the vocal cords, it is usually caused by superheated steam carried by water vapor into the lungs, or the inhalation of explosive gasses, which may occur during inhalation anesthesia, and is almost always fatal.

Management of airway edema is intubation as soon possible.

### Chemical Injury

Smoke inhalation often causes chemical injury to the lower airways. The acids and aldehydes in the smoke are likely to damage the lung parenchyma. They attach to carbon particles contained in smoke, which is heavier than air and inhaled. The particles travel down to the bronchi and into the alveoli.

Chemical injury causes hemorrhagic tracheobronchitis, an increase in edema, lowered levels of surfactant, and decreased function of pulmonary cells that are dust-phagocytic (macrophages). Within 24 to 48 hours, adult respiratory distress syndrome (ARDS) develops.

In the case of severe inhalation injury, the patient will have an increased need for fluids.

# MECHANISM OF INJURY

Burns, the application of more energy than the body can absorb without damage, occur in several forms: Heat/thermal, including scalds, flame, flash and contact; electrical, including shock and lightning; chemical, including contact and inhalation; nuclear; and frostbite.

Damage to the body ranges from minor to fatal. Accidents, motor crashes, industrial and residential accidents are the greatest sources of burns. For the most part, the longer the patient is in contact with the burning agent, the more severe the burn. The type and temperature of the agent inflicting the burn also affects the degree and extent of the resulting damage. If the patient has received other additional injuries, they may complicate the patient's recovery or contribute to his death.

# BURN INJURIES

## Thermal Burns

Comprising 60% of the burn injuries, thermal or heat mechanisms are flame, scalds, contact, steam, and flash burns. The seriousness of the burn is determined by five factors: Evaluating the depth/damage to the skin; calculating the total body surface area (TBSA); involvement of critical areas (hands, feet, face, genitalia); patient's age (very young or very old), the patient's general health and additional trauma status.

### Burn Depth

Burn depth is commonly referred to by degree: first, second and third. Another reference is skin thickness: superficial, partial and full. As stated before, burn depth assessment at admission is only an estimate, and the actual identification of the burn severity may take 3 to 5 days because of the status of Zone 2, stasis.

**First Degree:** Only the superficial epidermis is injured with minimal damage. The skin has mild erythema, no blistering, and there is no burning through the layers of skin. The epidermis may peel in small scales without scarring. Discomfort resolves in a day or two. Sunburn is a good example of a first-degree burn.

**Second Degree:** Also known as a partial-thickness burn, the entire epidermis and layers of the dermis are damaged. The entire dermis is not destroyed, nor is there damage to the subcutaneous layer. The skin is erythematous, edematous, and painful. Blisters will form. The burn heals in 7 to 14 days as the epithelial layer regenerates. Scalds most commonly are second-degree burns.

Middle and deep burns extend to the deeper dermal layers, leaving little tissue intact. Less painful than more superficial burns because of some nerve damage, blisters are not usually seen. The skin is reddened and has extensive weeping of plasma. Spontaneous healing may take from weeks to months to resolve, often leaving dense scarring.

**Third Degree:** Full-thickness of the epidermis and dermis is destroyed, and damage may extend through or beyond the subcutaneous fat. The burned area may appear waxy; dry; leathery; or discolored brown, white, or charred. Clotted blood vessels may be seen under the burned skin. Subcutaneous fat may be exposed. Ability for this area to spontaneously reepithelialize is destroyed. The contact burn area (Zone 1) is not painful because superficial nerve endings and blood vessels have been destroyed. However, the surrounding, less severely burned area will be extremely painful. The affected area requires debridement and skin grafting in order to heal.

Associated injuries often happen when people are trying to escape from a burning structure. Although easily missed, orthopedic injuries are common. Explosions may cause blunt chest and abdominal injuries. Other injuries occur after jumping or falling from heights. Evidence of inhalation injury should be looked for, especially if the patient was in a closed space. Look for possible injuries that may have occurred related to the circumstances of the patient being burned.

### Total Body Surface Area (TBSA)

**Rule of Nines:** The extent or amount of body surface area affected by thermal or chemical burns is calculated by using the Rule of Nines *(see Figure 14-2)*. Using this formula permits rapid, accurate assessment. The system divides the body into sections, each representing approximately 9% of the total body surface area. Obviously, because of different body proportions, the rule is modified in infants and small children, pregnant women, and some other patients.

Electrical injuries are more difficult to evaluate, due to the fact that surface area may be considerably less than the underlying damage.

The general formula for determining the TBSA:

Each upper extremity is counted as 9%.

Each lower extremity is considered 18%.

The torso front is 18%; the back is 18%.

Genitals and perineum are 1%.

When assessing small burns, an area comparable to the size of the patient's hand is equal to 1%.

### Involvement of Burn Areas

According to *Emergency Care and Transportation of the Sick and Injured:*

**Minor Burns:** Third-degree burns involving less than 2% TBSA or second-degree burns involving less than 15% TBSA fall into this group.

**Moderate Burns:** Although not critical, these burns are serious injuries. Included are third-degree burns involving 2–10% TBSA (excluding hands, feet, face, or genitalia); second-degree burns involving 15–25% TBSA; and first-degree burns involving 50–75% TBSA. Children with a second-degree burn of 10–20% TBSA or first-degree burns involving 50–75% TSBA are in this category.

**Critical Burns:** This is the most serious category, and includes all burns complicated by fractures or any respiratory damage. Any third-degree burn involving hands, feet, face, or genitalia over more than 10% TBSA or a second-degree burn over more than 25% TBSA is considered critical. In children, any third-degree burn or a second-degree burn involving more than 20% TBSA is also considered critical. A moderate burn in a critically ill or elderly patient is also considered to be in this category.

### Scald Burns

Scalds are the most common of all burns. Water at 140°F for 3 seconds will cause a deep partial or full-thickness burn. Liquid temperature of 156°F will cause the same burn in only 1 second. To illustrate with everyday liquids used in the home, just-brewed coffee is 180°F, as are soups and sauces. Liquids of thick consistency stick to the skin longer and, therefore, burn longer. Cooking oil and grease can reach temperatures of up to 400°F.

In the case of an immersion burn, such as a bath, even though the water may be cooler than 140°F, the contact with the skin lasts longer.

## FIGURE 14-2
## Characterization of Burns and Their Prognosis

### Abbreviated Burn Severity Index*

The Abbreviated Burn Severity Index (ABSI) is a five-variable scale that may be used as a quick reference for evaluation of burn injury severity. The five variables are patient sex, age, presence of inhalation injury, presence of full-thickness burn, and percentage total body surface area burned. The score, which may be calculated in less than one minute, is derived by summation of the coded values for each of the five variables. The total score may then be related to severity of burn injury and to probability of survival. An ABSI score of six or greater, high-voltage electrical burns, burns associated with other major injuries, or full-thickness burns to the face, axillae, joints, hands, feet, or genitalia should be considered for treatment in a hospital with special expertise in burn care. Aids for evaluation of depth of burn and percentage of total body surface area burned are located on the back of this card.

| Sex | Female | 1 |
| | Male | 0 |
| Age | 0-20 Years | 1 |
| | 21-40 Years | 2 |
| | 41-60 Years | 3 |
| | 61-80 Years | 4 |
| | ≥81 Years | 5 |
| **Inhalation Injury Present** | | 1 |
| **Full-Thickness Burn** | | 1 |
| **Total Body Surface Area Burned** | 1%- 10% | 1 |
| | 11%- 20% | 2 |
| | 21%- 30% | 3 |
| | 31%- 40% | 4 |
| | 41%- 50% | 5 |
| | 51%- 60% | 6 |
| | 61%- 70% | 7 |
| | 71%- 80% | 8 |
| | 81%- 90% | 9 |
| | 91%-100% | 10 |

### Total Burn Score

| Score | Probability of Survival | Score | Probability of Survival |
|---|---|---|---|
| 2-3 | ≥99% | 8-9 | 50-70% |
| 4-5 | 98% | 10-11 | 20-40% |
| 6-7 | 80-90% | ≥12 | ≤10% |

*Adapted from Edlich RF, Rodeheaver GT, Halfacre SE, Tobiasen JA, Boyd DR. Systems conceptualization of burn care on a regional basis. *Topics in Emergency Medicine* 3(3):7-15. 1961

### Clinical Diagnosis of Depth of Burn Injury*

| | Full thickness | Deep partial thickness | Superficial partial thickness |
|---|---|---|---|
| **Appearance** | Brown with thrombosed veins | White | Pink with blisters |
| **Hair** | Absent | Absent | Present |
| **Biomechanical properties** | Depressed and leathery | Elevated, soft and pliable | Elevated, soft and pliable |
| **Sensation** | None | Pressure | Light touch, pinprick, and pressure |
| **Pain** | Painless | Painful | Exquisitely painful |

*Adapted from Tobiasen JM, Hiebert JM, Sacco WJ, Edlich RF. Burn injury severity scoring systems. *Current Concepts in Trauma Care* 4(1) 5-8. 1981

### Percentage of Total Body Surface Area Burned

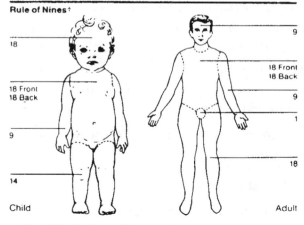

Rule of Nines†

† Adapted from Edlich RF, Haynes BW, Larkam N, Allen MS, Ruffin W Jr, Hiebert J, Edgerton MT. Emergency department treatment, triage and transfer protocols for the burn patient. *Journal of American College of Emergency Physicians* 7(4): 152-158. 1978

*Reprinted with permission from* Edlich, R. F., Glassberg, H. H. & Tobiasen, J. A. (1994). *Current Concepts in Trauma Care, 7*(1), 20.

### Flame Burns

The second most frequent cause of burns is flames. While residential fires have decreased due to public education, detectors and improved fire codes, careless smoking, clothing ignited by stoves or space heaters and motor vehicle crashes still contribute to a significant number of flame burns. Outdoor flame burns are often secondary to improper use of camping stoves, smoking in a sleeping bag, use of lanterns in tents and the use of gasoline or kerosene on a charcoal fire.

### Flash Burns

Flash burns are caused by explosions of natural gas, propane, gasoline or other flammable liquids. There is brief, intense heat. The burns are mostly partial thickness, but the depth of the burn is related to the amount and kind of fuel involved.

### Contact Burns

Direct contact with a hot object or a vapor such as steam can cause a serious burn. The burns are not usually extensive but can be deep. Examples of mechanisms of injury are machine-press burns, often also associated with crush injuries; hot tar; hot tools; and burners on a stove. Children may put their hand on a stove burner, hot steam iron, curling iron, or hair dryer.

## Light Burns

Exposure to extreme light focuses on the retina, significantly damaging the sensory cells. Infrared rays, laser beams and looking directly at the sun, even during an eclipse, can cause an injury resulting in permanent damage.

Ultraviolet rays from an arc welding unit, prolonged exposure to a sunlamp, or the reflection of sun on snow (snow blindness), can cause a superficial burn of the eyes. Although not painful at the time of the burn, 3 to 5 hours later extreme pain from corneal damage will be felt by the patient. The patient develops severe conjunctivitis, swelling and excessive tearing.

Each eye should be covered with a sterile, moist pad.

## Chemical Burns

Toxic substances in contact with the skin or inhaled result in chemical burns.

### Topical Burns

Chemicals cause denaturing of the protein (protein loses some of its chemical and physical properties, just as cooking an egg white denatures the albumen) in tissues, or a desiccation (drying) of the cells. In chemical burns, the type of chemical, concentration, and length of time of exposure all affect the extent of the burn.

Most chemical burns are caused by strong acids or alkalis coming in direct contact with the skin or through clothing.

Alkali burns cause more damage than acids because they are corrosive and are able to combine with water. With their ability to combine with water and action on fatty acids, alkaline burns cause rapid, deep destruction of tissue. Tissue is "gelatinized," turning grayish in color, with a soapy, slippery feel.

While acids can be washed off the skin's surface, alkalis combine with the water and continue burning until the chemical itself is totally removed from the patient. If the alkali is powdered, such as lime, it should be brushed off the skin before beginning to flush. A dry alkali chemical activated by the addition of water will cause more damage to the skin than when dry.

In order to stop the chemical burning process, the chemical has to be removed from the areas of contact with the patient. Flooding of the area should begin as soon as possible. The water used for flushing should be contained and not allowed to empty into the general drainage system. A forceful stream of water will further damage the tissues, so gentle flushing is best.

Clothing should be removed immediately, taking care not to get the chemical on the caregiver. The patient will feel better as soon as the flushing begins, but flooding should continue for at least 10 minutes to ensure all of the chemical is removed. The affected area should be flushed until a litmus test is neutral. Following the flushing, the burned area should be covered with sterile, dry dressings.

In most cases, the flushing of chemicals will be started either in an industrial area especially equipped with showers or hoses for this purpose or by the prehospital emergency crew en route to the emergency department.

### Inhalation Injuries

Inhalation of chemical fumes can cause serious problems. As discussed earlier in the section on pathophysiology, carbon monoxide is particularly dangerous and often occurs when a person is trapped in a closed building. Other sources of carbon monoxide inhalation are auto fumes and heating appliances.

Carbon monoxide inhalation is different than smoke inhalation. It is a deadly poisonous gas, without smell or taste and can be inhaled without the victim's awareness.

Early in carbon monoxide poisoning, while in the fire situation or just after, the patient feels few symptoms that he perceives as serious: some muscle weakness and mild dyspnea. The patient may become confused. Later signs of carbon monoxide poisoning are pink to cherry red skin, tachycardia, tachypnea, headache, dizziness and nausea.

Blood gasses should be drawn to measure the level of carboxyhemoglobin, the compound formed by carbon monoxide and hemoglobin in carbon monoxide poisoning. Levels below 15% rarely have symptoms and are often seen in heavy smokers. Symptoms such as headache and confusion are seen in levels ranging from 15–40%. Greater than 40% blood levels may result in coma. If the patient is thought to have carbon monoxide poisoning, 100% oxygen should be given, and hyperbaric chamber treatment may be ordered. Watch the patient carefully; as he may suddenly develop respiratory arrest.

Other chemical inhalation problems were discussed earlier in the pathophysiology section.

## Electrical Burns

### Electric Shock

Electrical burns are caused by low- or high-voltage contact, ranging from ordinary household current to utility power lines. Most electrical burns in the home are from the careless use of appliances or faulty equipment. Small children stick their fingers into electrical outlets or bite into electrical cords. Storms downing power lines that are lying in water or across an automobile is another example.

In order to cause a burn, electricity must enter the body at one point and exit at another point. As electricity passes through the body, it meets resistance from the body tissues and is converted to heat. The heat generated is in direct proportion to the amperage of the current and the electrical resistance of the body parts.

As electricity passes through the skin, it leaves a burn at the entry and exit sites. There may be extensive internal injury between these sites. The amount of internal tissue injury is usually more extensive than indicated by the appearance of the skin wound. Severe damage may be done to the deeper tissues.

The heart, lungs and brain can be damaged immediately after the body receives a shock. A burn may be followed by cardiac arrest due to a disruption in the normal electrical rhythm of the heart. Nerves, blood vessels and muscles are less resistant and more likely to be damaged than bone or fat. The nervous system is particularly vulnerable to electrical burns. Damage to the brain, spinal cord and myelin-producing cells can cause transverse myelitis, an acute form of myelitis involving the entire thickness of the spinal cord.

Electric current may cause violent muscle contractions resulting in fractures or dislocations. The shock may also cause the patient to fall to the ground and incur additional injury. High-voltage electricity can cause such severe destruction to muscles and skin that amputation is necessary.

Cardiopulmonary resuscitation may be the first intervention necessary with a patient who has sustained an electrical shock. If CPR is not necessary, further interventions can be initiated. Dry, sterile dressings should be placed on the burn wounds, and fractures should be immobilized. Further burn and trauma management is relative to the damage the patient has incurred.

*Lightning*

Lightning is a specific form of electrical burn. It has a force of thousands of volts. The strike lasts only for a fraction of a second and is not always fatal.

The high-voltage lightning strike involves the whole body. A superficial characteristic burn is usually on the skin at the site of the strike, but the burn itself, is rarely deep. However, many body systems are affected, especially the nervous and cardiovascular systems.

Most persons struck by lightning are immediately knocked unconscious and have no memory of being hit. Patients may experience numbness, tingling, partial or complete paralysis, blindness, loss of hearing, difficulty speaking, or being unable to speak at all. These problems usually resolve themselves.

The greatest concern with a lightning strike is the electrical disturbance causing a severely disrupted heart rhythm leading to ventricular fibrillation or full cardiac arrest. The absence of a heartbeat indicates vigorous resuscitation attempts should begin, because an arrest caused by dysrhythmia is often reversible. Patients can be successfully resuscitated with immediate and correct CPR techniques.

## Nuclear Radiation Burns

Nuclear reaction energy causes several types of injuries. Solar radiation causes burns similar to thermal burns. The heat from atomic explosions also produces burns similar to thermal burns. Exposure to radioactive chemicals and materials that result in acute burns have accompanying problems, including chronic illness or death.

*Radiation Burns*

Ionizing radiation from the sun passes through the ozone layer of the atmosphere and is able to cause a burn injury. The burns are not often serious and rarely worse than a first-degree burn. If a large portion of the body is affected, discomfort may develop, along with mild hypotension.

*Nuclear Radiation Exposure*

We are all exposed to some nuclear radiation through cosmic rays and natural radioactive materials.

Since the development of nuclear power, many people work with highly radioactive materials. Transportation of radioactive materials also provides an opportunity for accidental exposure.

The main concern regarding radiation accidents is to remove the radiation source from the patient or move the patient or patients away from the radiation source. If radioactive material has been spilled on clothing, it should be removed and stored in special containers. Then the patient should shower in a designated area. Care should be taken to contain the radioactive material.

Any other injuries should be assessed and appropriate interventions taken.

Hospitals are required to have policies and procedures regarding hazardous material treatment and disposal.

# ASSESSMENT

## Assessment Principles

- A detailed history; is essential. It should always be assumed that burn patients have associated blunt injuries.

- Assume burn patients have an inhalation injury. If in doubt, intubate early.

- Remember that formulas for the calculation of fluid requirements are only estimates. The best gauge to estimate adequate volume replacement is adequate urine output.

- Do not give glucose in replacement fluids.

- Avoid subcutaneous injections; they are not effective.

Throughout this chapter, assessment and management points relevant to specific kinds of burns have been included with relevant burn information. Included below is general advice for the evaluation of burn patients.

Neck stabilization and the ABCs should be conducted and followed with continuous monitoring because of the burn patient's potential for airway edema and respiratory and cardiac arrest. Immediately assess the patient for pulmonary/inhalation problems.

## Assessing a Burn Injury

### Seriousness of the Burn is Determined by Five Factors:

**Depth of Burn:** Evaluate the depth/damage of the burn. Estimate first-, second- or third-degree burn injury; partial- or full-thickness burn depth. Definitive burn severity can only be identified after 3 to 5 days when the status of Zone 2, stasis, has stabilized.

**Extent of Burn Injury:** The extent of thermal and chemical burn injuries is quickly and accurately assessed by using the Rule of Nines. Keep in mind that adjustments are made for infants and small children, pregnant women and other specific patients.

**Involvement of Critical Areas:** Determine the involvement of critical areas affected (percent of TBSA, hands, feet, face and genitalia) along with the factors of fractures and respiratory injury, plus the degree of burn depth.

**Patient Age:** Very young and very old patients tend to have more complications and are more adversely affected by burns.

**Patient Status:** Observe and gather information regarding the patient's general health status and the presence of other injuries either previous to, or along with, the burn injuries.

The patient's temperature should be taken initially and monitored serially.

Assess all other injuries the patient has, including respiratory difficulty and fractures.

Examine for full-thickness burns surrounding the chest. Look for tight, leathery eschar, or sloughing, encircling the chest, causing inadequate chest expansion.

If the source of the burns was flames, carbon monoxide poisoning or smoke, inhalation damage should be suspected. Inspect the oropharynx and vocal cords for edema, redness, blisters and carbon particles. Observe the patient for restlessness; confusion; muscle weakness; dyspnea; difficulty swallowing; increasing hoarseness; and rapid, shallow respirations.

Arterial blood gasses should be drawn for carboxyhemoglobin levels.

Be aware of the potential for the development of adult respiratory distress syndrome (ARDS), although it is not likely to develop until at least 18 hours after the burn. Signs of ARDS are decreased oxygenation, increased secretions, tachypnea, confusion, and increasing patchy infiltrates.

Assess for other injuries or problems that may affect breathing: pneumothorax, tension pneumothorax, hemothorax and flail chest. They may occur in conjunction with an explosion or motor vehicle crash.

Evaluate for circulatory problems such as decreased capillary refill, lack of distal pulses and paresthesias. A Doppler can be used to check the distal pulses. Because burn tissue cannot stretch, the edema beneath the burned tissue will compromise circulation.

Obtain the history as time and the patient's condition permit. When possible, document the circumstances of the incident.

Additionally,

- What preexisting medical problems does the patient have?

- What medications is the patient taking?

Allergies?

- When was the patient's last tetanus shot?

- Are there toxic materials on the patient or his clothing?

# NURSING STRATEGIES FOR THE PATIENT WITH BURN INJURIES

If the patient has been exposed to radiation or toxic materials, strictly follow policies and procedures regarding safety practices.

In the prehospital situation, it is extremely important to stop further burning from occurring. Either the patient should be removed from the cause of the burn, or the burning agent should be removed from the patient. Immediate transport to the emergency facility is top priority after neck stabilization and the ABCs.

If the patient arrives at the emergency department via rescue unit, he will have received a preliminary assessment, an intravenous line running, 100% oxygen, and he may be intubated. The patient should be on a continuous electrocardiogram.

Other injuries may have occurred in addition to the burn. For instance, when a person tries to escape a burning building, he may jump from a height, sustaining one or more fractures, or a spinal cord injury. Blunt chest and abdominal injuries may occur from an explosion, jumping or falling from a height. Depending upon the severity of the other injuries compared to burn severity, set priorities to stabilize and manage the other injuries. Consider the patient a trauma victim with a serious burn injury and the trauma injuries are not as likely to be missed.

## Airway

Signs of respiratory difficulties and impending obstruction call for early intubation, before complete obstruction occurs. Tracheostomy is not advised because edema adds to the difficulty of the procedure.

## Breathing

Burns of the chest may limit the ability of the chest wall to expand. Gas exchange will be inadequate. If the patient has eschar, or sloughing, surgical incisions in the tissue are made by the physician to release the eschar and expose the underlying subcutaneous tissue. There will be immediate improvement in the chest wall expansion. Because the eschar is a full-thickness burn, the nerve endings are burned and general anesthesia is not necessary for the eschar release. Escharotomy is conducted with intravenous narcotic analgesia. Significant bleeding may occur with escharotomy, which is controlled with cautery or hemostats. After completion of the procedure, topical antibacterial agents are applied, followed by light pressure dressings. After an extremity has an escharotomy, elevate the limb slightly (Newberry, 1998).

When a patient with carbon monoxide intoxication does not respond to high-flow oxygen within an hour or hour and a half, hyperbaric oxygen therapy may be necessary.

Adult respiratory distress syndrome is acute pulmonary congestion and atelectasis with hyaline membrane formation. If the patient develops ARDS, interventions include intubation and ventilation with positive end expiratory pressure. Bronchodilators may be administered. Corticosteroids should not be given to patients with burns and smoke inhalation; they can increase morbidity and mortality.

## Circulation

All patients with full-thickness burns are monitored for circulatory problems. Hypovolemia in the burn patient occurs due to fluid loss and fluid movement from vasodilation and increased capillary permeability.

One or two large-bore intravenous catheters should be placed, preferably not in the leg because of the risk of thrombophlebitis. Peripheral IVs may be inserted into burn tissue if no other access is available, but only as a last resort.

Isotonic salt solutions are recommended for IV administration (Peitzman et al., 1998). Glucose solutions should not be given, because burn patients can be hyperglycemic and glucose intolerant.

There is no standard formula for calculating fluid resuscitation in patients with electrical injuries. It is important to increase the urine output in order to excrete myoglobin. Mannitol® may be given to increase urine flow once urine output is confirmed. Ringer's lactated solution is the IV fluid used.

If the patient has signs of circulation compromise, escharotomy may be indicated.

## Temperature Regulation

Skin is the main organ for regulation of body temperature. A burn can disrupt or destroy this function. Further heat loss can occur from the flushing of burned tissue, administration of intravenous fluids, and the cool environment of the emergency department.

Keep heat loss at a minimum by covering the patient with sterile sheets, using warmed IV fluids, increasing the room temperature or using an overhead warmer.

## Wound Care

Remove jewelry and constrictive clothing, but delay wound care until the patient's status has stabilized. Emergency departments have burn packs containing sterile sheets. Cover the patient with the sterile sheets.

Superficial burns are painful but do not require any special wound care. Topical or oral analgesics may used.

Partial and full-thickness burns require a variety of interventions, depending upon the burn: topical antimicrobial agents, such as Silvadene®, Sulfamyalon®, silver nitrate solution, gentamicin, and bacitracin; excision and primary closure; and excision and grafting.

Thermal burns are cleaned with clean or sterile water with 0.25 strength Betadine® using clean cloths or coarse gauze dressings. If directed by the physician, blisters larger than a half-dollar are broken and removed, except on the hands and soles of the feet. Hair should be shaved from burns and nearby areas, followed by covering with topical antibiotic ointment, such as Silvadene® or bacitracin.

Chemical burns, as discussed earlier, are irrigated immediately with tap water or saline for at least 10 minutes, or until the chemical is completely removed from the skin. Include irrigating areas adjacent to the burns, as they may be injured but will not show signs of pain, blistering or erythema. After complete flushing, treat the same as a thermal burn.

Chemical burns of the eye are a serious emergency. The eye must be irrigated thoroughly with copious amounts of water or saline. An ophthalmology consult is required immediately.

Tar or asphalt burns range from superficial to deep injuries. Immediately cool the tar, but do not peel from the skin. Mineral oil, petroleum jelly, antiseptic ointment or a solvent will loosen the tar.

Electrical injuries may have muscle injury but little external tissue loss. However, electrical burns can be ugly. Cleanse the wounds gently with water or saline with Betadine. Debridement usually is not required immediately. Light dressings may be used to cover the wounds, but should not get in the way of circulatory assessment. The extremities can have considerable damage and tissue swelling, putting the patient at risk for compartment syndrome, which is indicated by pain, pallor, paresthesia, pulselessness and paralysis. Use extreme care handling the limbs, as the large vessels can tear, leading to massive hemorrhage. Monitor electrocardiograms for dysrhythmias.

Do not give the patient anything by mouth. Surgical intervention may need to be immediate and the risk of aspiration should be prevented.

# EXAMPLES OF NURSING DIAGNOSES RELATED TO BURN INJURY

- Potential for hypovolemia related to increased capillary permeability, edema, insensible fluid loss, and fluid shift

- Impairment of tissue perfusion related to vascular fluid shifts, increased capillary permeability, edema and decreased oxygen availability to the tissues

- Inadequate airway clearance related to upper airway obstruction caused by intrinsic or extrinsic edema and tissue damage

- Impaired gas exchange related to carbon monoxide intoxication

- High risk for hypothermia related to burn injuries, flushing of burned tissue, administration of intravenous fluids and a cold environment

- High risk for infection related to wounds open to bacteria and foreign bodies

- Intense pain related to injury sustained from burns

- Disfigurement and loss of function related to burn damage

- Anxiety related to pain and fears of damage from burn injury

# SUMMARY

Burns are potentially the most painful and serious injuries that a person can sustain. They are defined as occurring when the body receives more energy than it can absorb without damage.

Burns have a variety of causes: thermal, including scalds, flame, flash and contact; light; electrical, including shock and lightning; chemical, including contact and inhalation; nuclear; and frostbite.

The seriousness of the burn is determined by five factors: evaluation of the burn's depth and damage; extent of injury; involvement of critical areas; patient age; and the patient's general health and current injury status.

Associated injuries are common, including falls from a height, fractures and violent muscle contractions. Infections are a high risk with open wounds and foreign bodies. Pulmonary disorders from inhalation damage lead to many deaths. Disfigurement from burns can be grotesque and change or destroy the quality of the patient's life.

Actions taken by medical personnel have tremendous physical and emotional impact on the burn patient. Solid knowledge of assessment and management priorities can prevent further damage and potentially save the patient's life.

# EXAM QUESTIONS

## CHAPTER 14
### Questions 66–70

66. The skin

    a. is a true organ.

    b. functions as the main regulator of the body's temperature.

    c. serves to protect the body with its water-tight quality.

    d. does all of these things.

67. Pulmonary response to smoke inhalation

    a. causes bronchial asthma.

    b. causes a syndrome with three specific problems of carbon monoxide intoxication, upper airway obstruction and chemical damage to lower airways.

    c. is easily cleared with 100% oxygen administration.

    d. is only a problem in the elderly patient.

68. Which of the following assessment principle applies to burn victims?

    a. A detailed history is essential; it should always be assumed that burn patients have associated blunt injuries.

    b. Only thermal burn patients have inhalation injuries.

    c. Glucose is the intravenous solution of choice in burn patients because of hypovolemia.

    d. All burn patients have myoglobin damage.

69. A patient who has been in an industrial explosion is brought in to the emergency department. He is burned on his entire front torso, both legs, genitals and arms. What percent TBSA has been burned?

    a. 73%

    b. 49%

    c. 18%+18%

    d. None of the above

70. Which of the following statements is true?

    a. Signs of respiratory difficulties occur 18 to 24 hours after the patient has been burned.

    b. It is only necessary to have an electrical burn patient on continuous electrocardiogram until the ABC assessment is completed.

    c. If a patient with carbon monoxide intoxication does not respond to 100% oxygen within an hour and a half, hyperbaric oxygen therapy may be necessary.

    d. ARDS develops immediately after inhalation exposure.

# CHAPTER 15

# PEDIATRIC TRAUMA AND CHILD MALTREATMENT

## CHAPTER OBJECTIVE

Upon completion of this chapter, the reader will be able to identify the important strategies in management of pediatric patients suffering traumatic injuries.

## LEARNING OBJECTIVES

Upon completion of this chapter, the reader should be able to:

1. Identify normal vital signs and some unique characteristics of children.

2. Identify mechanisms of injury seen in children.

3. Recognize the hallmarks of child maltreatment.

4. Identify appropriate basic nursing strategies in pediatric trauma.

5. Indicate examples of nursing diagnoses for potentially life-threatening conditions caused by pediatric injuries.

## INTRODUCTION

It is often said in the field of pediatrics that children are not little adults. This **is** true. Children do have unique anatomic and physiologic characteristics. There are biophysical, psychosocial, and cognitive differences that distinguish them from grown-ups.

Trauma deaths in children and adolescents have now exceeded infectious diseases as the leading killer in ages 1 to 19 years old, causing over half of all the childhood deaths. These deaths are a major public health issue because most of them are preventable.

Each year in this country, 16 million children are seen in emergency departments. Of these, 15,000 die, 200,000 are temporarily disabled, and 30,000 to 100,000 are permanently disabled (Soud & Rogers, 1998; Peitzman et al., 1998).

In the United States in 1993, motor vehicle crashes were the leading cause of death in children and adolescents from ages 5 to 19 years old. Homicide was the leading cause of death for children 0 to 4 years old and young adults 20 to 24 years of age. Statistics in 1994 showed that the most common victims of violent crime were young people from 12 to 17 years of age. The crimes included rape, robbery, and assault, which occurred five times as often as in adults over 35 years old.

Child maltreatment seems to be increasing dramatically. Whether the statistics are due to better identification and reporting or an actual increase in abuse and neglect is unclear. A survey in this country in 1992 by the National Center on the Prevention of Child Abuse (NCPCA) found that approximately 3 million child maltreatment cases were reported to Child Protective Service (CPS) agencies, an increase of 6% over the previous year. The agency (NCPCA) reports that between 1985 and 1992 there was a 50% increase in cases reported to Child Protective Service agencies.

Medical expenses are in the billions of dollars, not to mention the costs to society. Pediatric trauma care is more costly than trauma care for adults, including hospitalization, resources for rehabilitation, mainstreaming the child back into society, and the years of potential work loss. Prevention is less expensive and more beneficial.

A visit to the emergency department for the child and his family is emotionally and physically challenging, regardless of the severity of the illness or injury. Sudden illness or injury, especially if serious, along with diagnostic and therapeutic interventions can be very stressful and anxiety producing. The environment is often chaotic and frightening. The equipment is frightening. Personnel usually have little time to comfort the patient and family. All of these factors further complicate the treatment and care of the pediatric patient.

On the other hand, the emergency department staff must have the ability to quickly identify potentially life-threatening situations. In order to conduct a rapid, accurate and effective clinical assessment of the injured child, the caregiver must have a thorough knowledge and understanding of the normal growth and development processes. The initial approach and continuing care of the child and adolescent are guided by the developmental level of the patient. The family or guardian should be included in this process.

In addition to interventions and management of the patient's injuries, a nurse's comprehensive knowledge of hospital and community resources that are able to help meet the patient and family's needs, will make a significant difference in how the patient handles treatment and recovery.

# EPIDEMIOLOGY AND MECHANISMS OF INJURY

The major declines in death rates during childhood are related to immunization, detection and improved management of diseases and medical disorders. Deaths from injuries have not shown the same dramatic declines because injuries have traditionally been thought of as unavoidable accidents or behavioral situations rather than health problems.

Until recently, relatively little money and resources have been allocated or received a high priority to deal with other than medical problems. It has only been in recent years that "accidental" deaths from motor vehicle crashes, drowning, burns, firearms, poisonings, sports injuries and so forth have been perceived as preventable. It is now recognized that pediatric trauma is not an "accident" or random occurrence, but the result of predictable behavior or a potentially dangerous environment.

Motor vehicle accidents are the leading cause of deaths for children from 5 through 19 years old. Although the gender distribution is equal from 5 to 14 years, after that age, young men are two to three times more likely to die in vehicular crashes.

At least 43% of youngsters are unrestrained or improperly restrained in vehicles. Car seats have been found to be used only 41% of the time with toddlers. In a vehicular accident, when unrestrained, young children are thrown around inside the vehicle, receiving injuries to the head, abdomen, chest and extremities. They are at high risk of being thrown through a window. Head injuries are the leading cause of death among unrestrained children. When children are held on the lap of an adult, they can be crushed between the adult and the dashboard or steering column, or against the front seat if they were backseat lap passengers.

Young children can sustain certain seat belt-related injuries due to their body size and proportion. A greater percent of a child's body size is above the safety belt than with an adult, which allows forward motion and an increased chance of head and neck injury. Children can also jackknife over restraints, causing an airway or hanging injury.

Air bags have contributed to serious injuries and deaths of infants and young children because they are deployed when the unrestrained child is thrown against the dashboard during rapid deceleration before impact. Air-bag deployment then propels the child against the structures inside the vehicle. Infants riding in rear-facing safety seats should never ride in the front seat of a car or truck with a passenger-side air bag.

All-terrain vehicles (ATVs), snowmobiles, farm equipment and riding lawn mowers can be dangerous vehicles and all cause serious injuries and deaths. Whether a young child is riding as a passenger or an older child is operating these vehicles, terrible injuries or death can occur either from carelessness or lack of skill.

Injuries to the head are the most frequent and cause the most fatalities in bicycle-related accidents. Of more than 2,300 children under 14 years old with bicycle-related injuries that were reported to the National Pediatric Trauma Registry (during a 3 year period), 54% sustained head injuries. In the past few years, education and legislation mandating helmet use has held a high focus of attention. In many cities, anyone riding a bicycle without a helmet will receive a law enforcement ticket and/or other punishment.

Skateboarding and rollerblading contribute to multiple injuries. Physically, children have a high center of gravity, which interferes with their ability to break a fall. Pediatricians recommend that children under 5 not use skateboards because they do not have a well-developed neuromuscular system.

Additionally, they have poor judgment and are unable to effectively protect themselves from injury. Skateboarders should always wear the proper protective equipment and stay out of traffic.

Pedestrian injuries in 5 through 9 year olds are the second greatest killer. Walking, running, crossing a street and entering or leaving a school bus make up most of the injuries, and occur most often in the afternoon and early evening. When children are struck by a vehicle, a triad of injuries, known as Waddell's triad, occur: thoracic abdominal damage from the bumper, extremity injury from hitting the vehicle and the ground, and head injury from landing on the ground. One way to determine the speed of the vehicle is that if the child's shoes have been knocked off, the vehicle was traveling at least 40 miles per hour.

Falls are the most common cause of head injury and trauma-related hospitalization in the young and elderly. Young children receive most fall-related injuries in the home, with cluttered homes, infants in walkers, open windows, stairs, climbing, bunk beds and a myriad of other situations. For children younger than 13 years old, falls from a window, jumping from a bed, stairs and low heights during rough play are the most common mechanisms of injury.

Depression and suicidal behavior are increasing dramatically, and for the adolescent population, has more than doubled in the past few years. Even though depression and suicidal emotional problems may overlap, they are not necessarily synonymous (Soud & Rogers, 1998). Females are more likely to use nonlethal methods such as pills, in suicide attempts, while males are more likely to be successful with lethal means such as firearms and hanging. The most affected group is white males. Unsuccessful attempts are eight times greater than successful attempts.

Homicide is the biggest killer of children from infancy through age 4 and from 20 to 24 years of age. Rates are nearly five times higher in the African-American population than among white children. The youngest children are mostly killed by physical brutality, while the older youths die from firearms. Recently, firearm slayings by children and youth have been increasing at an alarming rate. It is estimated that more than half of all the homes in this country has at least one firearm. Firearms range from traditional urban weapons and military weapons, to recreational pellet guns. Newberry (1998) states that one pediatric trauma center has seen penetrating trauma increase from 20% to 35% over a 7-year period, with an increase from 45% to 66% in the 12 to 15 year age group.

Violence by adults against children and children against children in the home, schools and community is reported on a daily basis. Incidents happen anywhere, within the family or gangs, with or without drugs; nowhere is immune to violence.

The problem of child abuse and neglect is also on the upswing, having tripled from 1976 to 1994. Newberry states that in 1994, over 3 million incidents of suspected child abuse and neglect were reported to Child Protection Services, with nearly half of the cases involving children under 1 year old. On a daily basis, the media reports terrible incidents of abuse, perpetrated by parents, drug addicts, trusted friends, teachers, and members of the clergy.

Child abuse is characterized by torture, injury, maiming, or unreasonable emotional or physical force. Specific markings, bruising patterns and fractures have been identified as hallmarks of physical abuse. Two types of abuse seen with increasing frequency are shaken baby syndrome and Munchausen syndrome by proxy. Neglect is just as much a crime as abuse. Currently, nearly half of all abuse cases also involve neglect.

Available research details the evaluation of events surrounding specific injuries and reveals information that can be used in planning and con-

ducting prevention strategies, education and activities.

# ANATOMY AND PHYSICAL CHARACTERISTICS OF CHILDREN AND ADOLESCENTS

## Physical Growth

The field of pediatrics includes children and adolescents over five developmental stages:

1. Infant development (0–1 year)

2. Toddler development (1–2 years)

3. Preschool development (3–5 years)

4. School-aged development (6–10 years)

5. Adolescent development (11–18 years)

The first year of life sees tremendous changes in growth and development. Average birth weight doubles in 6 months and triples by the end of the year. After that time, weight gain slows to about 2.5 kg (1 kilogram is equal to 2.2 pounds) a year during the preschool and school years. During adolescence, growth spurts occur.

Body proportions vary greatly. The midpoint of an infant's height is the umbilicus and in an adult it is the symphysis pubis. The child, therefore, has a higher center of gravity. The infant's head is large in relation to his body, allowing a significant amount of heat to be lost through the scalp. The combination of a large head and high center of gravity causes the infant and young child to have poor balance control and be predisposed to falls.

## Metabolism, Fluid and Electrolyte Balance

Fluid distribution in infants is different than that of the adult. Seventy-five percent of the infant's weight is water, compared to 60% to 70% in the adult. The infant also has a greater proportion of extracellular fluid than the older child or adult, with a daily turnover of water being more than half of his extracellular volume.

Infants and young children have a metabolic rate two to three times greater than older children and adults. Therefore, their caloric, fluid, and oxygen needs are greater. Increased fluid needs and fluid turnover can bring about rapid deficits during periods of decreased fluid intake or increased fluid loss. Dehydration quickly follows.

Greater metabolic demands of the young child, along with immature organ development, affect the ability to metabolize and excrete drugs and toxins. The immature liver of the infant may not metabolize drugs, such as acetaminophen, as quickly as in the older child.

After the neonatal period, normal serum electrolyte and blood gas levels are about the same in children and adults. Some imbalances in children tend to be more common and potentially cause more problems.

## Thermoregulation

Increased heat loss from the relatively large body surface area-to-weight ratio and the limited ability to produce heat make it difficult for infants and small children to maintain their body temperatures. The large head size accounts for a high percent of surface area and heat loss. Infants under 6 months old are not able to shiver. Non-shivering thermogenesis in the production of heat increases oxygen consumption and can lead to hypoxia.

Additional complications of hypothermia are lactic acidosis, hypoglycemia, pulmonary vasoconstriction and left to right cardiac shunting.

## Respiratory System

Newborns normally have adequate pulmonary structures to support oxygenation and ventilation. However, the small airway size and an immature immune system increase the possibility of obstruction and respiratory disorders.

### Airway

The upper and lower airways of the infant and small child are considerably smaller than an adult's, with the trachea only being the size of the infant's pinky finger. The neck is short and the tongue is large. It takes just a small amount of mucus, a small foreign object or slight tissue edema to close off the airway.

Infants are nose breathers for the first few months of life and nasal congestion can bring on signs of respiratory distress.

A jaw thrust or chin lift will open the infant or young child's airway. Nasal airways are usually not effective because of the infant's small air passages.

A child's ribs are flexible and do not adequately support or protect the lungs. Blunt trauma to the chest usually results in rib contusions instead of fractures. When there are rib fractures, severe internal trauma is also likely.

### Breathing

Children under 7 or 8 years of age breathe with their diaphragms or abdomens. The diaphragm is the child's primary muscle of respiration because the intercostal muscles are poorly developed and contribute little to chest wall movement. In respiratory distress, the diaphragmatic breathing and pliable ribs cause the chest wall to move inward, or retract, during inspiration.

Crying children tend to swallow air, causing gastric distention. The thin chest wall transmits breath sounds easily, making accurate respiratory assessment difficult.

Respiratory rates and oxygen consumption in children is higher because of their faster metabolic rates. Infants and young children have fewer and smaller alveoli than adults, consequently, less pulmonary reserve. Due to diminished respiratory reserve and higher oxygen requirements, untreated respiratory distress can rapidly turn into respiratory failure.

---

**TABLE 15-1**
**Normal Ranges of Vital Signs in Children**

| Age | Pulse (beats per minute) | Respiration (breaths/min) | Blood Pressure (mm Hg) |
|---|---|---|---|
| 0–2 months | 120–140 | 30–50 | 50–60 systolic |
| 2 months–1 year | 110–130 | 25–40 | 70–80 systolic |
| 1–3 years | 100–110 | 20–30 | 80 systolic |
| 3–5 years | 90–100 | 20–30 | 80–90 systolic |
| Above 5 years | 80–100 | 15–30 | 90–100 systolic |

*Reprinted with permission from* Kitt, S. & Kaiser, J. (1995). *Emergency nursing: A physiologic and clinical perspective.* Philadelphia: Saunders.

---

## Cardiovascular System

The child's normal cardiovascular system has anatomic and physiologic differences from the adult's that affect the child's response to stress.

Blood volume, while actually small in the child, is relatively greater than the adult's. It does not take a great deal of blood loss in the child to impair perfusion and decrease circulating volume. Even with serious blood loss, large cardiac reserve and catecholamine response will maintain a normal blood pressure (catecholamines, are active amines, epinephrine and norepinephrine that have a marked effect on the nervous and cardiovascular systems, metabolic rate, temperature, and smooth muscle). Not until 20% to 25% of the circulating volume is lost does hypotension become evident. Hypotension is a late sign of hypovolemia and indicates impending cardiac arrest.

Higher metabolic and oxygen demands in children require higher cardiac output per kilogram. When oxygen decreases, tachycardia is the response. If tachycardia does not increase oxygen delivery, tissue hypoxia and hypercapnia develop. Bradycardia follows, which is an ominous sign.

As a rule, blood pressure increases with the age of the child. A neonate usually has a systolic pressure of 50 to 60 mm Hg. The same pressure in a child indicates hypotension. A neonate's heart rate is usually 120 to 160 beats per minute and decreases as the child grows older. Normal pulse and blood pressure rates are presented in *Table 15-1.*

Congenital heart defects include impairments in circulatory status, dextrocardia (right-sided heart), situs inversus (transposition of all thoracic and abdominal organs), and functional and nonfunctional murmurs.

## Neurologic System

Major neurologic structures are present but incompletely developed at birth. Primitive Moro and Babinski reflexes are present due to immature corticospinal pathways. Temperature instability indicates incomplete development of the autonomic system. Infant sensitivity to parasympathetic stimulation is shown by bradycardia with defecation or deep suctioning. Uncoordinated movements and frequent tremors in infants are a reflection of incomplete myelinization of some motor nerves.

The infant's head is proportionately larger than the adult's. The bones of the cranium are soft and pliable, held together by fibrous sutures to allow for brain growth. This structure allows the skull to cope with increased intracranial pressure, but it is also less able to protect the brain. The large head and high center of gravity makes a child more prone to falls and head injuries.

Infants can have significant bleeding from a scalp laceration because of the increased vascularity and large surface area.

The cervical spine is vulnerable to injury. The vertebrae will not easily fracture, but the spine is vulnerable:

- Flexion-extension injuries are more likely because of the large, heavy head.
- Cervical muscles are undeveloped.
- Minimal force on the C1–3 joints can cause subluxation.
- Undeveloped C2–4 joints may not be able to tolerate flexion-rotation force.
- Lax spinal ligaments provide less support and more mobility for the spine.

## Musculoskeletal System

In a child, the periosteum (the fibrous membrane covering bones as a supporting structure for blood vessels to nourish bone and the attachment point for muscles, tendons and ligaments) is stronger, thicker and forms more bone tissue than in the adult.

Bones are pliable so that greenstick or incomplete fractures are common. The bone growth allows rapid callus formation, which permits bones to heal quickly. Although the bones are strong, fractures happen more frequently than muscle sprains or ligament tears because these structures are stronger than the bones.

The growth, or epiphyseal, plate is unique to children. New longitudinal bone growth is dependent on this cartilaginous area, which does not ossify until puberty. This characteristic allows a fracture to be present without radiographic detection.

## Gastrointestinal and Genitourinary Systems

Undeveloped abdominal muscles are weak and allow children's stomachs to protrude. The small

size of a child's abdomen holds the organs close together. These two factors make the abdomen vulnerable to blunt trauma, especially multiple organ injury. Further, pliable ribs not only are inadequate support for the lungs, they do not adequately protect the abdominal organs, which is another factor that places the child at risk for internal injuries.

Kidneys are likely to be injured because they are comparatively large, quite movable in the retroperitoneum, unprotected by perinephric fat, the abdominal muscles are weak, and the ribs are pliable. Congenital abnormalities such as ectopic kidneys make the child more vulnerable to renal trauma. As a matter of fact, some abnormalities are undetected until the child has had abdominal trauma and either undergoes extensive diagnostic procedures or has surgery.

Spinal flexibility can cause ureteral injury, but ureteral tearing is unusual. When the bladder is full, it takes the space equal to another abdominal organ, and at risk for rupture from trauma. While external injury may not appear severe, serious internal damage may have occurred and should be considered during assessment.

# PREDOMINANT PEDIATRIC TRAUMA

## Head Injury

Traumatic brain injury (TBI) is the most common cause of injury-related death in children. Sixty to 70% of the pediatric deaths by injury are from blunt trauma to the head caused by auto crashes, bicycle crashes, falls and maltreatment. Unrestrained children are thrown around the interior of a vehicle in motor vehicle crashes, or they land on their heads when they fall from a height because the large head tends to hit the surface first.

Thin cranial bones, open cranial sutures and a incompletely myelinated brain in the neonate and infant offer less protection than the adolescent or adult has. A thin cranium allows force to the head to be directly transmitted to the brain.

Severe head trauma is not as a common as mild to moderate injury, which comprises about 90% of the admissions to emergency departments.

Mild to moderate injuries to the head (GCS 13 to 15) require serial neurologic assessments to evaluate intracranial pressure. Level of consciousness, pupil response, motor and sensory response, and vital signs should be documented. Signs of increased pressure include persistent vomiting, post-traumatic seizure, and loss of consciousness. Be aware of neurologic dysfunction. Hemotympanum, cerebrospinal fluid otorrhea or rhinorrhea are indicators of a basilar skull fracture. Battle's sign, raccoon eyes and focal neurologic signs indicate significant cranial damage. Changes in the level of consciousness should be reported immediately as increased intracranial pressure could cause brainstem herniation.

Infants may have skull fractures along the suture lines. The fracture can "grow" in children under 3 years old, which is probably the result of cerebral tissue or arachnoid membrane herniation through a dural laceration. A pulsating mass may be palpated.

The child with a mild head injury may be discharged home with specific instructions to the parents to return to the emergency department if persistent vomiting; drainage from the nose or ears; changes in the level of consciousness, pupil size, and vision; drowsiness; seizures; or ataxia develop.

Recently, it has been discovered that children with mild to moderate head injury have more functional disabilities than previously thought. Minor limitations may not be clinically obvious but are significant enough to affect daily performance and function. Early aggressive management can limit these subtle disabilities.

Severe head injury signs are a decreased level of consciousness, posturing, combative behavior,

and abnormal neurologic responses. Shaken baby syndrome is characterized by retinal hemorrhages, seizures and decreased level of consciousness. If the cervical spine is intact, the Doll's eye maneuver will indicate brain stem integrity (see Chapter 5, "Head Injury"). A positive Babinski's reflex is abnormal and reflects severe neurologic damage in the child over 2 years of age. The airway will require rapid-sequence intubation, then hyperventilation because $CO_2$ is a potent vasodilator (Newberry, 1998). A drop in $PaCO_2$ below 30 mm Hg can cause vasoconstriction, cerebral ischemia and decreased perfusion to the brain. Glucose intravenous solutions should not be used because of the potential for cerebral edema.

Brain injuries are divided into primary and secondary phases. Primary injury is the result of a traumatic force to the brain, which causes the brain to hit the interior skull, or a foreign body causing direct brain injury. The consequence is diffuse axonal injury, skull fracture, contusion and hemorrhage. Secondary injury is the result of changes in the brain brought about by the initial injury. Examples are cerebral edema, hypoxia, increased intracranial pressure and decreased cerebral perfusion.

Closed head injuries include concussion; contusion; diffuse axonal injury; and intracranial hemorrhage, such as epidural hematoma, subdural hematoma, subarachnoid hemorrhage, and brain hemorrhages and lacerations.

Skull fractures include linear fractures, basilar fractures, depressed skull fractures, and compound fractures. It appears that children recover from head injuries better than adults. However, the exact reasons have not been identified.

## Spinal Cord Injury

Cervical injuries commonly occur with multiple injuries sustained from motor vehicle crashes, pedestrian vs. motor vehicle accidents and shaken baby syndrome.

*Chapter 15–*
*Pediatric Trauma and Child Maltreatment*

**215**

Young children rarely sustain cervical spine injuries. However, under 8 years of age, unique characteristics contribute to cervical injuries: larger head size; weak neck muscles and ligaments.

More common in children than adults is the spinal cord injury that does not show a radiographic abnormality. The pliability of the child's spine will allow cord injury without bony abnormality. Transient displacement of the spinal column is the result of a flexion-extension or acceleration-deceleration force. The head is hyperflexed or hyperextended and the cord stretches, causing injury or transection. This action is followed by the spinal cord returning to its normal length and the vertebrae realignment. The patient has signs of spinal cord damage, such as paralysis, without radiographic indication.

Signs and symptoms of cervical spinal cord injury can be hard to detect in the young child. Look for deformity, pain or tenderness on palpation, numbness or tingling in the extremities, decreased or no response to pain, decreased or absent motor response, and loss of bowel and/or bladder control (Soud & Rogers, 1998).

Even though cervical spinal cord injuries in children under 8 years old are unusual, the mechanism of injury will point to the likelihood of this type of damage. Therefore, any child in a motor vehicle crash, pedestrian injury or fall from a height should be fully packaged and immobilized immediately at the scene.

Indicators of any spinal cord injury are the same in the child and adult: numbness; tingling; weakness; flaccidity; and occasionally, priapism and perianal wink. There may be pain and tenderness. Aside from complete immobilization when a spinal cord injury is possible, a high cord injury will require intubation and mechanical ventilation. Lower cord injuries should be carefully monitored for respiratory problems. Serial neurologic assess-

ments should be done to determine any progression of cord edema.

Consequences of spinal cord injury range from mild neurologic deficits to complete paralysis. The child will probably be frightened and feel helpless. Providing information, tenderness and reassurance to the child and family is very important. Be sure to let them know what is happening and why.

## Thoracic Injury

Most pediatric chest injuries are the result of blunt trauma. Infants and young children usually are injured from falls, and older children are more often hurt in motor vehicle crashes, and as pedestrians or bike riders.

Adolescents are increasingly victims and perpetrators of penetrating trauma due to violence. Other predominant causes of thoracic injuries are recreation, sports and child abuse.

In children, energy from blunt force may be transmitted to the internal thoracic structures, the heart, lungs and great vessels. Because the ribs are undeveloped and flexible, blunt trauma usually causes a contusion rather than a fracture. When a fracture does occur, it is likely the result of considerable force, and there is a good chance of damage to the internal organs. Flail segments should raise suspicion of severe parenchymal injury (see Chapter 9, "Thoracic Trauma").

Common injuries are rib and pulmonary contusion, cardiac contusion, pneumothorax, hemothorax, tracheobronchial injury, and diaphragmatic injury. Life-threatening blunt injuries to the chest cause death in about 14% of all childhood trauma.

## Abdominal Injury

In bicycle injuries, the handlebars may strike the abdomen. Other mechanisms of injury are sledding, motor vehicle crashes, altercations, falls, child abuse and sports activities (Newberry, 1998). Violent penetrating abdominal trauma, as with thoracic injuries, is increasing.

As with thoracic trauma, blunt force is the most frequent cause of abdominal injury in children. Hemorrhaging from the energy force is the most common cause of death. Described before, the abdomen is small with the organs close together, so blunt force is liable to cause damage to more than one organ. In order of frequency of injury is the spleen, liver, pancreas and intestines.

Large liver lacerations may result in considerable blood loss and need surgical repair. Small lacerations of the liver without hypovolemia can be managed conservatively. Damage to the pancreatic tail and major ductal structures are usually managed with a distal pancreatectomy.

Signs and symptoms are pain and tenderness, distention, contusions and abrasions. If there is internal hemorrhaging, hypovolemic shock may occur. The location of tenderness indicates which organ is damaged, such as the upper left quadrant is associated with injury to the spleen.

Treatment of abdominal injury is according to hemodynamic stability. If the child is stable, a CT scan is a more accurate diagnostic tool than peritoneal lavage. Surgical intervention is necessary if the patient is hemodynamically unstable and does not respond to fluid replacement.

Any child with high-velocity abdominal trauma, such as a gunshot wound, should be prepared for surgical exploration and repair. Low-velocity trauma, such as a stab wound, is treated according to the patient's status. The child is usually admitted to the hospital for observation.

## Genitourinary Injury

Genitourinary injuries in children mostly occur from blunt trauma. Mechanisms are motor vehicle crashes, falls, sledding, altercations and sports. About 40% of the injuries are associated with abdominal, musculoskeletal and central nervous system injuries. Blunt trauma is the cause of about 80% of all renal injuries and is also the cause of most bladder and urethral injuries. Genitourinary injuries are often the result of pelvic fractures. Most of these injuries are minor, but increases in violent crime causing penetrating injuries have led to more serious genitourinary trauma. Penetrating injuries from gunshot and knife wounds usually cause ureteral injuries.

Female genitalia injuries result from straddle falls, sexual abuse or assault. Female genitalia injuries involve hymenal tears, vaginal hematomas and bleeding, tears of the perineum, inability to urinate, hematuria, rectal bleeding and abnormal sphincter tone. There may be abrasions, lacerations or hematomas.

Male genitalia are injured by straddle falls, adolescent altercations and sports. Infants may have a tourniquet injury from threads, hair or bands lodged in the coronal groove, which forms a constricting ring, lacerating the penile shaft. Degloving injuries and penile amputations are uncommon in children.

Sexual abuse should be considered for any child with genital trauma whose history is inconsistent with his type of injury.

The genitourinary system of the child is more vulnerable to some injuries than the adult. A child has proportionately larger kidneys with less perinephric fat than the adult. The kidneys are not well protected because of the pliable rib cage. The ureters of the child have greater elasticity and the torso is more mobile, making them more vulnerable to injury. Young males are at greater risk for urethral injury than females because of the length and position of the urethra.

The bladder is located in the abdomen, and when full, takes up more space and is more susceptible to rupture. A full bladder may rupture when crushed between the seat belt and the pelvis or the spinal column.

Patients with abnormalities, such as Wilms' tumor, ectopic kidneys and hydronephrosis, are more susceptible to trauma.

Signs of renal trauma are flank and abdominal tenderness. There may be contusions, abrasions or hematuria. The degree of hematuria does not indicate the severity of injury. Renal injury should be considered when the child has lower rib fractures or a fracture to the transverse process of the vertebrae. Interventions range from observation and bed rest to surgery.

Ureteral injury is uncommon. The child may exhibit hematuria, urinary leak, flank mass or iliac pain, which may not occur until 7 to 10 days after the incident. Because ureteral injuries are most often the result of penetrating trauma, urine may leak at an entrance or exit wound. If there is no wound, signs of retroperitoneal abscess, which is a palpable mass; chills; fever; lower abdominal pain; pyuria; and urinary frequency may be present. Surgical intervention is indicated.

Signs of bladder injury vary according to the type of injury sustained. A ruptured bladder will show signs of suprapubic tenderness, urgency with inability to urinate, hematuria and a palpable mass in the abdomen. An extraperitoneal rupture causes significant discomfort, and the child may be able to pass small amounts of urine. It is best to do a retrograde cystogram in male patients before placing a Foley catheter to determine if there is an urethral injury. Severe hemorrhaging will result in shock. If the injury is a contusion, patient observation and reevaluation are usually sufficient. Surgical repair may be necessary.

Along with bladder trauma, pelvic fractures are often associated with urethral damage. An indication of a pelvic fracture is blood at the urinary meatus. **Do not** insert a Foley catheter, as there may be a partial urethral tear that could be enlarged to a complete tear. The patient may also have an inability to void, urgency and ecchymosis of the genitalia. Conservative treatment for partial urethral tears consists of a suprapubic or an indwelling ure-

thral catheter inserted under fluoroscopy. Complete tears require surgical repair.

## Musculoskeletal Injury

Children sustain a wide range of musculoskeletal injuries, from strains and sprains to fractures. Long bones are broken in falls, sports and motor vehicle crashes. This type of trauma is rarely life threatening, so that the ABCs and neurologicals are almost always intact.

As a rule, bones stop growing for girls by the age of 14 and for boys by the age of 16. Children's bones are more porous than adult's. The epiphyseal growth plate at the end of bones is the source of long bone growth. Injury can retard or interrupt this function. The periosteum in children is strong and thick, which allows trauma to bend and only partially break bones (greenstick fractures) and bones to heal faster. Ligaments are strong, which accounts for bone fractures rather than ligament tears.

Musculoskeletal injury has point tenderness, soft tissue swelling and discoloration; limited range of motion and function; and may cause sensory deficits; decreased capillary refill and changes in pulses. Closed fractures may or may not have an obvious deformity. Fractures may be open, requiring reduction and suturing.

Radiographs include the joint above and below the injury and are used to confirm fractures and the degree of misalignment. Radiographs reveal previous fractures, a possible clue to maltreatment. Spiral fractures in lower extremities, femur fractures, in toddlers, and multiple "accidents" and injuries not matching the historical accounts all point to investigating child maltreatment.

Soft tissue injuries are treated with immobilization devices and rest. Nondisplaced fractures are treated with casts or other immobilization measures; displaced fractures require manipulation or open reduction.

## Burn Injury

Injuries from burns are the main cause of accidental death in the home for children under 14 years old. Most of the burn injuries to children occur in the home, and most death-related injuries result from carbon monoxide poisoning or smoke inhalation. Children account for about 30% of the burn-related hospital admissions (Soud & Rogers, 1998).

The types of burn-related injuries can be matched with age. Scalds are seen in older infants and toddlers who have become mobile without awareness of their environment. Electrical burns are caused from toddlers exploring electrical outlets and wiring. Older children, from the ages of 5 to 18, are most often burned by flames.

Burn injuries are the result of exposure to thermal, electrical, chemical and radiation sources. Chapter 14 discusses burns in greater depth.

# MALTREATMENT OF CHILDREN

Soud discusses the fact that different states have different definitions of child neglect and abuse. The terms "child abuse" and "child maltreatment" are used interchangeably to describe neglect and physical, emotional and sexual abuse. The manner of identifying and reporting maltreatment is directly related to the legal definitions and protocols of the state, city and hospital. Hospital staff must be well versed in this information and procedures. *Table 15-2* presents definitions of child abuse.

## Neglect

Neglect is defined as the "intentional or unintentional omission of needed care and support" or "a caregiver who is unable or unwilling to provide the most basic needs for a child." The definition of basic needs may differ geographically and legally,

but generally, the accepted definition includes food, shelter, clothing, medical care and immunizations, education, and emotional nurturing.

Some areas make a distinction between general neglect and severe neglect. Severe neglect involves willfully placing the child in imminent danger. General neglect can happen in families where the parents are unable to provide basic necessities because of limited means, including emotional resources.

Neglect has a wide scope of indicators. There may not be any signs of abuse, but neglect is just as damaging to the child, often leaving deep physical and emotional problems. The child may be dirty, inappropriately dressed for the weather, not have any record of previous medical care or inoculations, appear malnourished, seem to be emotionally lacking, be unable to demonstrate interpersonal communication, or have a diagnosis of failure to thrive.

It is thought that neglect is also involved in nearly half of the child abuse cases. Recognition is not easily or clearly defined and identified, particularly in a busy emergency department. However, signs and behaviors indicating neglect should be identified by the nurse, documented and reported to the physician.

## Physical Abuse

Physical abuse to a child **is not** an accident. It is the intentional infliction upon a child or children of physical injury, torture, maiming or unreasonable force, or omission/failure by an adult to protect the child from danger and injury. In the 1960s, Kempe (1962) described the battered child syndrome, which identified many manifestations of physical abuse to a child.

Specific behaviors and physical findings are found in physical abuse. The Oklahoma Department of Health in 1992 identified behaviors to include:

## TABLE 15-2
## Major Forms of Child Abuse

**Physical Abuse** - Any non-accidental injury to a child. This includes hitting, kicking, slapping, shaking, burning, pinching, hair pulling, biting, choking, throwing, shoving, whipping and paddling.

**Emotional Abuse** - Any attitude or behavior which interferes with a child's mental health or social development. This includes yelling, screaming, name-calling, shaming, negative comparisons to others, telling them they are "bad, no good, worthless" or "a mistake."

**Sexual Abuse** - Any sexual act between an adult and child. This includes fondling, penetration, intercourse, exploitation, pornography, exhibitionism, child prostitution, group sex, oral sex or forced observation of sexual acts.

**Neglect - Physical** - Failure to provide for a child's physical needs. This includes lack of supervision, inappropriate housing or shelter, inadequate provision of food, inappropriate clothing for season or weather, abandonment, denial of medical care and inadequate hygiene.

**Neglect - Emotional** - Failure to provide affection and support necessary for the development of emotional, social, physical and intellectual well-being of a child. This includes ignoring, lack of appropriate physical affection (hugs), not saying "I love you," withdrawal of attention, lack of praise, lack of positive reinforcement.

*Source:* Childhelp USA website, http://www.childhelpusa.org/child/abuse.htm. Childhelp USA 24-Hour National Abuse Hotline, 800-4-A-CHILD. Accessed 9/25/2000.

- Asks for or feels deserving of punishment

- Fearful of going home and attempts to stay at school or day care

- Overly shy and avoids physical contact with adults, especially parents

- Exhibits behavioral extremes such as being over-aggressive or withdrawn

- Cries excessively or sits and stares

- Reports injury by a parent or caretaker

- Gives unbelievable explanations for injuries

- Clings to health care worker rather than parent

### Physical Findings

- Unexplained bruises or welts found on the face, torso, buttocks, back or thighs, often reflecting the shape of the object used, such as a belt buckle, strap or fly swatter.

- Unexplained burns on palms, soles of feet, buttocks or back; burns from a cigarette, electrical appliance; or rope burn.

- Unexplained fractures or dislocations involving the skull, ribs and bones around joints, including multiple fractures or spiral fractures.

- Other unexplained injuries such as lacerations, abrasions, a human bite, pinch marks, clumps of lost hair, retinal hemorrhages or abdominal injuries.

## Sexual Abuse

Newberry quotes from the Nevada statutes, regarding child sexual abuse as "involvement of children in sexual activities that violate social taboos, is usually done for gratification or profit of a significantly older person. Children do not understand these acts and are not able to give informed consent." Soud (1998) also states, "Sexual abuse entails the involvement of children, adolescents or developmentally immature adults in some kind of sexual activity that they do not fully understand. This includes fondling, inappropriate kissing on the mouth, oral-genital or oral-anal contact, exposure of an adult's genitalia to a child; penetration of the vagina or anus and sexual exploitation such as pornographic activities." The definition varies from area to area, state to state.

In 80% of the situations, the child knows the adult offender. Coercion is usually involved, in the form of some kind of threat. Incest is sexual activity between relatives, such as father and daughter. Acute sexual assault implies sexual contact within the past 48 to 96 hours. Chronic sexual abuse lasts over an extended period of time.

The emergency department is the primary facility for sexually abused children to be identified and cared for. Physicians may be reluctant to commit to a diagnosis of sexual abuse for fear of further involvement and feeling uncomfortable dealing with this type of social issue. The nurse should remember that the community depends upon the medical examinations, diagnosis and referral to children's services through the emergency department in order to help stop sexual abuse to children.

## Emotional Abuse

The most difficult form of abuse to identify and prove is emotional abuse. The child usually does not present with physical injuries. Examples of this form of abuse are bizarre forms of punishment, humiliating or belittling comments to or about the child that he hears and making the child feel he is a failure and will never be good enough to succeed in anything.

## Significant Clinical Findings

BRUISES are the most commonly seen injuries.
Unintentional bruises generally are over bony prominences such as the knees, shins, forehead and elbows. The bruises are uniform color and shape and on one plane of the body.

The abused child's bruises have specific characteristics. It is unusual for accidental bruising to be on the cheeks, behind the ears, abdomen,

lower back and buttocks, upper and inner thighs and genitalia. The shape of the object of abuse may be seen in the shape of the bruise. There may be several different shapes to the bruises, particularly if the child has been injured with a variety of objects. Multiple bruises in different stages of healing and coloring suggest repeated trauma inflicted to the child.

BITE MARKS are considered deliberate and found in both the physically and sexually abused child. Seen alone or with a suck mark, adult marks are considerably larger than animal or children's teeth.

BURNS happen to infants, toddlers and young children because they are inquisitive and unaware of potential dangers. Burns are also the result of neglect or abuse.

Intentional burns are frequently identified because the history and injury are inconsistent. For instance, a history of a child turning on a hot water faucet while briefly left alone is inconsistent with glove and stocking burns that occur when hands and feet are held under the faucet. Accidental burns do not have a symmetrical pattern with a specific line of demarcation; there will be splash marks. Intentional burns often occur during the period of toilet training when a child soils his pants and is picked up, put into hot bath water, and scalded.

A child will not burn his arms and legs with a cigarette, which causes deep circular burns. In particular, a child will not burn himself repeatedly unless he has a severe emotional disorder.

FRACTURES are suspicious when they occur in a young child, especially if they are spiral fractures. Other signs of abusive fractures are: extremity bone breaks in children under 1 year old; a metaphyseal or midshaft fracture of the humerus (which takes considerable force); a caregiver who cannot remember the incident

---

**FIGURE 15-1**
**Indications of Possible Abuse**

- Repeated responses to provide care for the same child or children in a family.

- Indications of past injuries. This is why you must do a physical examination and why you must remove articles of clothing. Pay special attention to the back and buttocks of the child.

- Poorly healing wounds or improperly healed fractures. It is extremely rare for a child to receive a fracture, be given proper orthopedic care, and then show angulations and large "bumps" and "knots" of bone at the "healed" injury site.

- Indications of past burns or fresh bilateral burns. Children seldom put both hands on a hot object or touch the same hot object again (true, some do…this is only an indication, not proof). Some types of burns are almost always linked to child abuse, such as cigarette burns to the body and burns to the buttocks and lower extremities that result from the child being dipped in hot water.

- Many different types of injuries to both sides or the front and back of the body. This gains even more importance if the adults on the scene keep insisting that the child "falls a lot."

- Fear on the part of the child to tell you how he was injured. The child may seem to expect no comfort from the parents and may have little or no apparent reaction to pain.

- The parent or care giver at the scene who does not wish to leave you alone with the child, tells conflicting or changing stories, overwhelms you with explanations of the cause of the injury, or faults the child may rouse your suspicions and cause you to assess the situation more carefully.

---

occurring; or describes a minor incident with a major injury. A delay in seeking treatment or several unwitnessed injuries should put the staff on alert.

Rib fractures are uncommon because the ribs are so pliable in children under 5 years old. Therefore, in order to fracture the ribs, substantial force must be used. Fractured ribs from cardiopulmonary resuscitation is not considered abuse.

It is important not to jump to conclusions regarding abuse. Weird accidental breaks do happen. The nurse should also be careful when taking the patient's history to ascertain any underlying bone diseases, such as osteogenesis imperfecta or bone cancer.

**HEAD INJURY** is the most frequent nonaccidental trauma seen in infants under 1 year of age. Serious damage from a fall from a height should arouse suspicion. Bilateral scalp hematomas or fractures in children, any skull fracture in an infant, cerebral edema, subdural hematoma, subarachnoid bleeds, retinal hemorrhages, and traction alopecia related to hair pulling are all hallmarks of abuse and the history of the incident should be carefully evaluated.

Shaken baby syndrome produces a triad of head injuries resulting from the infant being either intentionally shaken severely or in rough play. Acceleration-deceleration motion causes subdural hemorrhage, retinal hemorrhage and altered level of consciousness.

**MUNCHAUSEN SYNDROME BY PROXY** is a syndrome that has recently received considerable public attention because of some media-related cases. Complex factors are involved when a child is deliberately kept ill by the parent or caretaker, who benefits from recognition as the one who is "saving" the child from further illness or death. The illness is drawn out by the caretaker through various means, including poisonings, introduced pathogens or other means. Medical histories may also be falsified to make it appear the child is more seriously ill than is actually true.

**FAILURE TO THRIVE** is a condition seen in children under the age of 5 whose growth continues to significantly fail to meet the norms for age and sex based on national growth charts. These children fall below average in measurements for height, weight and head circumference. The condition may be the result of a medical condition such as a Giardia infection, celiac disease, lead poisoning or malabsorption. The condition may also be psychosocial, such as neglect, but not in every case. Aggressive treatment and follow-up is essential to prevent developmental and behavioral problems resulting from nutritional deprivation of the nervous system and other systems.

A multidisciplinary approach for family counseling, nutritional counseling, medical intervention and family support is the best approach to intervention.

# ASSESSMENT

In order to properly assess and stabilize the child, the nurse must know the developmental and physiologic differences between infants, children, and adolescents.

There are several scoring mechanisms used in pediatrics to determine the injury status of a child.

In the field, the Trauma Score (TS) and the Revised Trauma Score (RTS), which uses a recalculation of the Glasgow Coma Scale (GCS), are generally used. However, emergency department staff may not be experienced in adopting the score of a nonverbal child with the GCS, making the RTS method time consuming and difficult to conduct quickly.

The Pediatric Trauma Score (PTS) tends to be the method of choice both in the field and emergency department. The PTS uses the child's size plus five physiologic parameters to determine injury severity and potential morbidity and mortality. The components include the evaluation (normal +2, maintainable +1, and unmaintainable -1) of airway, central nervous system, weight, systolic blood pressure, open wounds and fractures. Scores range from -6 to +12. Those with scores of +8 or less have a serious injury, with a decreased chance of survival. These patients are acutely injured and should be treated in a pediatric trauma center as soon as possible (Soud & Rogers, 1998).

Start with introducing yourself to the child, if he is alert, and whoever is with the child. Identify whoever is accompanying the child and their relationship with the child. Explain that you are there to help the child and will let the child and family know what is being done and why.

## Initial Assessment

The initial assessment has two components: primary and secondary (Newberry, 1998).

### Primary Survey

**Airway:**

- Check for patency; look for loose teeth, vomitus, edema or other obstruction.

- Note the position of the head.

- With multiple injuries, immobilization of the neck is necessary because of potential cervical trauma. Maintain neutral alignment. Check the effectiveness of the cervical collar and other immobilization on a periodic basis until the patient is cleared by the physician.

**Breathing:**

- Auscultate breath sounds in the axilla for presence and quality of ventilation. Effectiveness is evaluated using the following criteria (Soud & Rogers, 1998):

  — Are respirations spontaneous?

  — What is the respiratory effort: use of accessory muscles, retractions, nasal flaring?

  — Are grunting, wheezing, and crackles present?

  — What are the rate of respirations?

  — Are the neck veins distended?

  — Is the trachea midline or deviated?

  — What is the integrity of the chest wall and evidence of trauma?

  — Is there symmetry of chest movement?

  — Note skin color (pale, dusky, cyanotic) and neurologic status for signs of hypoxia, agitation or decreased level of consciousness?

**Circulation:**

- Check apical pulse for rate, rhythm and quality; compare apical and peripheral pulses for quality and equality.

- Evaluate capillary refill; it should be less than 2 seconds.

- Check skin temperature and color.

- Note open wounds or uncontrolled bleeding.

**Disability:**

- Assess level of consciousness, orientation to person, time and place x3 in the older child.

- In a younger child, evaluate the level of alertness, interaction with the environment or caregiver and ability to follow commands.

- Check the pupils for size, equality and reaction.

**Expose:**

- Remove clothing and inspect the entire body.

*Secondary Survey*

**Head, Eyes, Ears and Nose:**

- Check the scalp for abrasions, lacerations and open wounds.

- Palpate the scalp for step-off defects, depressions, hematomas and pain.

- Palpate the forehead, orbits, maxilla and mandible for crepitus, deformities, step-off defects, pain and stability.

- Reassess the pupils; check for extraocular movements; ask the child if he has any visual difficulties. Look for raccoon eyes or Battle's sign.

- Note if the ears or nose has rhinorrhea or otorrhea.

- Evaluate for malocclusion by asking the child to open and close his mouth; note open wounds and loose, chipped, broken or missing teeth.

- Check for orthodontic appliances, and note if they are intact.

- Evaluate facial symmetry by asking the child to smile, grimace, and open and close his mouth.

- Do not remove impaled or foreign objects.

**Neck:**

- Carefully open the cervical collar, while another person maintains neck alignment, to reassess the anterior neck for jugular vein distention and tracheal deviation. Note bruising, open wounds, edema, crepitus, debris or chemicals under the collar.

- Check for hoarseness or changes in the voice by speaking to the child.

- Note pain.

**Chest:**

- Note respiratory rate; reassess breath sounds for quality.

- Palpate the chest wall and sternum for pain, tenderness or crepitus.

- Observe inspiration and expiration for symmetry or paradoxical movement.

- Note use of accessory muscles.

- Reassess apical heart rate, rhythm, and clarity.

**Abdomen, Pelvis, Genitourinary:**

- Look for bruising and distention of the abdomen; auscultate bowel sounds in all four quadrants; palpate the abdomen gently for tenderness; assess the pelvis for tenderness and stability.

- Palpate the bladder for tenderness and distention; check the urinary meatus for injury or bleeding; note priapism, genital trauma, lacerations or any foreign bodies.

- Have physician examine the rectal sphincter tone and look for lacerations.

**Musculoskeletal:**

- Assess extremities for deformities, swelling, lacerations, or other injuries.

- Palpate distal pulses for presence, quality, rate, and rhythm and compare to central pulses.

- Ask the child to wiggle toes and fingers; evaluate strength of hand grips and foot flexion/extension.

**Back:**

- Logroll the patient, being careful to maintain spinal and neck alignment, to inspect the back; look for bruising and open wounds; palpate all vertebrae for tenderness, pain, deformity and stability; assess the flank area for bruising and tenderness.

If conscious, the child may not be particularly cooperative because of pain, fear and a variety of other factors.

## History

The history is important in assessing the patient and preparing him and his family for needed interventions. Information may be unavailable or inaccurate if the incident was not witnessed or the child is nonverbal.

Information is gathered on the principle of who, what, where, when and why the injury occurred. Detailed information is particularly important when the mechanism of injury is a passenger/MVC, pedestrian/MVC, bicycle crash, fall, gunshot or stab wound or there is suspected neglect or abuse.

Be sure to find out if the patient had a loss of consciousness, for what duration and if it was followed by vomiting and visual changes.

# NURSING STRATEGIES FOR THE PEDIATRIC TRAUMA/CHILD MAL-TREATMENT PATIENT

The goal with pediatric trauma or maltreatment cases is to prevent further injury or disability and prevent the loss of life. Nursing strategies depend upon the nurse's knowledge and understanding of growth and development of the infant, child or adolescent as it relates to the injury.

Do not move the child who has fallen from a height unless it is necessary to establish an airway. In that case, follow the instructions given in Chapter 8, "Trauma to the Spine."

Uncuffed endotracheal tubes are usually used for infants and children under 8 years of age. The problem with uncuffed tubes is they are more easily dislodged than cuffed tubes. After intubation, always auscultate for breath sounds. Use age-appropriate stethoscopes for greater auscultation. Listen in the midaxillary line as listening in the midclavicular line allows the nurse to hear reflected sounds. If endotracheal tubes are inserted too far, they may enter the right bronchus, thus only ventilating the right lung instead of both lungs. If both lungs are not ventilated, the morbidity and mortality potential increases substantially.

Do not use an esophageal obturator airway on children, particularly if they are less than 12 years old. If the child is able to be distracted or comforted, it is a sign he is alert and has adequate cerebral perfusion.

It is essential to remember that bradycardia is a warning of severe hypoxia. A pulse rate of 80 is normal in an adult, but in a newborn, it is serious and immediate action must be taken to prevent death. Consider CPR if child is symptomatic.

Apply pressure to bleeding sites.

Improper stabilization of a fracture can lead to permanent deformity and disability.

Hypothermia should be prevented. Cover the child or place a cap on the infant to prevent heat loss. Remember the infant has a large head and loses a considerable amount of heat through the scalp. Hypothermia depresses cardiac function, increases oxygen consumption by using energy to make heat and decreases the delivery of oxygen to the tissues.

Do not give the patient anything by mouth until he has been cleared from surgery or other tests and interventions. The patient may have nausea, in which case, nothing should be given by mouth.

Infants and children may become frightened, restless, agitated and pull out lines and tubes, or run from the examining room in an attempt to escape the emergency department. Lines and tubes should be secured well, and those with the child informed the child should not remove these treatment aids.

When there is an opportunity for the child to make a choice regarding an intervention or procedure, such as which arm to insert the intravenous, allow him to participate.

If a procedure must be done, don't ask the child if you can do it; he will probably just say, "NO." Explain, in a pleasant but firm manner, what you are going to do and why is it necessary.

If no one accompanies the patient to the emergency department, make every effort to contact the family or guardian. Tactfully confirm this is their child and let them know he is in (the name of) your emergency department. However, your hospital probably has specific protocols for contacting the family or guardian that should be followed.

Try not to let the child see other patients, especially those who are acutely ill or injured. It adds to his anxiety and fears.

Remember the needs of those accompanying the child whenever you can. Inform them of what is happening and, if necessary, offer to put them in contact with appropriate social services or police authorities.

Try not to vent your frustration on the child if he is uncooperative and obnoxious. If it is possible, stop what you are doing for a moment and involve the family in the patient's care, such as letting a parent hold the child during a procedure.

# EXAMPLES OF NURSING DIAGNOSES FOR PEDIATRIC TRAUMA/CHILD MALTREATMENT PATIENTS

- Fear and anxiety related to the injury and the unfamiliarity of the emergency department

- Communication deficit related to children who are nonverbal or who have an impairment in their ability to communicate

- Aspiration related to teeth, foreign bodies and emesis in the mouth entering the lungs

- Hypovolemia related to the loss of blood from hemorrhage due to trauma

- Ineffective airway clearance related to small air passages, foreign bodies and edema

- Pain related to injury

- Fear related to an abusive parent accompanying the child to the emergency department

- Abuse related to an adult having inappropriate contact with the child

# SUMMARY

The pediatric patient has unique characteristics and problems for the trauma nurse. Potentially life-threatening injuries must be quickly and accurately identified within the relationship of the trauma to the infant's, child's or adolescent's growth and development.

Trauma is a growing threat to young people, one that is basically not accidental and usually preventable. The growing violence in the child and adolescent populations is increasing the serious penetrating injuries and deaths.

Child maltreatment encompasses neglect and emotional, physical and sexual abuse. The problem has long-lasting and often tragic consequences. Fortunately, there is growing public awareness and education, along with legal and community resources aimed at identifying neglect and abuse and helping the child.

Trauma to the infant, child and adolescent is more costly than that of the adult in actual dollars and other resources, ranging from initial interventions to continuing treatment and rehabilitation.

Most injuries are preventable.

# EXAM QUESTIONS

## CHAPTER 15
### Questions 71–80

71. About _____ children with traumatic injuries are seen annually in United States emergency departments.

    a. 16,000
    b. 160,000
    c. 16,000,000
    d. 160,000,000

72. Trauma deaths in infants, children and adolescents now

    a. exceed infectious deaths as the leading killer in this country.
    b. are accidents and not preventable.
    c. are not a public health issue.
    d. should all be evaluated by the medical examiner.

73. The leading cause of death for children from 5 through 19 years of age is

    a. influenza.
    b. lack of immunizations.
    c. child abuse.
    d. motor vehicle accidents.

74. Hypotension is a late sign of hypovolemia and indicates

    a. higher cardiac output.
    b. impending cardiac arrest.
    c. normal pediatric response to injury.
    d. congenital cardiovascular defects.

75. Traumatic brain injury is the most common cause of injury-related death in children. Which statement is true?

    a. Thin cranial bones in a neonate provide more flexibility to the skull during blunt trauma.
    b. There are more severe head injuries than mild to moderate injuries in children.
    c. 60% to 70% of the pediatric deaths by injury are from blunt trauma.
    d. Children with a mild head injury do not have functional disabilities.

76. You can recognize shaken baby syndrome by

    a. the triad of retinal hemorrhage, decreased level of consciousness and brain hemorrhage.
    b. discolored hematomas to the back of the head and neck.
    c. a primary injury.
    d. linear fractures that grow along the cranial sutures.

77. Pediatric chest injuries are usually the result of blunt trauma. Which statement is true?

    a. Children's ribs are pliable and do not fracture easily.
    b. children's ribs are pliable and have greenstick fractures.
    c. Because children's ribs are pliable, blunt injury reflects off the body.
    d. Children's ribs are not pliable.

78. Physical abuse to a child is not an accident. Which of the following findings would be considered significant?

    a. Bruising over bony prominences such as knees, shins and the forehead.

    b. Frequent fractures known as osteogenesis imperfecta.

    c. Fractures to the distal radius and ulna.

    d. Bilateral scalp hematomas.

79. The pediatric history is important because it

    a. is important in the assessment and planning of trauma management.

    b. makes patient care more interesting.

    c. is necessary for the insurance companies.

    d. is required by medical records.

80. Munchausen syndrome by proxy has received recent national recognition in the media. Which of the following is true?

    a. It is a cluster of symptoms produced by artificial means.

    b. It is a set of symptoms resulting from head injuries.

    c. Is not related to child maltreatment.

    d. It occurs after functional disabilities form.

# CHAPTER 16

# ELDER TRAUMA, ABUSE, AND NEGLECT

## CHAPTER OBJECTIVE

Upon completion of this chapter, the reader will be able to recognize signs and symptoms of elder trauma, abuse and neglect.

## LEARNING OBJECTIVES

Upon completion of this chapter, the reader should be able to:

1. Identify anatomic and physiologic changes that take place with aging.

2. Identify mechanisms of injury common to elder persons.

3. Recognize hallmarks of abuse and neglect seen in the elderly.

4. Identify appropriate basic nursing strategies related to trauma, abuse and neglect seen in the elder person.

5. Indicate examples of nursing diagnoses regarding elder trauma, abuse and neglect.

## INTRODUCTION

In 1990, the United States had nearly 31 million people over the age of 65, about 12.5% of the total population. It is estimated that by the year 2020, the number will rise to 52 million, with 6.7 million over the age of 85.

Older persons are living longer and with better health than ever before. Reasons vary from medical advances to personal awareness of nutrition, fitness, prevention and care, along with societal support for improved quality of life. Numerous older adults continue to pursue many of the same activities that they did at a much younger age, but at an increased opportunity and risk for injury.

Trauma in the older patient is likely to be more serious than the same injury in the younger person. They develop more complications that are potentially more serious, are hospitalized longer and have less certain prospects for survival. For example, most spinal cord injuries occur in males between the ages of 16 and 30 years of age. When the same trauma happens to an elder person, it is more likely to be devastating. A study cited in a 1996 *American Journal of Nursing* stated that of patients who suffered spinal cord injuries between the ages 16 to 30 years, 95% survived at least 2 years, compared to only 59% who were 61 to 86 years of age.

Although the elder population (over 65 years old) represents only 12% of the trauma patients, they make up nearly one third of the trauma-related health care expenditures in this country and account for more than one quarter of the deaths.

Elder abuse and neglect is increasing. There are many reasons, including more older persons today and complex problems regarding the caregivers. Changes in managed care are decreasing the types of care provided and do not include custodial care. Nursing care facilities are under-staffed and salaries tend to be low. Qualified and committed personnel are difficult to find, as evidenced by the large number of classified advertisements to recruit staff. Abuse is found in all socioeconomic backgrounds. Women are more abused than men. Females tend to suffer abuse from their children, whereas men suffer neglect from their wives.

Newberry (1998) states that the incidence of elder abuse is reported to affect between 1.5 to 3.2 million individuals. Data are difficult to collect and validate because much of the abuse is subtle, hard to identify; and so many cases are reported as falls and other "accidents." There is also considerable shame and embarrassment associated with this problem, so abused individuals often keep from reporting incidents to the physician or others.

The American Medical Association defines elder abuse and neglect as "actions or the omission of actions that result in harm or threaten harm to the health and welfare of the elderly." There are five primary categories of maltreatment: physical abuse, neglect, psychological abuse, violation of personal rights and financial abuse.

# EPIDEMIOLOGY AND MECHANISMS OF INJURY

As stated in the introduction, older adults continue to participate in many of the same activities they did at a younger age because they are in better condition than ever; society now includes them in more activities; and probably, also in defiance of their age. This age group incurs a higher population-based death rate from trauma than any other age group.

## Falls

For those over the age of 75, falls are the most frequent cause of accidental trauma and the second most frequent cause for people between the ages of 65 and 74 years.

Many falls result in an isolated orthopedic injury, such as tripping and fracturing a hip. However, falls from a height have a significant energy transfer and can be particularly damaging. Continuing activities such as climbing trees, roofs and ladders have a high degree of risk.

When an elder has a fall injury, the cause should be investigated thoroughly. Frequently, falls occur because the aging process causes postural instability, poor balance, alteration in gait, and decreased muscle strength and coordination. Acute or chronic associated conditions such as syncope, cardiac dysrhythmias, hypoglycemia, anemia and transient cerebral ischemia or other gait-altering disorders must also be considered as precipitating factors for falls. For example, an episode of bradycardia may bring on syncope, resulting in a fall. Orthostatic hypotension occurring when an older person rises from a lying or sitting position is another common factor in falls.

Abuse and neglectful care for safety measures should not be forgotten in the search for causes of falling.

## Motor Vehicle Crashes

The number of licensed drivers over 65 years of age is increasing. Currently, those over 65 with driver's licenses represent about 13% of the drivers, and their crash rate is second only to the 16- to 25-year-old group. Persons over 75 years have the highest rate of fatal crashes.

Although falls are more frequent, a motor vehicle crash is the most common presenting trauma to the elderly seen in the emergency department. Most of the crashes occur in the daytime, good weather and close to home. Alcohol intoxication is much less frequent than in younger persons.

Contributing factors to automobile accidents by the elderly are decreased coordination and reac-

## TABLE 16-1
### Passenger Vehicle Driver Deaths per 100,000 Licensed Drivers, 1998

| Age | Male | Female | All |
|-----|------|--------|-----|
| 16-19 | 33 | 16 | 24 |
| 20-24 | 26 | 10 | 19 |
| 25-29 | 16 | 7 | 12 |
| 30-34 | 13 | 6 | 9 |
| 35-39 | 13 | 6 | 10 |
| 40-44 | 12 | 5 | 8 |
| 45-49 | 12 | 5 | 9 |
| 50-54 | 11 | 5 | 8 |
| 55-59 | 11 | 6 | 8 |
| 60-64 | 11 | 5 | 8 |
| 65-69 | 14 | 7 | 10 |
| >=70 | 23 | 12 | 17 |

©2000, Insurance Institute for Highway Safety, Highway Loss Data Institute.

tion time, visual impairment, alterations in hearing processing, deficits in cognitive functioning and antecedent medical conditions. Studies have been conducted to determine what percent of accidents occur first and cause a fatality, and what percent of fatalities occur first from conditions such as stroke or myocardial infarction and cause the driver to have an accident.

## Pedestrian vs Motor Vehicle Accidents

Pedestrian vs vehicle accidents are the third most often seen injuries to those over 65 years, and result in nearly a quarter of all fatalities due to this mechanism.

Many aging conditions such as osteoarthritis, change pace and gait, and alterations in sight and hearing may contribute to these accidents.

## Burns

About 8% of the injury-related deaths to older persons are from burns. Burn injuries in the elderly, compared to the younger population, are larger and deeper, and result in a greater mortality rate. Factors involved in elderly burns are altered mobility limiting muscle strength and coordination, which cause spilling and scalding; neurosensory changes, including peripheral neuropathy and vascular disease causing alterations in sensation perception that allow prolonged contact with heat; forgetfulness and poor judgment regarding safety issues; and altered gait, limiting escape.

Decreased dermal cell production causes thinner skin, which allows burning to be more severe and susceptible to infection.

## Injury Related to Violence

From 4% to 14% of the elderly trauma victims admitted to the nation's emergency departments have injuries resulting from shootings, stab wounds and blunt assaults. The infirmities that develop with older age also make this group vulnerable prey for criminals. Decreased agility, speed, coordination and strength make it difficult to ward off attacks or flee from attackers. Poor vision and hearing compound the problem.

## Abuse and Neglect

Abuse is a problem gaining more recognition, and elder injuries must be carefully documented and investigated. Frequent visits for "minor" injuries, multiple bruises in various stages of coloration and healing, unkempt appearance, poor nutrition and poor hygiene are all signals of possible abuse or neglect.

Newberry cites four main theories that may explain elder abuse: role theory, transgenerational theory, psychopathology theory and stressed caregiver theory.

### Role Theory

When the parent ages and becomes more dependent and childlike, the child takes on the parental role. Now, the child gives orders to the elder, which has a tremendous psychological impact. As role conflicts develop, the potential for abuse increases significantly.

### Transgenerational Theory

Many think that violence is learned behavior. A child growing up in a highly aggressive environment will exhibit similar behaviors as an adult. A parent who abuses his or her child is likely to be abused by the child in return.

### Psychopathology Theory

A caregiver with altered impulse control due to mental health problems or substance abuse or dependence has considerable potential for inflicting emotional and/or physical abuse. The typical elder abuser is a middle-aged, white woman living with the older person; and has a substance addiction, long-term financial difficulties and high stress levels. The victim is perceived as the source of the abuser's stress.

### Stressed Caregiver Theory

Whether the caregiver is a family member, friend or professional, providing long-term care to the elderly can be extremely stressful and frustrating. Any of these persons are subject to giving in to abuse when their internal resources are exhausted. The stress in the health care environment combined with personal stress can bring about expression in terms of abuse. The caregiver may have marked fatigue from handling too many tasks.

# CHANGES IN AGING

With aging, anatomic, physiologic, and mental changes occur. Resources diminish. Potential for healing diminishes.

## Cardiovascular System

Fibrosis causes progressive stiffening of the myocardium that results in diminished pump function and lower cardiac output. Blood pressure grad-

ually increases. Blood vessels tend to harden. The cardiovascular system has less reserve.

Decreasing sensitivity to catecholamines, such as epinephrine and norepinephrine, causes an inability to develop appropriate tachycardia. Therefore, there is a decreased ability to increase cardiac output in response to hypovolemia, pain, and stress.

Peripheral atherosclerotic disease has a tendency to reduce blood flow to vital organs and diminish physiologic reserve. It also diminishs peripheral pulses, which can cause misinterpretation of pulse characteristics, and results in inappropriate treatment.

Commonly used prescription medications, such as digoxin or beta blockers, may mask normal response to injury and stress. Some long-term medications, such as daily aspirin or Coumadin® may exacerbate the patient's injuries such as increased hemorrhaging.

## Respiratory System

Teeth usually are replaced by dentures, crowns, or partial plates, which can become a foreign object that lodges in the airway during trauma or intubation. A patient without teeth is difficult to ventilate with a bag mask because the lack of teeth leaves the cheeks without shape and air leaks around the mask.

Diminished pulmonary compliance and reduction of the ability to cough effectively are the result of decreased lung elasticity and progressive stiffening of the chest wall. Vital capacity of the lungs decreases.

Coalescence of alveoli and a reduction of small airways support lead to a decrease in surface area for gas exchange. The reduced efficiency in gas exchange decreases arterial oxygenation.

Atrophy of the lining of the bronchi contributes to a decrease in the ability to clear foreign materials and bacteria.

# FIGURE 16-1

## Changes in Physiologic Function with Age in Humans (Expressed as a Percentage of Mean Value at Age 30 Years)

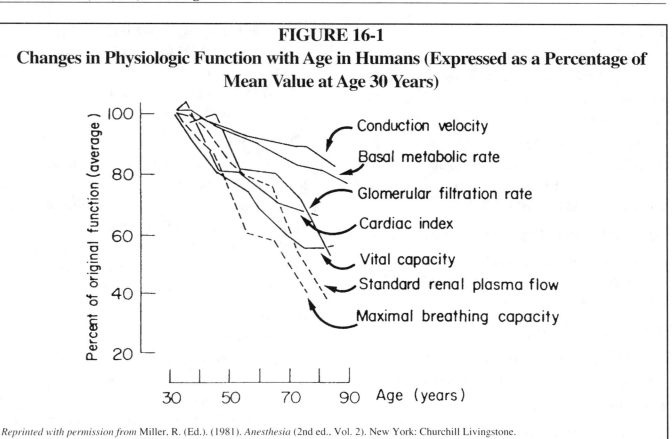

*Reprinted with permission from* Miller, R. (Ed.). (1981). *Anesthesia* (2nd ed., Vol. 2). New York: Churchill Livingstone.

The upper airway tends to have chronic colonization with gram-negative bacteria and Hemophilus species, which predisposes the patient to pneumonia.

## Nervous System

Starting in the 40s, the brain begins to atrophy. By the 70s, there is a 10% reduction in the size of the brain. As a result, the space between the surface of the brain and the skull increases and stretches the dural bridging veins. The stretching of the veins makes them more vulnerable to disruption and bleeding.

Functional deterioration increases the potential for accidental injury:

**Cognition:** Poor memory, impaired judgment and deficient data acquisition.

**Hearing:** Decreased auditory acuity, particularly with high-frequency sounds. Lack of or inadequate hearing devices due to financial limitations or limited access to health care.

**Eyesight:** Decreased visual acuity and peripheral vision; intolerance to glare; and outdated, inadequate or inappropriate eyeglasses.

## Musculoskeletal System

Loss of bone density from osteoporosis brings about a predisposition to fractures, even with minor traumatic energy transfer. Osteoporosis is more pronounced in women but occurs in most elderly, leaving them prone to fractures of the hip, wrists, and ribs. Pelvic fractures can be life threatening and all fractures are slow to heal. Complications are not uncommon.

Osteoarthritis and diminution in vertebral body height contribute to significant spinal changes. Examples are kyphoscoliosis and spinal stenosis due to osteoarthritis.

Fibrosis and decrease in muscle mass diminishes agility and strength.

## Renal

Renal mass and function declines. By the age of 65, a 30% to 40% loss is not uncommon. Remaining nephrons show aging and deterioration on the tubules and glomeruli.

Sodium tends to be lost, and potassium tends to be retained. Potentially nephrotoxic agents, such as iodinated contrast solutions, aminoglycosides and diuretics, should be used judiciously.

## Metabolic and Hepatic Changes

The basal metabolic rate slows, along with the liver's ability to clear toxins. Effects of hypoxia are more pronounced.

## Thermoregulation

Older persons are more prone to heat loss, chilling, and dehydration than younger persons.

## Comorbid Conditions

Along with the anatomic and physiologic changes that occur in aging, significant diseases commonly develop and may seriously affect the older person's response to injury and stress.

It is essential for the nurse to find out concurrent diseases and medications in order for appropriate interventions and treatment to be administered. The information is important, and affects patient management, from resuscitation strategies to continuing care.

The more common conditions include cardiac disease, hypertension, neurologic disorders, liver disease, pulmonary disease, renal disease, diabetes, malignancy, and obesity.

# ELDER ABUSE AND NEGLECT

## Primary Categories of Elder Mistreatment

### Physical Abuse

Pain, injury and/or physical confinement; an act of violence that results in bodily harm or mental distress; includes sexual abuse. **Clinical findings:** Bruises, welts, lacerations, fractures, burns, rope marks, medication overdose, inadequate or inappropriate medication, unexplained sexually transmitted disease or genital infection.

### Neglect

The most common form of abuse, deliberate refusal to meet basic needs, withholding assistance vital to performance of activities of daily living, behavior that causes mental anguish or failure to provide nutrition and medical care. **Clinical findings:** Dehydration, malnutrition, decubitus ulcers, poor personal hygiene; lack of compliance with medication schedule.

### Psychological Abuse

Verbal aggression and berating; intimidation and humiliation; harassment threats to deprive the elder of property or services, place him in a nursing home, or remove his financial support; unreasonable demands; deliberately ignoring the elder. **Clinical findings:** Left alone for long periods; ignored or given "the silent treatment;" failure to provide companionship or a change in routine or activities. Isolation from human contact, pets or sensory stimulation. Caregivers speak harshly or disrespectfully to the elder.

### Violation of Personal Rights

Deprivation of inalienable rights: for example, personal liberty, free speech, personal property, and privacy.

### *Financial Abuse and/or Neglect*

Unauthorized use of money and/or goods for personal gain; includes petty theft or declaration of the elder as incompetent in order to confiscate property, and failure to pay the elder's bills. **Clinical findings**: Denial of a home or shelter. Coercion to enter contracts, invest, give up money, assign durable power of attorney to the caregiver and change the elder's will. Financial or material neglect, such as lack of substantial care in the home despite adequate financial resources, and sudden transfer of assets from the elder to a family member.

## Risk Factors Associated with Elder Abuse

- Advanced age, over 65

- Multiple chronic diseases or disorders

- Incontinent or unaware of the need to use the toilet. He may need to be led to the toilet and then not know what to do when he gets there.

- Inability to feed himself without spilling and making a mess

- Dementia, forgetfulness, or other organic brain disease

- Insomnia or walks in his sleep, wanders during the night and even may leave the house.

- Increasing dependency on the caregiver

- Alcohol abuse in either the caregiver or the elder

- Child abuse by parent may lead to a role reversal and the child then abuses the parent.

- Past history of abuse is a great risk for future abuse in the same setting.

- Caregiver inexperience or indifference

- Economic stress

- Caregiver mental illness

- Caregiver stress from effects of "the sandwich generation" i.e., being squeezed between the demands of dependent parents and dependent children.

- Lack of support systems or practical help for the caregiver.

- Unrealistic expectations of the caregiver

- Sudden, unwanted, or unexpected dependency of the elder on the caregiver

- Cramped living conditions

## Signs and Symptoms

The elderly are abused and neglected nearly as often as children. However, this problem has only recently been given the visibility it deserves. Unfortunately, there are no specific definitions, so the abuse diagnosis is usually only given when there is visible battering. Assessment and identification of elder abuse is neither quick nor easy. Neglect is even more difficult to prove.

In order to identify abuse of the older person, the nurse must have a high degree of awareness and observation during the assessment. There are clues the patient may project that may indicate he is either being abused or neglected:

- Depression

- Fearfulness

- Extreme mood changes

- Poor personal hygiene

- Old and new bruising

- Unexplained injuries, including many falls

- Sexually transmitted diseases

- "Shopping" for health care

- Overconcern with the cost of health care

- Serial missed medical/dental appointments

A typical victim is a white woman over 75 years old, who has a mental or physical impairment and is living with a relative.

# ASSESSMENT

## Assessment Principles

- An accurate history is fundamental and particularly necessary for the elder patient.

- Intubate sooner than later. If there is doubt, intubate (Peitzman et al., 1998). Remember that older trauma patients are different than younger patients and require different approaches to trauma management. The best approach is immediate invasive monitoring and mechanical ventilation, aggressive volume monitoring, special attention to identifying complications and early mobilization to a trauma center.

- Older people as a group have more complications, are hospitalized longer and are likely to need repeat hospitalization. Many will need long-term care.

- Discussions with the family regarding protection and safety are essential.

## Resuscitation and Initial Assessment

As in any trauma patient, resuscitation should begin as early as possible. The ABCs protocol should be followed, control the airway, ensure adequate ventilation, and restore any loss in volume.

Even though the patient may not be hemorrhaging, the elderly are often hypovolemic due to dehydration. Preexisting disease and senescence can lead to the body's inappropriate response to hypovolemia: failure to develop tachycardia or a drop in blood pressure. Fluid resuscitation, while often necessary, should be done with care, especially with the cardiac patient.

It is important to contact the family, caregiver, or care facility to identify the patient's preinjury level of function, state of health, comorbid conditions, allergies and whether or not a living will exists.

*Disability:* Determine the neurologic status, which is especially important and often difficult in the geriatric patient. If possible, any preexisting neurologic disorders should be identified. Mental dysfunction such as Alzheimer's disease, dementia, or previous cerebrovascular accidents may exist, causing patient response to be confused. Answers to questions may make no sense although the patient seems to be alert.

Chronic disease may be misinterpreted during assessment as an acute state, bringing about potentially harmful overtreatment. On the other hand, a patient with a "normal mental status" after a blow to the head may actually have a lethal intracranial injury that has not had time to be manifested due to the patient's extensive cerebral atrophy. Part of the evaluation for the patient with a head injury should include CT scanning.

The Glasgow Coma Scale should be frequently reevaluated. Suspicion of certain types of trauma, such as spinal cord injury, may often need to be based on the mechanism of injury as much as physical indicators.

*Expose:* The patient should be fully disrobed and physically examined, both back and front, while protecting his privacy and dignity and while keeping him warm. Scars will indicate previous surgical interventions and some medical history. In particular, look for a medial sternotomy scar or signs of peripheral vascular surgery that are indicative of systemic arteriosclerotic disease.

## Secondary Survey

The initial assessment is a systematic search for serious injuries. The secondary assessment involves special attention to the history before the injury. This is crucial to appropriate management of the patient, possibly preventing inappropriate treatment or contributing to a potentially preventable event.

- Did a motor vehicle crash occur under "normal" situations, or was there an antecedent episode, such as a cerebrovascular accident, a transient ischemic attack, or a myocardial infarction that caused the accident?

- Have more than one of these incidents or similar incidents occurred in the recent past? If so, there may be an untreated condition contributing to the incidents.

- Has the patient recently begun a new medication or had a change in the dosage of a regular medication? Is there a new diagnosis, such as diabetes?

- Each category of elder abuse or neglect has associated diagnostic or clinical findings, which were included previously under the primary categories of mistreatment. When assessing the patient, look for any of these findings as part of the whole picture.

# NURSING STRATEGIES FOR THE ELDER TRAUMA OR MALTREATMENT PATIENT

## Trauma

- Identify yourself to the patient and let him know what you are doing.

- Speak slowly, clearly, and in easy-to-understand terms. Use a pleasant voice and try not to communicate urgency. Be reassuring. Don't shout because the patient is elderly.

- Evaluate the patient's mental status.

- Begin oxygen immediately or intubation if indicated.

- Look for loose teeth or dentures and appliances. Look to see if an airway has broken or dislodged any teeth or dentures. If there seems to be an obstruction, look for a foreign body and if there is, sweep it from the mouth and check periodically.

- If the patient needs to be ventilated with a bag mask, leave the dentures in place in order to provide form and firmness to the jaw and face and help form a seal around the mask. Be sure the dentures are securely in place. If endotracheal intubation is necessary, remove, save and label the dentures.

- Monitor the EKG frequently, looking for arrhythmias, tachycardia and bradycardia.

- Remember that beta blockers may diminish sympathetic response to trauma.

- Get a list of all the patient's medications, dosages and times of administration as soon as possible. If no one has a list, try to obtain all the patient's medication containers or call his pharmacy for a list.

- Carefully document the patient's medical history, including allergies. He may have a list of his medications, particularly if he is brought in from an extended care facility. He may also have a Medic Alert® bracelet or necklace.

- Check tissue perfusion carefully. Note if it is altered.

- Look for peripheral edema; it may indicate pre-existing cardiovascular problems.

- Check skin turgor.

- Hip fractures are usually not painful, and the patient is often unaware the injury exists. Careful examination of a patient who has fallen is essential.

- Be sure the patient is warm but not overheated. Heat loss hampers resuscitation efforts.

- Keep the patient NPO until the physician has cleared the patient for surgery and he is free of nausea and vomiting.

- If the patient is diabetic, find out what type and get blood glucose levels.

- The patient may become aggressive or violent due to the trauma, age, hypoxia, pain or fearfulness. Protect the patient and yourself. Be sure the side rails are up.

- Check for substance abuse and include this in the history.

## Abuse and Neglect

- Be especially aware and observant of the patient if there is any chance he has been abused or neglected.

- Look at any bruising, abrasions or lacerations for coloration, location and age. Bruises on the upper arms may indicate the patient has been clutched and shaken. The patient may also have a whiplash injury from being shaken. Bruises on the trunk may indicate being beaten or kicked. Bruises on the wrists or ankles indicate the patient may have been tied down.

- Look for any other clinical indicators of abuse, such as burns from rope or cigarettes. Determine if the burns are old or new.

- Does the patient appear dehydrated or malnourished? Are clumps of hair missing? Is there evidence of sexual abuse, indicated by difficulty walking, bruising or lacerations on the thighs or genitalia or tearing of the genitalia? Does the patient have subconjunctival hemorrhages or evidence of retinal detachment?

- Has anyone voiced his concern that the patient may be abused or neglected?

- Document any irregularities or uncommon observations and actions taken by all staff and agencies.

- Identify the patient's living conditions.

- If the caregiver is present, observe the interaction between the caregiver and the patient. Is the patient withdrawn, fearful or agitated? Is the caregiver complacent, unconcerned or hostile? Observe their verbal and nonverbal interactions.

- Do not communicate any suspicions to the caregiver, but do inform the physician. Abuse is a reportable offense and the appropriate authorities and agencies must be informed according to hospital policy and local, state and federal statutes.

# EXAMPLES OF NURSING DIAGNOSES RELATED TO THE ELDER TRAUMA OR MALTREATMENT PATIENT

- Ineffective airway clearance related to trauma or foreign objects such as dentures

- Ineffective ventilation related to delayed aggressive measures such as intubation

- Inappropriate physiological response to hypovolemia, pain and stress related to decreased sensitivity to catecholamines

- Confused or impaired verbal communication related to neurologic deterioration, which is compounded by the stress of trauma

- Predisposition to fractures related to aging bone density loss

- Premorbid illness seriously affecting response to injury related to the aging process

- Premorbid illness precipitating traumatic situations, such as motor vehicle crashes, related to the aging process

- Ineffective thermoregulation related to the aging process

- Physical and emotional deterioration related to elder abuse

- Malnutrition related to elder neglect

# SUMMARY

O lder persons are living longer and in better health than ever before. By the year 2020, the number of people in this country over 65 years of age will be at least 52 million.

The changes that occur with aging are anatomic, physiologic and mental. These changes make recovery more complicated and long-term.

Trauma in the elder person is likely to be more serious, develop more complications, be more costly and have more psychosocial ramifications than in the younger person. Falls are the most frequent cause of trauma for those over 75 years old, and the second most frequent cause for people between 65 and 74 years old. Motor vehicle crashes involving people over 65 years are increasing, second only to those between the ages of 16 to 25, because the numbers of people in this age group are rapidly increasing and many of them continue to drive. Crashes may result from a vehicular incident, or a premorbid medical condition may precipitate the crash.

The problem of elder abuse and neglect is increasing, but it is also getting more visibility and attention. Everyday, patients are seen in emergency departments with injuries that could be the result of abuse, but identification is difficult because there are no specific definitions. Neglect is even more difficult to diagnose. Unless there are obvious signs of battering or other kinds of abuse, it is difficult to make a definitive diagnosis.

Alert and aware emergency care staff can be key in picking up on the signs and symptoms of elder abuse and neglect, documenting and reporting their information to the appropriate staff and authorities. Staff observation and action can have a great deal of effect on the elder's well-being and quality of life, and may save a life.

# EXAM QUESTIONS

## CHAPTER 16
### Questions 81–90

81. The most common cause of accidental trauma in persons over the age of 75 is

    a. motor vehicle accidents.

    b. falls.

    c. gunshot wounds.

    d. ingestion of a foreign body.

82. Trauma in the older patient is likely to be

    a. less complicated than in younger persons.

    b. from abuse.

    c. the result of carelessness.

    d. more serious than the same injury seen in a younger person.

83. In the older person, the cardiovascular system

    a. is affected by fibrosis causing progressive stiffening of the myocardium.

    b. causes the blood pressure to gradually decrease.

    c. causes increased sensitivity to catecholamines.

    d. develops functional deterioration.

84. Assessment principles in elder trauma include

    a. contraindication of intubation because of dentures or broken teeth.

    b. elder patients are different than younger patients and require different approaches to trauma management.

    c. assumption that all injuries are the result of infirmity.

    d. determining the patient's type of insurance.

85. During resuscitation and initial assessment

    a. control the airway, ensure adequate ventilation, restore loss in volume, determine disability, and expose.

    b. pay special attention to the patient's pre-injury history.

    c. identify if the patient has been abused.

    d. get a list of the patient's medications and treatments.

86. Nursing strategies for the elder trauma or maltreatment patient includes

    a. Keep the patient cool because the elder's thermoregulatory system is dysfunctional.

    b. Give the patient a liquid diet to prevent dehydration.

    c. Giving oxygen immediately or intubate early if there is any question.

    d. Hip fractures require intravenous pain medication.

87. Beta blockers

    a. may diminish sympathetic response to trauma.

    b. cause peripheral vascular dilation.

    c. elevate blood pressure.

    d. constrict cranial blood vessels.

88. A patient presents with multiple bruises in various stages of healing. They are located on his upper arms. He also complains of neck pain. There are what appears to be round burn marks on his hands. His caregiver says he fell out of his wheelchair. The nurse should

   a. be especially aware to observe for indicators of abuse or neglect, and note these indicators.

   b. immediately report the caregiver to the authorities.

   c. call in the family and question them as to what they know about the situation.

   d. have social services put a seat belt on the patient's wheelchair for his safety.

89. Signs and symptoms of an abused or neglected elder are

   a. hostility and aggressiveness.

   b. dementia.

   c. depression, poor personal hygiene and poor skin turgor from dehydration.

   d. cramped living conditions.

90. Nursing strategies for the elder trauma patient include

   a. having the patient describe how he was abused by the caregiver.

   b. giving the patient oral fluids during the assessment to prevent further dehydration.

   c. monitoring the EKG frequently, looking for changes in rhythm and rate, and being aware the patient may not display the usual physiologic reaction to pain, stress, and hypovolemia with tachycardia.

   d. speaking loudly in case he has a hearing deficit.

# CHAPTER 17

# PSYCHOSOCIAL CONSIDERATIONS

## CHAPTER OBJECTIVE

Upon completion of this chapter, the reader will be able to identify the psychosocial issues affecting patients who have experienced a traumatic injury.

## LEARNING OBJECTIVES

Upon completion of this chapter, the reader should be able to:

1.  Describe what the term "psychosocial needs of the trauma patient" means.

2.  Identify a psychosocial response that a trauma patient may exhibit.

3.  Recognize posttraumatic stress disorder and how it may be manifested.

4.  Describe Dr. Elisabeth Kubler-Ross's five stages related to loss, potential loss, death and dying.

5.  Recognize the needs and concerns that family and significant others may have when a member of their family, friend or mate has an injury.

6.  Recognize and describe psychosocial concerns and needs of staff who care for trauma patients.

## INTRODUCTION

A caregiver should not care for any patient, and in this context, the trauma patient, without having a basic understanding of the psychosocial responses and needs the patient and significant others are likely to experience.

Psychosocial considerations of trauma and its resulting potential disabilities and disfigurement, loss or potential loss, stress, crisis intervention, patients with special needs, rehabilitation and adaptation to daily living are important in the patient's early management. The emergency nurse should take these considerations into account while conducting other interventions with the injured patient. Specific strategies can be used to support the patient and his family.

## A GENERAL PERSPECTIVE OF PSYCHOSOCIAL ASPECTS OF TRAUMA

Generally speaking, psychosocial describes the internal/psychological and interpersonal/social factors that determine one's emotional state. In trauma and emergency situations, psychosocial usually relates to responses and reactions resulting from situations or conditions. The term is not to be confused with the term "psychiatric," which relates to altered mental conditions.

For example, a 1993 study in Denmark researched cranial trauma and stroke patients. It showed that although the mechanisms of brain damage were different, psychosocial responses were essentially the same. There was psychosocial decline following the incident that improved following rehabilitation. Because of appropriate direction to resources, most patients had a decline in the need for assistance in their daily living situation following rehabilitation, along with a decline in the use of health services. The study did not discuss what was the optimal time for entering the rehabilitation program.

Another study conducted in Canada indicated that the recuperative ability of the trauma patient was equated with psychological well-being. It was thought there is the possibility that such resilience is better described as social-behavioral competency resulting in the ability to conceal emotional pain, due to childhood abuse. The conclusions were that findings are consistent with current concepts of trauma/abuse recovery as involving multiple dimensions of functioning, some of which are more observable than others. Some apparently resilient persons may have good social-behavioral competency while still experiencing psychological pain.

Because trauma patients require the nurse to have considerable anatomy, physiology and technical knowledge and skills, often requiring immediate physical assessment and interventions, the psychosocial aspects of taking care of the whole person can get lost in the rush. Aspects of communication with the patient can be uncomfortable for the nurse to deal with. However, providing quality care includes understanding the responses of the patient and family to trauma and providing access to needed resources. The ultimate goal is to ensure the multidimensional quality-of-life outcomes are as positive as possible.

In a study regarding hospital designation as trauma centers, Hollingsworth (1989) showed that nurses are usually the "glue" that holds the patient care interventions in the system together, integrating physical medicine, ancillary departments, psychosocial and other services.

# TRAUMA AND STRESS

Injury is disrupting to a person's life. Patients may react to trauma by becoming disorganized, dazed or overwhelmed by what has happened. Reality may become distorted.

Concerns are:

- Pain and disability
- Physiological response to emotional stress: hypertension, tachycardia, hyperventilation
- Loss or interruption of current relationships or roles
- Disruption in functioning
- Extent of treatment and rehabilitation
- Possibility of permanent damage, disfigurement, or dying
- Psychological shock
- Disbelief
- Acute anxiety and nervous behavior
- Volatile emotional state

All trauma causes stress, whether it is a sprained knee or a critical multiple trauma situation. Pain causes stress. A change in one's lifestyle, whether for a long or short period of time, causes stress. Anything that challenges a person's steady status produces stress. Stress affects the patient and family, often encompassing friends and coworkers.

Disruption to the patient's life can include family structure, function, routines, the living situation, and income.

There is a need to return to the point of equilibrium. In order to cope with stress, mechanisms that the patient has either previously developed or learns after the trauma, are used to adapt to the new situation. Not all patients or families have the means to adapt and may react inappropriately with emotions of anger or violence. There may be physiological signs such as tachycardia, hypertension, syncope, or tension headaches. The internal resources a patient has to cope with stress also vary with his status before the trauma. If he was already pushed to his maximum coping ability, he will have few resources left to handle the new situation.

# RESPONSES TO TRAUMA

The patient's response to trauma goes beyond the physical injury. In *Trauma and Recovery,* Herman (1992) states that the mind and spirit also react to the injury. "The ordinary human response to danger is a complex, integrated system of reactions, encompassing both the body and mind. Threat initially arouses the sympathetic nervous system, causing the person in danger to feel an adrenaline rush and go into a state of alert. Threat also concentrates a person's attention on the immediate situation. In addition, threat may alter ordinary perceptions: people in danger are often able to disregard hunger, fatigue or pain."

The patient may be so emotionally traumatized that he is crippled by posttraumatic stress disorder. This reaction received public attention with veterans of the Vietnam War. The disorder is also experienced by survivors of disasters, assaults and traumatic events.

In posttraumatic stress disorder, the indelible imprint of the traumatic moment causes intrusive thoughts. There is an altered state of consciousness, resulting in psychic numbing and surrender. A person in this state may feel as though the event is not happening to him, that he is observing the event rather than being a participant. Some trauma survivors may have "flashbacks" or a recurrence of the event. The experience is terrifying for the indi-

vidual. Immediate calm reassurance is necessary, along with long-term counseling. Specialists trained in treating posttraumatic stress disorder should be part of the intervention network.

Trauma may present the threat of potential loss and loss of limb and life. It also may cause the patient to feel threatened with the loss of control. In 1974, in her book *Questions and Answers on Death and Dying,* Dr. Elisabeth Kubler-Ross identified five stages of resolution for those facing potential loss or loss. Her work was an expansion of her 1969 research into death and dying. It focuses on the patient and his family as human beings and what they go through during these times of anxieties, fears, and hopes.

## Denial

During the first stage of resolution, the patient and/or family react with statements such as, "No, not me/us. This cannot be true." He may go to great lengths in order to support the possibility of loss as being incorrect. The reaction serves as a buffer to the reality, allowing the patient and/or family the chance to collect himself/themselves, and with time, mobilize less radical defenses. Denial is usually a temporary defense mechanism that will evolve into at least partial acceptance.

Staff should closely examine their reactions in these situations. Their reactions are often reflected in the way they respond to the patient and his family.

## Anger

The unrealistic world of denial usually cannot be maintained for very long. It then is replaced by anger, rage, envy, and resentment. "Why didn't this happen to…" This stage is difficult for the family and staff to cope with. The anger is displaced in every direction and at everyone. The patient finds fault with everyone and everything. It is hard for others to understand and accept where the patient's anger is coming from, and their response may only increase his anger. It is easy for the recipients of the anger to take the outburst personally, rather than understand the actual dynamics. If the patient's anger is met with anger, it feeds into the patient's hostile behavior. This stage may serve to push away all those who care about him. Reactions often take the place of responses. The staff may employ avoidance behaviors to cope with their discomfort with the situation.

## Bargaining

Often this stage is either overlooked or unknown by the caregivers. For the most part, this stage does not last long, but it is helpful to the patient. There is the psychological pull from past experiences that says if he cannot win one way, maybe he can maneuver a "deal" …just one more chance, just to be pain free for a while, just to do this one thing one more time… The bargaining is an attempt to postpone because the psychological reality is there that the loss will happen. Most bargains are made with a deity and include a promise of service or dedication. Psychologically, the promises may be associated with guilt about the current or past event. It is essential the staff does not make light of the patient's or family's attempt to bargain. At this point, an interdisciplinary approach may help the patient cope with feelings of guilt or other feelings.

## Depression

When the circumstances can no longer be denied, fought or bargained for, a great sense of loss will overcome the patient. The loss has many facets: physical appearance, function, control, independence and a myriad of other losses.

Remorse is deep, guilt may pervade, and the question of how the situation could have been prevented weighs heavy with the patient. Further, the depression may be compounded by immense expenses that he cannot recoup.

The initial reaction is to "cheer up" the patient. False reassurance is the worst thing that can be inflicted on the patient because the falseness or futility of the plight is evident to him. Telling the patient to look at the bright side of things or be grateful for what he has is not only ridiculous and insensitive but demeaning to the patient or family. The patient is in the process of great loss.

Encourage the patient to express his thoughts and feelings. Just holding his hand can be supportive. The caregiver should not be afraid to use appropriate humor with the patient. Laughter is therapeutic. So is warmth.

## Acceptance

When the patient/family has had enough time, they may reach the point of acceptance of the inevitable. This is not a sense of "giving up" or a "happy" state; the patient is neither angry nor depressed. There is almost a void of feelings. Communication is more likely to be nonverbal. At this point, the family may need more help, understanding and support than the patient.

Although these stages may seem to apply more to death and dying and to long-term care than to the emergency department, the nurse should have an understanding of them and know that at least some of the stages will occur with certain trauma patients in the acute, emergent environment. Further, it is necessary to understand what the patient and his family will be facing beyond his time in the emergency department.

# CRISIS INTERVENTION

Trauma is a sudden, unanticipated event that affects more than the patient's physical being and more than the patient. The trauma may be severe enough to precipitate a crisis situation. Some patients who come to the emergency department are already in a crisis state. A crisis is a circumstance of enough distress to disrupt the equilibrium of a person's life.

A crisis ordinarily has three phases: pre-crisis, impact of the crisis, and the post-crisis. The emergency nurse's function, along with the primary and secondary physical assessment, is to assess the emotional aspect of the patient. The nurse helps the patient define the immediate problem or crisis, and gives him the opportunity to express his feelings and fears.

Remember to view the patient as an individual rather than a stereotyped image. Be aware not to be influenced by a preconceived concept of certain types of traumatic situations, such as a drug overdose or suicide attempt.

Aguilera and Messick (1994) designed a crisis intervention model using a problem-solving approach. The model views people as beings in a state of equilibrium until a stressful event changes that state. In order to resolve this problem, specific balancing factors have to be present:

• The patient has a realistic perception of the event.

• Adequate situational support must be available.

• The patient has adequate coping skills to address the problem.

If all the factors are present, there is a good possibility of resolving the problem, reestablishing the equilibrium and preventing the crisis. The model also postulates that if one or more balancing factors are absent, the problem will be unresolved, the disequilibrium increases, and the crisis becomes imminent or occurs.

Steps in crisis intervention correlate with assessment and problem-solving. The assessment gives the nurse a basis for planning and therapeutic intervention in order to prevent escalation of the crisis. It is the point for including ancillary staff and other support resources in the patient's (and family's) care.

No one has the coping skills to deal with every kind of crisis, including the nurse. But the nurse is expected to, at least momentarily, deal with the patient's crisis and help him and his family through theirs. The nurse is also expected to avoid collapse and breakdown while being a resource for the patient and his family.

# SUICIDE AND SUICIDE ATTEMPTS

The second leading cause of death in the age range of 15–24 years is suicide. Suicide attempts and successful suicides are increasing, with 25,000 to 30,000 Americans dying each year of self-inflicted injuries. These numbers are an estimate because not all suicides are identified, including those involving drug overdose, firearms and single-car crashes.

The survivor of an attempted suicide and his family and the family of a successful suicide are immediately in a crisis state. They need prompt assessment, intervention and a link to experienced resources.

The nurse may find the suicide attempt or eventual suicide success conflicts with personal beliefs, and may find it difficult to empathize with the circumstances. However, the nurse's role is to provide care, be nonjudgmental and understand that the patient's situation is unique to him. If this role is too stressful for the nurse, it is better to have another nurse work in the situation and receive counseling at a later time to learn coping mechanisms for these situations.

# SPECIAL PATIENTS

Patients with special needs may be admitted to the emergency department at any time and in any condition. If the nurse is not able to communicate with a patient who has special needs, it is important to know how to call upon a resource who can help. The emergency department should have a list with the names and contact numbers of resources available at any time and any day. Inform other staff members of the patient's needs so they are prepared when they approach him.

## Hearing Impaired

When it is identified the patient is hearing impaired, find out his means of communicating with the hearing person. Does the patient read lips, have a hearing aid, sign? Is there a family member or friend who can interpret? If there is not a person available who can communicate with the patient, and the patient is able, he can use paper and pencil. Touch is reassuring. Touch and pointing can also indicate where the pain is located. Nonverbal communication can be informative. The nurse should be face-to-face with the patient as much as possible so they can "read" each other. Shouting accomplishes nothing but frustration, is ineffective, and inappropriate.

## Vision Impaired

If the patient cannot see well, or not see at all, verbal communication should be calm, descriptive, clear, and with patience. The nurse and all staff members should introduce themselves, identify what they are there to do and let the patient know about his status.

There is no need to keep a running line of conversation just to keep talking with the patient. However, it is important and helpful to the patient to let him know what is being done and why. Frequent updates should be provided.

Remember to keep the side rails up and a urinal or bedpan where the patient can reach it whenever necessary and without having to call anyone. Let him feel where the call bell is located and secure the bell so it won't fall from the bed.

## Other Disabilities

Physical disabilities are challenging, and the nurse may not be immediately aware that the patient has a problem. If the patient comes to the emergency department via a rescue unit or is sent from a care facility, there should be information regarding a disability preexisting to the trauma. It is also necessary to determine the degree of disability and the patient's limitations before the injury. For example, an elderly patient may have had a stroke or other disabling problem before the injury occurred.

If the patient is conscious and coherent, ask him if he needs any help physically and what you can do for him. This question does not need to be asked in a condescending manner but simply and directly stated.

## Non-English Speaking

Find out what languages the patient speaks and if there is anyone with the patient who can interpret. There may be someone on the hospital staff who can communicate in the patient's language. It is helpful if the hospital has a list of staff who speak foreign languages and what languages they speak. With the influx of refugees from foreign countries, it is increasingly likely that there will be more non-English speaking patients. The patient and his family may have been sponsored by a church or group who has an interpreter available, knows the patient and can help.

# NURSING STRATEGIES FOR MEETING PSYCHOSOCIAL NEEDS OF THE TRAUMA PATIENT

Stress is part of the trauma picture. Along with conducting primary and secondary physical assessments, the patient's psychosocial response to the traumatic event should be identified and documented by the nurse.

The nurse's understanding of the interrelationship between the body, mind and spirit helps to recognize and understand patient responses and gather

---

**FIGURE 17-1**

**Conveying News of Sudden Death to Family Members**

- Remember: the moment you stop resuscitative efforts on a person, you acquire a new set of patients—the family and loved ones.
- Call the family if they have not been notified. Explain that their loved one has been admitted to the emergency department and that the situation is serious. In general, survivors should be told of a death face-to-face, not over the telephone.
- Obtain as much information as possible about the patient and the circumstances surrounding the death. Carefully go over the events as they happened in the emergency department.
- Ask someone to take family members to a private area. Walk in, introduce yourself, and sit down. Address the closest relative.
- Briefly describe the circumstances leading to the death. Go over the sequence of events in the emergency department. Avoid euphemisms such as "he's passed on," "she is no longer with us," or "he's left us." Instead use the words "death," "dying," or "dead."
- Allow time for the shock to be absorbed. Make eye contact. Consider touching the family member and sharing your feelings. Convey your feelings with a phrase such as "You have my (our) sincere sympathy" rather than "I am (we are) sorry."
- Allow as much time as necessary for questions and discussion. Go over the events several times to make sure everything is understood and to facilitate further questions.
- Allow the family the opportunity to see their relative. If equipment is still connected, let the family know in advance.
- Know in advance what happens next and who will sign the death certificate. Physicians may impose burdens on staff and family if they fail to understand policies about death certification and disposition of the body. Know the answers to these questions before meeting the family. One of the survivors will surely ask, "What do we do next?" Be prepared with a proper answer.
- Enlist the aid of a social worker or the clergy if not already present.
- Offer to contact the patient's attending or family physician and be available if there are further questions. Arrange for follow-up and continued support during the grieving period.

---

the resources necessary to help the patient cope with his and his family's needs.

Strategies are helpful for meeting the psychosocial needs of the trauma patient:

- A professional approach can be enhanced with warmth and nonjudgmental recognition of the patient's reactions and responses.
- Initially, be clear and direct with the patient. Let him know you are there for him and what you will be doing. He will be concerned about his status related to his injury. His comprehension will be limited because of the stress. Communication should be brief, uncomplicated and may have to be repeated.
- Give frequent updates to the patient and family as to his status, interventions and tests that are planned, and why.
- You may need to call in other team resources to help the patient in crisis.
- Present the opportunity for the patient and his family to express their feelings and fears.
- Reassurance is important to the patient and family, provided it is reality based. False reassurance is destructive and demeaning for the patient.
- Be prepared for a wide range of emotions from the patient and family.

- Be aware of your own reactions and responses to the circumstances, patient and family.

- Have an understanding of the emotional process of potential loss, or loss. The patient and family may exhibit one or more of the stages of resolution while you are caring for him.

- Physical and emotional trauma interact with each other. Be alert for physical signs of emotional stress in addition to the physical damage caused by the injury. For instance, stress and pain may be manifested with hyperventilation, or restlessness may be a sign of hypoxia.

- Remember that you are taking care of the whole patient. Emergent skills and technology take precedence during the initial injury assessment and crisis, but even then your psychosocial communication skills can be used when you relate to the patient. He should respond better to the interventions.

- Involve the family and/or significant others with the patient and his care as soon as it is possible. They should not feel left out, and may be helpful in understanding the patient's responses and in utilizing appropriate psychosocial resources.

- Direct the patient and family to hospital social services personnel who have access to agencies and resources they will need during the patient's care and rehabilitation.

- Be aware of your own professional and emotional scope. No one can be all things to all people, and it is acceptable to call on other team members to participate in areas in where you are uncomfortable or unfamiliar with.

A characteristic of emergency department nursing is high stress, high activity, and high responsibility. There is a paradoxical role of wanting to care for critical patients and keep skills up on one hand, and on the other hand, not wanting people to be injured. Staff is geared for the adrenaline rush felt in the midst of an emergency and may feel let down when all the activity subsides. Burnout is well known to be a hazard of emergency department nursing. Symptoms are short tempers, cynicism, anger, depression and calling in sick frequently.

Critical incident debriefing gives the team an opportunity to review actions and reactions, learn and share *(see Figure 17-2)*. Issues such as ethical concepts and the appropriateness of interventions are discussed. Discussion and written evaluation helps the team reestablish their own equilibrium.

# EXAMPLES OF NURSING DIAGNOSES RELATED TO THE PSYCHOSOCIAL CONSIDERATIONS OF TRAUMA

- Fear of loss of body image related to damage sustained from the injury

- Pain and disability related to injury

- Emotional reaction to situational crisis related to trauma received by the patient

- Emotional stages related to the potential loss or loss of limb or life

- Knowledge deficit related to lack of awareness of community resources available for psychosocial support

- Posttraumatic stress disorder related to severe emotional disruption from a traumatic event

- Loss or interruption of current relationships or roles related to injury sustained

# SUMMARY

Injury is physically and emotionally disrupting for the patient and his family. Response to trauma goes beyond the physical injury. Because people are individual beings, they each

---

**FIGURE 17-2**
**Critical Incident Debriefing**

- The debriefing should occur as soon as possible after the event, with all team members present.
- Call the group together, preferably in the resuscitation room. State that you want to have a "code debriefing."
- Review the events and conduct of the code. Include the contributory pathophysiology leading to the code, the decision tree followed, and any variations.
- Analyze the things that were done wrong and especially the things that were done right. Allow free discussion.
- Ask for recommendations/suggestions for future resuscitative attempts. All team members should share their feelings, anxieties, anger and possible guilt.
- Team members unable to attend the debriefing should be informed of the process followed, the discussion generated, and the recommendations made.
- The team leader should encourage team members to contact him or her if questions arise later.

Reproduced with permission. *Advanced cardiac life support*, 1997. Copyright American Heart Association.

---

have a unique response based upon their internal and interpersonal makeup.

Care of the injured patient includes psychosocial considerations. The emergency nurse should take these considerations into account while con-

ducting trauma interventions. It is also important to include the family in support strategies. Often community agencies and other resources are necessary to bring the patient from the point of injury through the rehabilitation process.

When confronted with potential loss or loss, most patients experience stages of resolution during the process of coping. Dr. Elisabeth Kubler-Ross identified five stages of denial, anger, bargaining, depression and acceptance. Although the stages occur over a period of time, they may begin during the initial emergent care. The nurse's knowledge and understanding of these stages is essential in being able to recognize the patient's reactions and responses.

No one has the coping skills to deal with every kind of crisis, including the nurse. However, the nurse is expected to repeatedly deal with the patients' psychosocial crises along with carrying out physical interventions. Such professional demands are stressful.

In order to be the most value to oneself, the patient, his family and other team members, periodic debriefings for the staff are valuable. They help to prevent burnout, cope with actions and reactions, and review the appropriateness of interventions. Discussion and written evaluation helps the nurse and emergency department team to establish equilibrium.

# EXAM QUESTIONS

## CHAPTER 17
### Questions 91–95

91. The term "psychosocial" refers to

    a. psychiatric disability.

    b. psychological response to social events.

    c. crisis.

    d. internal/psychological and interpersonal/social factors.

92. In posttraumatic stress disorder

    a. the indelible imprint of the traumatic moment causes intrusive thoughts.

    b. there are five stages of resolution.

    c. critical debriefing is essential.

    d. there is a potential threat of loss of life and limb.

93. Five stages of resolution to loss identified by Kubler-Ross are:

    a. Denial, anger, bargaining, depression and acceptance.

    b. Crisis, anger, denial, bargaining and acceptance.

    c. Loss, anger, denial, depression and acceptance.

    d. Denial, anger, fear, depression and acceptance.

94. A patient's response to trauma

    a. affects the parasympathetic nervous system.

    b. goes beyond the physical injury.

    c. is initially physical.

    d. is categorized according to the severity of injury.

95. Critical incident debriefing

    a. should be conducted with the patient immediately after the primary and secondary assessment.

    b. is conducted only after mass disasters.

    c. is required by the American Hospital Association.

    d. gives the emergency department team an opportunity to reestablish their equilibrium.

# CHAPTER 18

# ORGAN DONATION

## CHAPTER OBJECTIVE

Upon completion of this chapter, the reader will be able to describe the process of organ donation and tissue transplantation.

## LEARNING OBJECTIVES

Upon completion of this chapter, the reader should be able to:

1. Describe the process used to identify organ and tissue donor candidates.

2. Recognize and describe the appropriate approach to families being requested to donate their loved one's tissues or organs.

3. Describe the steps in organ procurement.

4. Identify the statutes and regulations regarding organ transplantation.

5. Recognize the need for organ and tissue donation and identify the most likely recipients.

## INTRODUCTION

Perhaps there has been no greater incident to call the world's attention to the need for and benefit from tissue and organ donation than the shooting and death of little 7-year-old Nicholas Green in Italy.

Although Italy is a country that had not been aggressively involved in organ donation and despite the fact that Nicholas was killed by an Italian, Nicholas' family donated his tissues and organs to save Italians. This unprecedented act in Italy, of kindness and understanding, captured the attention and hearts of people around the world when they were introduced on television to the seven persons whose lives were saved by Nicholas's tissues and organs. None of these people would be alive today without the benefit of transplantation.

Italy has honored the family of Nicholas and now has an effective organ and tissue transplantation program in operation. Organ and tissue transplantation enhances and extends lives of all ages, from the infant receiving a heart transplant so he can live, to the elder once more independent and productive because corneal transplants allow him to see clearly. A transplant is truly a gift of living.

Medical and scientific advances now allow more types of tissues and organs to be transplanted with fewer complications and failures. Unfortunately, the numbers of donors are not keeping up with the need. Although about 55 people in the United States each day receive life-enhancing organ transplants, another 10 people die who are waiting on the national list (the United Network of Organ Sharing [UNOS], 1998) to receive an organ or tissue.

In 1996, a total of 20,319 organ transplantations were performed in this country, while only 19,592 procedures took place in all of Western

Europe. In March 1998, more than 54,500 people were on the list, which grows by about 500 every month. Worldwide, the kidney is the most sought-after organ, followed by the liver, heart, heart-lung combination, bowel and pancreas. Patients in the United States wait an average of 842 days to receive a kidney. Ironically, patients waiting for a heart have the shortest wait: 213 days.

While philosophically most Americans approve of organ donation, too few actually take steps to give this gift of life to others.

# HISTORICAL BACKGROUND

**M**an has always been concerned with being able to extend his life span. The replacement of diseased or damaged tissue or organs has been intriguing for ages.

Historical literature describes Meekren's attempt in 1682 to replace part of a soldier's skull with the skull of a dog. In 1800, Wolf attempted corneal graft surgery, and in 1881, skin grafting was tried as a temporary means of treating a burn. In 1893, Williams transplanted a sheep's pancreas into a human.

The concept of tissue transplantation was explored earlier than whole-organ transplantation. In the 1940s, Sir Peter Medawar used skin grafts treated with cold refrigeration. He was awarded the Nobel Prize for his work in the rejection phenomenon and immune response, which was later used during further studies in transplantation. Immunosuppression therapies have been used and have greatly increased the potential for success in many transplantation procedures hindered by rejection complications.

Graham used his wooden hoop dialyzer to attempt dialysis as a treatment mechanism for renal failure in the 1860s. Then in the 1940s, Kolft designed a dialysis machine, which is the prototype for dialyzers to this day. In 1954, Peter Bent Brigham Hospital in Boston, Massachusetts, instituted dialysis as a therapy program based on Kolft's findings that dialysis was the treatment of choice for end-stage renal failure. Now there are dialysis programs all over the world.

However, dialysis is still a lengthy, expensive and limited treatment mechanism. The patient who is dialyzed frequently, often encounters problems with the shunt used for access and constantly lives with stress, disruption of lifestyle and the fear of death.

In 1902 Ullmann attempted the transplantation of goat kidneys. Others soon joined his research in response to the increasing numbers of patients with end-stage renal disease.

The first kidney was transplanted at Peter Bent Brigham Hospital in 1954 between living, identical twins. These autografts were successful and led to further work with siblings, related donors, and cadaveric donors.

The more successful kidney transplantations became, the more there was expansion into other whole-organ possibilities. The first liver was transplanted in 1963 in Denver, Colorado. The first lung was transplanted in 1963 at the University of Mississippi, and the first kidney and pancreas transplantation was conducted at the University of Minnesota in 1967. The most dramatic transplant was the first heart, in Cape Town, South Africa, in 1967, by Dr. Christiaan Barnard. Shumway did the first heart-lung procedure in 1981 at Stanford University.

Although early extrarenal transplants were limited in the degree that they restored life and activity for the patient, they all added to the new technologic era of extending life through the organs of others.

As transplantation activities and innovative research progressed, new areas of concern arose. Of major importance was the prevention of infection and rejection. Research continues to expand into related areas, such as the efficacy of xenografts, genetic manipulation of some animal models and using mechanical bridges to keep the patient alive until an organ or medical alternative is available.

# LEGISLATIVE BACKGROUND

An anatomical gift is a donation of human organs and tissues. The success of transplantation medicine goes beyond medical and surgical technique. It involves significant legal and ethical concerns. The rapid advancement of technology has exceeded education and social attitude adjustment. In many instances, an individual recognizes the consequence of transplantation but has not emotionally bridged the distance to the possibility of being a recipient or a donor. Individuals, professionals and institutions grapple to adjust their thinking to advanced concepts and possibilities.

The legal system also has had problems with the rapid advancement of transplantation medicine. Two key issues requiring legal involvement are the definition of brain death and the development of donation guidelines.

Transplantation began to be a growing medical treatment in the 1960s. Advancements in medicine have made it possible to transplant 25 different organs and tissues, including corneas, skin, kidneys, hearts, livers, lungs, the pancreas and bone. Aside from human transplantations, donations may also be used for research related to diseases, injuries and disabilities.

Two important documents were developed in 1968. One document was legislative and the other professional regarding effective medical practice. These documents were called the *Uniform Anatomical Gift Act of 1968* and the *Harvard Criteria for Determination of Brain Death.*

The *Uniform Anatomical Gift Act of 1968,* in which organ and tissue donation became accepted legal and medical practice, was enacted as law in all 50 states. The law allows a person over 18 years of age and of sound mind to decide to become a personal organ or tissue donor or on the behalf of another. A minor may choose to donate organs and tissues with the consent of a parent or legal guardian.

The donor may specify the donee and may carry a card or have the notice put on his driver's license indicating his donor intent. This notification serves as communication to the emergency medical personnel and family. However, hospital facilities also require consent for donation to be signed by the next of kin as a matter of procedure.

The act not only provides a person with the legal ability to donate tissues and organs, but also protects a person if he chooses not to be a donor.

Over the years, the *Uniform Anatomical Gift Act* has been amended to adjust to the growing needs of transplantation. A congressional investigation in the early 1980s, led by Senator Albert Gore (D, Tennessee), regarding the problems a patient might have obtaining an organ because of the shortage of organs and lack of third-party funding, led to the concept of "required request." The most significant amendment to the act is the "required request" clause. Its purpose is to give every individual the right to be offered the opportunity of tissue and organ donation. It also requires hospitals to designate an individual within the institution to request anatomical gifts when a suitable candidate has been identified. As a result of recommendations, required request legislation took the form of amendments to state anatomical gift acts in 44 states. Every state's laws have their own requirements and peculiarities, but all have the same basic goal. The goal of the required request law is to increase the number of organs and tissues available by providing a family with the option of donating their family member's tissues and/or organs to give the gift of life and function to patients of all ages.

Ethicist Arthur Caplin, PhD, described the required request legislation as indicative of the collective acceptance by society that people should be given the option of organ and tissue donation as a last act of respect for the dead and their families and as an expression of concern for those who will die unless more organs and tissues are made available.

Other shortcomings and inequities of the transplantation process were also looked into. The result was the *National Organ Transplantation Act of 1984* (PL98-507), which mandated a national transplantation system to be operated by transplant professionals, with oversight by the Secretary of U.S. Department of Health and Human Services (DHHS). The purpose is to ensure an equitable allocation system in the public's interest. The act created the Organ Procurement and Transplantation Network (OPTN), a nonprofit private sector network to be operated by a contractor to DHHS. The act also set up the Organ Transplantation Task Force.

Originally, OPTN membership and policies were voluntary. However, with the enactment of the Omnibus Budget Reconciliation Act of 1986, adding Section 1138 of the Social Security Act, all hospitals that perform transplants and all organ procurement organizations (OPOs) were required to abide by the rules and requirements of the OPTN in order to receive Medicare and Medicaid reimbursement. In December 1989, DHHS placed a *Federal Register* notice indicating that all OPTN rules and requirements would remain voluntary until the Secretary promulgated regulations to define the roles and policy-making procedures of OPTN and DHHS. After extensive hearings and comment periods, DHHS announced the final rule to be published in the *Federal Register* in March, 1998. The rule provides the framework within which the OPTN, its members and other partici-

pants in organ procurement and transplantation will operate.

The OPTN is to be operated by a private-sector nonprofit agency called the United Network for Organ Sharing (UNOS). It functions as the network, serves as a clearinghouse and carries out the objectives of the Secretary. UNOS is located in Richmond, Virginia, and provides information regarding transplantation at 1-800-24-DONOR. Their web site is http://www.unos.org.

Ten UNOS regions have been designated as procurement areas. Each region has a designated Organ Procurement Organization (OPO) that advises hospital administration, nurses and medical professionals about issues, and provides services necessary for recovery and placement of organs and tissues. In some areas, the OPOs share responsibility, which eliminates competition. As soon as a potential donor is identified, the hospital should notify the OPO. *Table 18-1* is an extrapolation from data on the UNOS web site.

# THE DONATION PROCESS

Organ donation is still the major obstacle to transplantation. Most donated organs are from cadaveric donors, most of whom are trauma victims declared brain dead but have some cardiac function until the organ is removed. In order to ensure the organ's viability for transplantation, the organ must be obtained as soon as possible after brain death occurs.

Issues accompany the requests for donor tissues and organs. Families may resent being approached for organ donation while struggling with the news of a loved one's death, especially if it is sudden and traumatic. The family may not be educated in the need for and process of transplantation. Even if the deceased signed a donor card, the family may refuse to sign the consent. Family refusal is by far the greatest obstacle to organ dona-

## TABLE 18-1
## U.S. Organ Donors by Organ and Donor Type: 1988–1997

| ORGAN/DONOR TYPE | 1988 | 1997 |
|---|---|---|
| KIDNEY | | |
| Cadaveric | 3,876 | 5,079 |
| Living | 1,812 | 3,695 |
| Total | 5,688 | 8,774 |
| LIVER | | |
| Cadaveric | 1,833 | 4,590 |
| Living | 0 | 68 |
| Total | 1,833 | 4,658 |
| HEART | | |
| Cadaveric | 1,784 | 2,427 |
| Living | 7 | 0 |
| Total | 1,791 | 2,427 |
| LUNG | | |
| Cadaveric | 130 | 836 |
| Living | 0 | 31 |
| Total | 130 | 867 |

*Source:* UNOS Annual Report, September, 1998. www.unos.org/data/anrpt98/or98.

tion. This is truly a time when psychosocial considerations are paramount.

Additionally, although transplantation technology, technique and supporting drug therapy have developed rapidly over the past 20 years, a consistent U.S. policy on the collection of organs along with informed public opinion lags way behind.

Spain has achieved the most significant improvement in compliance with organ donation in Europe. Over a 2-year period, donations doubled from 14 to 28 per million, most of which is credited to emergency room and intensive care practitioners stepping up their efforts.

In an attempt to increase procurement, Sweden adopted the "Surgical Transplants Act." The act switches from the previous assumption of non-consent to a presumed-consent system. Unless the citizen states otherwise, tissues and organs are automatically donated after his death. They may be used for transplantation or other medical purposes.

## Recognition of Donors

The nurse should be aware donors are not only able to give organs, but can also give tissues such as corneas, skin, heart valves, bone, cartilage and veins.

Early recognition of a potential donor is essential. The best donor candidate is a person who was in good health before the traumatic event that brought him to death or brain death. Many donors are victims of head trauma. Nontrauma donors may have had a cerebral hemorrhage, been a victim of smoke inhalation, or have brain hypoxia from drowning.

Most emergency departments have a Death/Organ/Tissue Donation checklist that the nursing staff completes and places on the patient's medical record. The checklist functions as a tracking mechanism for documenting compliance with the statutes regarding death and required request. *Figure 18-1* is an example of a general checklist.

Additionally, the emergency department may have a Worksheet for Organ and Tissue Donor Referral. This worksheet is not required to be kept on the medical record but is used for staff information and tracking. The information in *Figure 18-2* is likely to be included.

Some states require that the medical examiner or coroner must evaluate victims of fatal trauma. There may also be an age restriction for donors. The transplant team will know the parameters. Physiologic condition of the donor rather than the chronologic age is usually of greater significance to

---

**FIGURE 18-1**
**Death/Organ/Tissue Donation Checklist**

Patient Name _____

Time and Date of Death _____

Current Date _____

|  | YES | NO | TIME |
|---|---|---|---|
| Patient identified as donor | _____ | _____ | _____ |
| Routine inquiry form signed | _____ | _____ | _____ |
| Organ procurement agency called* | _____ | _____ | _____ |
| Death report completed | _____ | _____ | _____ |
| Medical examiner approval obtained | _____ | _____ | _____ |
| Donor consent signed | _____ | _____ | _____ |
| Autopsy consent signed, if necessary | _____ | _____ | _____ |

*organ procurement coordinator and/or eye bank phone number or contact number

---

the transplant team. Donors are frequently evaluated on a case-by-case basis.

When a patient dies in the emergency department, he is considered a donor candidate. Three items must be documented on the patient's medical record:

1. Determination and declaration of death

2. State law requires the medical examiner's approval

3. Consent from the next of kin

In the donation process, the next of kin gives final permission for donation. The order of priority to identify the next of kin is spouse, adult child, parent, sibling and guardian. The next of kin must be at least 18 years of age.

## Criteria For Donors

At a minimum, the potential donor should have

- Cessation of brain functions

- Heart continues to beat; intact circulation. A heartbeat is not absolutely necessary for all

transplants; some tissues will be viable for several hours after circulation stops.

- Cessation of respiration, causing the patient to be dependent on a respirator

## Determination of Death

A patient must be declared dead in order for the donation process to begin. The following are commonly accepted criteria that have been adopted as the standard of practice:

I.  A person with irreversible cessation of circulatory and respiratory function is dead.

   A. Cessation is recognized by an appropriate clinical examination.

   B. Irreversibility is recognized by persistent cessation of functions during an appropriate period of observation, trial of therapy, or both.

II. A person with irreversible cessation of all functions of the entire brain, including the brain stem, is dead.

## FIGURE 18-2
## Worksheet for Organ and Tissue Donor Referral

(800) 24 HOUR HOT LINE (Phone number for Organ Procurement Organization [OPO])

Name of Patient _____

Medical Record Number _____

Age_____ Date of Birth_____ Admission Date _____

Time of Death_____ Cause of Death _____

Brief Medical History_____

_____

Ocular History, Including Surgeries _____

_____

Anticoagulation Therapy: _____

   Date and Type of Therapy: _____

History of Positive Blood Culture: Date:_____ Organism: _____

   Treatment: _____

Cancer History: Type:_____ Metastasis:_____ Date Diagnosed: _____

Treatment Type:_____ Date: _____

Social History: _____

Next of Kin: _____

Attending Physician: _____

Emergency Department Physician: _____

Medical Examiner Case: Yes____ No____ Time Called: _____

24 HOUR CONTACT NUMBER: _____

Approve Donation:_____

Disapprove Donation:

Comments: _____

_____

A. Cessation is recognized when the evaluation discloses two findings:

- Cerebral functions are absent.

- Brain stem functions (pupillary reflex, corneal reflex, gag reflex) are absent.

B. Irreversibility is recognized when evaluation discloses three findings:

- Cause of coma is established and is sufficient to account for loss of brain functions.

- Possibility of recovery of brain functions is excluded.

- Cessation of all brain functions persist for an appropriate period of observation, trial of therapy, or both.

Neurologists and other specialists are often called upon to confirm brain death. Once brain death is confirmed, the patient is considered dead. Standards advise that the physician confirming brain death not participate in the removal or transplantation of tissues or organs from the patient. At this time, it is essential the family understand that the patient is not alive or being kept alive by machines. The patient is not actually functioning or living.

Until not too long ago, the traditional concept of death was "when the heart stopped beating." When technology brought the world to the point of being able to maintain a patient's functions with mechanical support, determination of death by brain death criteria became necessary. Many neuroscience groups attempted to determine the criteria for defining brain death. One of the most notable papers was the *Harvard Criteria for Determination of Brain Death,* published in the late 1960s.

The development of criteria for determining brain death, and when it is applied, have become more specific. This is because of experience with the application of criteria and the need for clarity,

along with the need for an increased comfort level on the part of physicians and medical personnel.

## Donor Evaluation

Once death has been determined, the time and date must be documented and signed by the physician on the patient's medical record. If the patient has not previously been identified as a donor candidate, once the death has been documented on his record, the patient's potential as a donor is evaluated.

Criteria used in determining whether the patient is a suitable donor candidate are subject to frequent modification. The organ procurement agency staff will apply the most current criteria as they determine suitability for donation; **which should be completed before medical personnel speak to the family.**

Certain medical contraindications prevent the donation of organs and some tissues:

- Any transmittable disease such as bacterial, viral or fungal infections: septicemia, hepatitis, or if the patient is a high risk for human immunodeficiency virus.

- Other disorders generally thought to prohibit donation are diabetes mellitus, history of chronic or intravenous drug abuse, severe pre-existing hypertension and prolonged hypotension. However, the procurement agency will determine if these or any other disorders preclude the patient from qualifying as a donor.

All others can be considered potential candidates for donation. Frequently an error is made in determining that a patient diagnosed with metastatic cancer is ineligible for tissue donation. Nearly any person with most forms of cancer, including metastasis, is eligible to donate corneas for transplantation and/or research. Eligibility of a candidate should be discussed with the procurement agency before approaching the family.

Emergency nurses referring potential donors to the procurement agency are required to adhere to the referral policies established by their respective hospitals. A copy of the policies should be available in the emergency department. If the policy needs revision or has not yet been written, the procurement agency is able to help design a program that complies with state and federal statutes and is suitable for the hospital.

## Medical Examiner Evaluation

Although statutes and regulations may vary in each state, the medical examiner must be notified when a donation is to occur under some circumstances, including:

- Homicide victims
- Suicide victims
- Victims of accidental death
- Patients who die within 24 hours of admission
- Patients admitted with a loss of consciousness followed by death
- Patients who are 18 years of age and under

Each state's laws are specific regarding when a hospital should refer to the medical examiner includes the donation of tissues and organs. The hospital should have current written guidelines available in the emergency department for reference. Documentation of medical examiner notification is part of the medical record and required for the transplantation process to proceed.

## Hospital Requirements

The laws mandating required request resulted in hospital policies for carrying out the statutes. Rules and regulations of the law dictate documentation of all aspects of the donation request, including a solid administrative policy and education of all staff regarding the law and the importance of required request.

Three forms must be documented:

- **Consent form** that indicates whether the family agrees to the donation of tissues and/or organs must be signed by the next of kin or witnessed over the telephone.

- The **hospital's internal reporting form** should document the request for organ or tissue donation and the next-of-kin's response and is usually required for legal compliance. This document must be completed for every person who dies in the hospital regardless of the family's decision about donation.

- Some states may require a **state reporting form** that is a summary of the hospital's annual tissue and organ donation activity.

## Obtaining Consent

After the procurement agency determines eligibility for donation, the family can be approached regarding transplantation. Fortunately, because of continuing public information and education, some families may approach the staff first.

Before the family is approached for donation, they have to be told the patient has died. They need to be reassured everything was done to save the patient and death was inevitable. Of major importance, if at all possible, is having kept the family informed about the patient's status during his injury treatment. Then family members need to know the team worked hard to save the patient and, most likely, they will have anticipated the patient's death.

The family may be at the hospital at the time of the patient's death or choose to come to the emergency department to see the patient who has just died. Especially if the death is sudden, it is best to give the family an opportunity to go through some of the steps of death and dying to begin to cope with their loss. Being able to view the body is a vital step in the grieving process. They need time to say good-bye and make plans and arrangements.

The family is usually offered the opportunity to be comforted by the hospital chaplain. A private room or a quiet, private space that is comfortable, where they can share their feelings of grief and loss, should be made available. The thought that one of their family has died and will no longer be a part of their daily life can be devastating. They should also have access to a telephone.

Timing is everything. What the family knows or has been told is very important as to when to offer the option of donation. If they have not yet accepted that the death has occurred, it is not appropriate (at that time) to ask them to donate tissues and organs. Give the family some time to adjust to their crisis.

Referring to the patient as "not having any hope," "having passed," or "gone on," is an error that staff commonly makes; as these terms are too indirect and may sound insincere. It is essential the family hear the word "death" or "dead." These words are straightforward and leave no room for misinterpretation. The family's shock-denial mechanism should not be fed by misunderstanding.

Clarity is of particular importance when telling the family the patient is brain dead. The concept that the patient is not alive when the heart is still beating is a difficult one to grasp, particularly in the midst of a crisis.

An assumption should not be made by emergency staff about the family's name or apparent ethnicity that their religious or cultural background will preclude them from wanting to agree to donation. The choice should be offered to the family and belongs to the family.

There may be a designated team or physician trained in the psychosocial aspects of working with families of patients who have died.

It is never comfortable to be the one who offers the next of kin the opportunity to donate tissues or organs for transplantation. However, if the staff person designated to request donation is properly trained and keeps the perspective that others will live because of the donation, he will understand the rewarding responsibility of helping the family con-

sent to donating tissues and organs. This is particularly important if the patient had wanted to be a donor and made his wishes known.

A good person to speak with the family about donation is the staff member who has developed rapport with the family. Unfortunately, with trauma cases, there may not have been the chance to establish rapport. Whoever is designated to carry out the request should have a comprehensive understanding of the donation process and be comfortable with his own feelings about death. A great degree of thought, perception and knowledge is necessary.

The nurse should first discuss the potential for donation with the physician. The physician may or may not be comfortable with being in the position of requesting donation. At this time, it is decided who will discuss donation with the next of kin. Most likely, the hospital will have a written policy and protocol to follow.

Often the coordinator from the procurement agency is the one who obtains the signatures on the documents.

It is supportive for the family to know:

- The donor's condition and care is always the first priority, he will be treated with the utmost respect.
- There are no expenses to the donor's family related to transplantation. These costs are paid by the recipient.
- Recovery of tissues and organs is conducted under sterile surgical conditions, no different than any other surgical procedure.
- Once the tissues and organs are recovered, the ventilator is turned off, wounds are closed, and the body is released to the morgue and then the funeral home.
- There is no disfigurement from the recovery process, so that if the family wishes, they can still have an open casket at the funeral.

- Identities of the donor and recipient are not disclosed. The donor's family will be told general information about the recipient, such as age, sex, and general geographic location.

The first step in the process of consent for donation is to identify the next of kin. This can be straightforward or complicated, depending upon the family situation. It should be remembered that there may be a difference between the next of kin and the family spokesperson. The next of kin may be at the hospital at the time of death, or it may be necessary to obtain consent over the phone. With phone consent, two witnesses must verify that the next of kin gave permission. Exactly what they give permission for must be obtained and documented. The witnesses' signatures should be dated and timed.

Whoever approaches the next of kin about donation should make it clear that the law requires the hospital to offer the next of kin the choice of donation, and it is just that, a choice. He should also be given correct information upon which to base his choice, including whether the patient signed a donor card or indicated his consent on his driver's license.

If the next of kin member refuses donation, it is his choice. Not everyone is comfortable with the concept of donation. He should be allowed to feel comfortable with his decision, no matter what it is.

# THE PROCUREMENT PROCESS

Procurement for tissues and for organs is managed differently. The tissue donor is declared dead and has no heartbeat. The potential organ donor is considered brain dead, meaning the heart is still beating, often by mechanical devices. Tissues may also be obtained from this donor.

Once donated organs are procured, if they are to be used for transplantation, they must be immediately placed in a preservative solution to prevent deterioration.

Following placement in preservative solution, the tissue is typed. Tissue typing helps to determine the compatibility with potential recipients. Dr. Jean Dausset won a Nobel Prize in medicine in 1980 for discovering human leukocyte antigen (HLA) molecules, which are organ donor antigens critical to tissue typing.

After the typing, each donated organ is cross-matched with approximately 100 potential recipients on waiting lists. After a recipient is selected, the organ is shipped to the recipient's transplant center.

The length of time allowed before transplant varies among organ types, which may limit the distance the organ can be shipped. The quality of organ preservation is directly related to the organ's viability.

Even after collection, allocation and surgery have been accomplished, successful transplants still face hurdles. Rejection is the predominant cause of transplant failure. In order to fend off rejection of the transplanted organ, the recipient must begin a life-long regimen of immunosuppressive drugs immediately after surgery. In the past few years, a group of drugs have been introduced that allow the physician to customize immunosuppressive therapy for the patient. Consequently, there has been a drop in organ rejection to 25% to 35%. A year after transplantation, the graft survival rate is 91.5% for a kidney from a living donor and 81.1% for a cadaveric kidney.

## Tissue Procurement: Eyes, Corneas, Heart Valves, Bone and Skin

Tissue retrieval is not as complicated as internal organ procurement. The coordinator from the procurement agency arranges for the recovery team and works with the operating room nurses to set up procurement times.

Approximate maximum time allowed to recover tissue after the heart stops, depending on the procurement agency's protocols and availability of refrigeration, is

- 10 hours for bone
- 6–10 hours for heart valves
- 24 hours for corneas and skin

Obviously, the sooner the retrieval, the better.

### Bone

Bone is recovered under sterile conditions. Ordinarily, all four extremities, including both femurs, proximal tibia, fibula and humerus are recovered. On occasion, the mandible; hemipelvis; every other rib; and other limb tissues such as tensor fascia lata and Achilles tendon with a block of calcaneus are obtained.

The procedure lasts from $1\frac{1}{2}$ to 4 hours, depending on how many tissues are recovered. After the bones are extracted, prosthetic devices are inserted to retain the shape of the limb. The only evidence on the exterior of the body is incisions made along the side of the limbs.

Bone is stored in a freezer at -70°F, freeze-dried or processed into chips. There are many uses for bone, such as replacement of bone where it had been invaded by tumor and replacing bone removed in neurosurgical cases.

### Eye and Corneas

Technical staff for recovering eyes must be specially trained and, in some states, certified because the techniques are so precise.

If the eyes and corneas are to be donated, the patient should be kept in a refrigerated area with the head elevated and the eyes taped shut with paper tape. Cool compresses over the eyes prevent swelling, making procurement easier.

Recovery is a clean procedure using sterile technique and takes about 30 minutes. The whole eye or just the cornea may be recovered. Tissue in a preservative solution is placed on ice in a cooler. Eyes and corneas are sent to the eye recovery center for processing. Corneas generally are transplanted within 24 to 48 hours. They are used for the treatment of diseases of the cornea.

When the globe is recovered, the orbit is filled with cotton and a cap to maintain its shape.

### Heart Valves

The entire heart is removed in order to procure the aortic and pulmonary valves. Aortic root replacement, tetralogy of Fallot and pulmonary atresia repair can be done using valve parts.

After the heart is removed, it is placed in Ringer's lactated solution, packed in a sterile container, sterilely double-bagged and packed in ice to be shipped to a processing center. When the valves are removed, they are examined for their integrity and the heart is examined for pathologic conditions. Serology tests are done and, after a 40-day quarantine, the valves are released for homograft transplant.

Removal of the heart leaves only a single incision on the chest and no obvious disfigurement to the body.

### Skin

Skin recovery is not conducted everywhere. Where it is available, the procedure can take place in the morgue in a clean room using sterile technique. A dermatome procures skin from the buttocks, thighs, back, and abdomen. Tissues removed are split-thickness grafts (part of the skin's thickness) and are barely visible, unless the donor had a dark tan or deep pigmentation.

Recovered skin tissue is treated with antibiotics, prepared surgically for grafting, and stored at -70°F. Skin tissue is used for temporary grafts on burn patients to protect the patient from infection, fluid shifts and other burn-related complications.

## Solid-Organ Procurement: Heart, Lungs, Liver, Kidneys and Pancreas

Solid-organ procurement may be complex. Transplant team members represent many different disciplines. Along with working with the donor's family to respond to their concerns and fears, the transplant coordinator works with the intensive care unit staff to manage the donor until the time of procurement.

Once declared dead by brain death criteria, organ preservation management begins. Before the actual transplantation takes place, there may be several hours of hemodynamic maintenance. Management includes keeping fluids and electrolytes balanced, use of pressors such as dopamine and treatment of diabetes insipidus if it develops. Herniation can bring on diabetes insipidus and an imbalance of fluids and electrolytes. The donor's blood pressure is extremely labile. The pulmonary status must be carefully monitored for blood gas levels. Hematocrit is watched to determine if oxygen is being delivered at a sufficient level and not being lost due to hemorrhage from the trauma. All lab values are carefully monitored to ensure hemodynamic stability. The hemodynamic maintenance of the patient is far more complex than the brief description here.

Once the patient is declared a donor and all the organs to be recovered are assigned to recipients, the recovery teams meet at the agreed-upon time. The host hospital has the option of setting the procurement time. Most retrievals occur late at night to avoid disrupting daytime operating schedules. The hospital is asked to provide operating room, staff and anesthesia support.

When the donor is transported to the operating room he is completely supported by mechanical means and hemodynamically supported according to previously decided guidelines. He is maintained throughout the entire organ dissection and tissue mobilization and until they are ready for immediate removal and preservation.

Once the last steps of the dissection are finished, the aorta is clamped and the heart stops. Then, quick cooling and in situ flushing of the organs are conducted. After the organs have been flushed, they are removed, individually examined in a sterile basin, usually flushed again and packed in a sterile container. The organs are then transported for transplant.

If followed carefully, the parameters for maintenance of the donor will allow the retrieval of healthy organs for transplant. This rule is the same for adults and children.

## ETHICAL CONSIDERATIONS

Once transplantation became a viable medical treatment, numerous ethical issues arose. Some issues relate to medical professionals and others relate to the family.

Decision making at a time when a loved one has died is extremely difficult. When the decision extends to giving away parts of that loved one, it may be excruciating. Families may become confused about what to do. Fighting can erupt between family members, further increasing the stress. Some families have discussed donation at a previous time, some have not. If the patient has expressed the desire to donate organs or tissues, it may take the decision-making pressure off the family. However, although a patient may have wanted to be a donor, hospitals will follow the next of kin's wishes, even if they go against the donor's wishes.

Medical personnel are not all at the same point of education and acceptance regarding asking the next of kin to donate a loved one's tissues and organs.

Many issues are raised concerning declaration of brain death. Families and some medical professionals have great difficulty coming to terms with when to call brain death and when the possibility of the patient "waking up" will no longer occur. There are also ethical and emotional struggles concerning maintaining a patient for organ donation, even though others will live because of the organs transplanted.

Additional concerns are the determination of who will receive the tissues or organs, selling live organs for transplantation, required request versus presumed consent and is there any limit to what can be transplanted and what should be transplanted?

Controversy continues to confront the transplantation process. Every year, thousands of people die waiting for organ transplant. Poor planning, bad communication, lack of information, and denial and mistrust of the medical system are some of the reasons more people do not commit to donation. Even if the patient has committed to donation, his wishes can be blocked at the hospital by the next of kin for a variety of reasons, none of which support the donor's original intent.

The demand-and-supply gap continues to grow. It has been presumed that cadaveric donation has always been based on altruism. At this time, the Pennsylvania State Health Department is considering paying up to $3,000 toward hospital and funeral expenses of the donor, which is hoped will act as an incentive toward donation. Realism may have to accompany altruism in order to save lives.

Then there is the question of how some people seem to jump up on the waiting list. The governor of Pennsylvania received a heart and liver quickly, and Mickey Mantle and Larry Hageman quickly received livers. Questions arose about how some people appear to obtain organs more quickly than others. These questions also pointed out the immense and growing need for more tissues and organs and helped to serve as an education and discussion tool for the public.

# FINANCIAL CONSIDERATIONS

Donation and transplantation is extremely expensive. In this country, third-party payers are the most common source of transplantation payment. In 1972, the Bennett Amendment to the Social Security Act included the extension of Medicare coverage for people with end-stage renal disease for dialysis and kidney transplantation. All people are to be given the opportunity for treatment essential to life.

With liver and heart transplantation, most third-parties pay for the transplantation surgery and post-operative care. In some states, heart and lung, pancreas and lung transplants are not eligible for reimbursement because they are still considered experimental.

The costs involved in transplantation are under considerable discussion, with emphasis on the number of people helped and cost and life expectancy after the graft and transplantation. Now, with cost containment and managed care, many entities have difficulty justifying the costs of transplantation, although the demands are growing. For instance, Oregon has reallocated transplantation dollars, with the exception of kidneys and corneas.

# THE FUTURE OF TRANSPLANTATION

Organ allocation is the most controversial issue facing the future of transplants. The system for procurement and disbursement has improved since 1984 when the National Organ Transplantation Act made the allocations more fair. The law mandated a national waiting list of recipients, equitable distribution of organs and a national transplantation registry. Discrepancies still exist. New criteria for establishing waiting list priority are currently under consideration.

Despite the great need for, and considerable lack of organ and tissue donations, there is still reason to be hopeful. Today, more than 25 different tissues and organs are able to be transplanted. In this country, there are 69 organ procurement organizations serving 278 transplant centers.

Clinical results are improving because of new treatment options. The transplant community is persistent in lobbying for the "gift of life" and overall donor compliance is improving.

In an effort to increase the pool of suitable organs, researchers are experimenting with xenotransplantation (animal transplants). Additionally, surgeons are "cutting down" livers in half and sewing them into children because livers usually regenerate within 3 months and readjust to the recipient's body.

Public policy reflects officials' and interest groups' efforts to increase organ and tissue donations. Celebrities lend their names to support national programs. There is international focus with the World Transplant Games. The event fosters competition among athletes who are transplant recipients in order to showcase healthy post-transplant lifestyles and encourage donation.

Economically, Medicare now covers anti-rejection drugs for 36 months for kidney transplant recipients who are covered by Medicare, a raise from 12 months. Some members of Congress are pushing for further expansion of benefits.

# NURSING STRATEGIES FOR ORGAN DONATION

- Have a thorough familiarity of the hospital's policies and procedures regarding required request for organ and tissue donation.

- Have a comprehensive understanding of the donation process in order to be able to inform the family before they make their decision about donation.

- Recognize that the required request is required by law and the next of kin has the right to make his own choice.

- Know how to immediately contact the organ procurement coordinator.

- Be sure to fill out all required documents completely and place them on the medical record.

- Know the criteria for brain death and how to explain what brain death is to the family.

- Have an awareness of your own feelings about death and organ transplantation.

# SUMMARY

Organ and tissue transplantation enhances and extends lives of all ages. Medical advances now allow 25 different tissues and organs to be transplanted with constantly improving rates of success. However, the gap between the need and the supply is growing. Thousands die waiting for their transplant.

The Uniform Anatomical Gift Act of 1968, in which tissue and organ donation became accepted legal medical practice, was enacted as law in all 50 states. The National Organ Transplantation Act of 1984 set into motion a nationwide system to be operated by transplant professionals with oversight by the Secretary of the Department of Health and Human Services. The purpose of the act is to ensure an equitable organ and tissue donation system that operates in the public interest.

The donation process includes the recognition of donors, criteria for donors, determination of death, donor evaluation, medical examiner evaluation, hospital requirements and obtaining consent.

Procurement for tissues and for organs is managed under different criteria and guidelines. The tissue donor is declared dead and has no heartbeat. The potential organ donor is considered brain dead, meaning the heart is still beating, often with mechanical assistance.

Many ethical considerations are involved with transplantation. Issues involve the family of the dead patient, medical professionals, the selling of organs, live donors, and means of allocation. Some recipients, particularly if they are rich and famous, seem to rapidly move up the recipient list, causing controversy and damaging the credibility of the system.

The future of transplantation, while rife with problems, appears to be improving. Today there are 69 organ procurement organizations serving 278 transplant centers in this country. Some members of Congress are pushing for further expansion of Medicare benefits. Many well-known people and events are becoming involved in educating the public in order to increase the number of organ and tissue donors.

# EXAM QUESTIONS

## CHAPTER 18
### Questions 96–100

96. The process of identifying tissue and organ donor candidates includes

    a. finding out what diseases the patient had before his injury.

    b. asking the family if they want the patient to be a donor if he dies.

    c. notifying the nursing supervisor.

    d. notifying the organ procurement agency to determine the suitability for donation.

97. The family should be approached for required request of donation

    a. after the procurement agency determines the eligibility for donation.

    b. immediately after brain death has been determined.

    c. after the nurse has evaluated their feelings regarding donation of organs.

    d. by the medical examiner.

98. The procurement process

    a. is supervised by the medical examiner.

    b. is conducted after the body has been transported to the receiving facility.

    c. is managed differently for tissues and organs.

    d. is determined by the next of kin.

99. The legislation in which organ and tissue donation became accepted legal and medical practice is the

    a. Medicare Bill of 1968.

    b. National Organ Transplantation Act of 1984.

    c. Uniform Organ Transplant Act of 1964.

    d. Uniform Anatomical Gift Act of 1968.

100. The most likely recipients for tissues or organs are

    a. those who are covered by Medicare payments.

    b. whomever is at the top of the transplant list and has the closest tissue type.

    c. whomever can pay for the transplant.

    d. whomever is well known and has made the public aware of the need for transplantation.

**This concludes the final examination. An answer key will be printed on your certificate of completion so that you can determine which of your answers were correct and incorrect.**

# GLOSSARY

**Battle's Sign:** Ecchymosis over the mastoid area that may indicate a fracture at the base of the skull.

**Blunt Trauma:** Damage to the body without penetration of the skin, caused by rapid deceleration and sudden impact with an object.

**Brain Death:** Cessation of all functions of the entire brain, including the brain stem. Cerebral functions are absent. Brain stem functions are absent. The heart is kept beating by mechanical support, but the patient is not alive or being kept alive by the machines. The patient is not actually functioning or living.

**Burn:** Tissue injury resulting from excessive exposure to thermal, chemical, electrical or light mechanisms; smoke inhalation; or radiation. Effects vary according to the type of burn, duration of exposure, intensity of the agent, and the part of the body involved.

**Cardiopulmonary Resuscitation:** An emergency technique used in the attempt to save the patient's life when he is in cardiac or respiratory arrest. The goal is to provide oxygen quickly to the brain, heart and other vital organs until definitive medical treatment is able to restore cardiac and pulmonary functions.

**Cardiovascular System:** A system comprised of the heart and blood vessels, including the aorta, arteries, arterioles, capillaries, venules, veins and venae cavae. The system keeps the body running by delivering oxygen and nutrients and disposing of cellular waste and carbon dioxide through a complex arrangement of systemic circulation and pulmonary circulation.

**Central Nervous System:** The portion of the nervous system made up of the brain and spinal cord. The brain is the controlling organ of the body and the spinal cord transmits messages back and forth between the brain and the body.

**Child Maltreatment:** Although different states' definitions vary to an extent, the terms child abuse and maltreatment are used interchangeably to describe neglect and/or physical, emotional, and/or sexual abuse to the child.

**Choroid:** The dark-brown vascular coat of the eye between the sclera and retina. The choroid is made up of blood vessels united by connective tissue containing pigmented cells and five layers. It is a part of the uvea or vascular tunic of the eye.

**Comorbid Conditions in the Elderly:** Diseases that commonly develop, along with the anatomic and physiologic changes occurring in aging, that seriously affect the elder's response to injury.

**Cranial Nerves:** Twelve pairs of nerves originating in the brain stem, each having a separate name, Roman numeral identifier, and anatomical and physiological function. The nerves have unconscious control over sensory, motor or both activities.

**Death:** Irreversible cessation of circulatory and respiratory function, evidenced by persistent cessation of these functions. Time and date must be documented on the patient's medical record and signed by the physician.

**Diffuse Head Injury:** A head injury that involves the entire brain.

**Displaced Fracture:** A fractured bone that has been pushed out of alignment, causing deformity and requiring reduction before immobilization.

**Embryo:** The stage in prenatal development between being the ovum and becoming the fetus, lasting from the 2nd to the 8th week of gestation.

**Epidemiology:** The distribution and determinants of disease frequency in man. Epidemiology is relative to trauma in the collection of data such as age, gender, race/ethnicity and geographic characteristics that form frequency and distribution patterns of injury, morbidity and mortality due to trauma.

**Failure to thrive:** A condition seen in children under the age of 5 when growth continues to significantly fail to meet the norms for age and sex based on national growth charts.

**Fetus:** The developing child in utero from the 3rd month of pregnancy to birth.

**Focal Head Injury:** A head injury having a specific area of involvement.

**Foot Pound:** Work expended when one pound is moved a distance of one foot in the direction of the force.

**Gestation:** The period of time from conception to birth, usually from 38–40 weeks.

**Golden Hour:** Refers to the occurrence of death following injury as a function of time. There are three peaks of the occurrence of death after injury: immediate, early and late. It is "early" deaths, occurring within the first few hours, that the "golden hour" refers to. Modern trauma centers are often able to save these patients. Survival of seriously injured or ill patients is the highest when intervention takes place within the first "golden hour" after the injury occurs.

**Inhalation Injury:** Damage to the air passages caused by the inhalation of toxic fumes, hot air or carbon monoxide.

**Level I Trauma Center:** A hospital providing the highest level of trauma care and services 24 hours a day, 7 days a week.

**Level II Trauma Center:** Emergency department capabilities similar to Level I centers. The trauma team is not necessarily in-house 24 hours a day but must be able to meet the severely injured patient when he arrives in the emergency department.

**Level III Trauma Center:** Hospitals that are not immediately accessible to Level I and II centers. In-house surgical coverage on a 24-hour basis is not required and staffing may be on an on-call basis. Accessibility to higher level facilities should be timely and is usually by helicopter transportation.

**Manual Techniques to Clear the Airway:** Techniques used to open the patient's airway, which include jaw thrust, head tilt-chin lift and chin lift maneuvers.

**Mechanical Methods for Airway Control:** Used in the semiconscious or unconscious patient when basic manual techniques do not clear the airway. Use of these mechanisms requires special training for professionals. Devices include: oropharyngeal airways, nasopharyngeal airways, esophageal obturator airways, pharyngo-tracheal lumen airways, and endotracheal tubes.

**Meninges:** Three vascular layers of membranes that surround and protect the brain and spinal cord.

**Neglect:** Intentional or unintentional omission of needed care and support, or the caregiver being either unable or unwilling to provide the most basic needs for the person in his care.

**Nursing Diagnosis:** A clinical nursing judgment about individual, family or community reactions or responses to illness or injury, problems or life processes. The diagnoses serve as a basis for nursing interventions that have outcomes for which the nurse is accountable. The physician does not have to give an order for these interventions.

**Orbital Complex:** A bony pyramid-shaped cavity in the skull that contains and protects the eyes, comprised of the frontal bone, zygoma and maxilla.

**Organ Donor:** After death has been pronounced, it is determined by the organ procurement agency, according to specified criteria, as to the patient's suitability for the donation of organs (and/or tissues) to be used in transplantation.

**Orthopedic Injuries:** Musculoskeletal injuries, including soft tissue strains and sprains; damage to the skin, tendons, ligaments, cartilage and associated vessels and nerves; and dislocations, subluxations and fractures that are a significant cause of short and long-term disabilities.

**Pathologic Fracture:** A fracture in a diseased or weak bone that can occur with minimal force. Pathologic fractures frequently occur in the spine without the patient being aware of the fracture; he "just gets shorter."

**Penetrating Trauma:** Injury caused by an object hitting the body with such force that it pierces the skin, and, which may leave tissue and organ injury or destruction along its path.

**Peripheral Nervous System:** Linking cables of nerve fibers reaching outside the central nervous system. The system includes the nerves that enter and leave the spinal cord and those that connect the brain and organs without passing through the spinal cord. There are 31 pairs of peripheral nerves called spinal nerves and 12 pairs of cranial nerves.

**Peritoneal Space:** A cavity that is really a potential space between the layers of the parietal and visceral peritoneum. It contains a small amount of fluid so that the viscera can glide easily on each other or against the wall of the abdominal cavity.

**Physical Abuse:** Intentional infliction of physical injury, torture, maiming or unreasonable force, or omission/failure to protect the individual from danger and injury.

**Prehospital Care:** The part of the emergency medical services system beginning at the point of discovery of a person's illness or injury, access to the system and professional medical care until the patient reaches the emergency department. There are two levels of care provided by prehospital personnel: basic life support (BLS) and advanced life support (ALS).

**Priapism:** Abnormal, painful and continued erection of the penis due to disease or may be due to lesions of the cord above the lumbar region.

**Primary Assessment:** Rapid and accurate initial assessment of the patient's condition that is conducted on every patient. Primary assessment includes determination of the status of the ABCs: airway, breathing, and circulation. Included are: Providing resuscitation and stabilization on a priority basis; determination of critical injuries and the level of care the patient needs.

**Psychosocial:** The internal/psychological and interpersonal/social factors that determine a person's emotional state. Psychosocial conditions should not be confused with psychiatric or altered mental conditions.

**Raccoon Eyes:** Black eyes or discoloration under the eyes that may indicate a basilar skull fracture.

**Respiratory System:** A system consisting of air passages and organs: nasal cavities, oral cavity, pharynx, larynx, trachea, and lungs, including bronchi, bronchioles, alveolar ducts, and alveoli. The system functions to bring in and distribute oxygen to nourish the body and to rid the body of the waste products of respiration.

**Response to Trauma:** Response to trauma going beyond the physical injury and including the mind and spirit's reactions; a complex, integrated system of reactions.

**Retinal Detachment:** The pigment layer of the retina, remains attached to the choroid and the rest of the retina detaches from it. Occurs with or without a tear.

**Retroperitoneal:** Located behind the peritoneum and outside the peritoneal cavity, containing the kidneys, bladder, ureters, reproductive organs, inferior vena cava and abdominal aorta.

**Saddle Nose:** A nose with a depressed bridge—usually congenital—due to the absence of bone or cartilidge support; due to disease; or it may be a deformity secondary to trauma causing a septal hematoma.

**Secondary Assessment:** Conducted after the primary assessment, or survey, is completed and the ABCs are stabilized. The purpose is to thoroughly evaluate and document additional injuries and illnesses, including stopping any bleeding and administering supplemental oxygen. The patient is reassessed frequently, and a history is obtained, along with recording the patient's current medications and allergies.

**Shock:** A clinical syndrome that is a series of reactions to mental or physical upset of the body's internal balance.

**Thermoregulation:** The regulation of temperature, and physiologically, body temperature.

**Trauma:** Physical injury caused by an external action, such as an assaulting force, thermal or chemical agent that is strong enough to potentially threaten limb or life.

**Trauma Center:** A hospital facility designated according to the level of trauma care it provides. Determination is made according to established criteria regarding the numbers and qualifications of the surgeons who staff on a 24-hour-a-day basis and specialty services provided. Levels of trauma centers are I, II, and III. Trauma centers have a team activation system that operates according to triage criteria with its members having defined roles and responsibilities to provide systematic and coordinated care.

**Triage:** Injury assessment using defined criteria. Triage means sorting. In emergency medical services, it means assessment to sort the patients by severity of illness or injury. The process is used in a prehospital situation where the patient is assessed and directed to the most appropriate level of hospital emergency services. In the emergency department, triage is used to sort the severity of illness or injury in order to determine the priority of care the patient receives. Triage is also used during mass casualties and military operations.

**UNOS:** United Network for Organ Sharing (UNOS) is a private, nonprofit agency that operates the Organ Procurement and Transplantation Network by serving as a clearinghouse and carrying out the objectives of the Secretary of the Department of Health and Human Services in accordance with the National Organ Transplantation Act of 1984.

**Urinary System:** Controls the elimination of specific toxic waste products filtered from the blood, along with managing the body's water and electrolyte balance. Other functions include the stimulation of red blood cell production, activation of vitamin D and insulin degradation.

# BIBLIOGRAPHY

ABC News Internet Ventures. (1999). *Paradox in Pennsylvania: How much is too much for a human organ?*

Aguilera, D. C. & Messick, J. M. (1994). *Crisis intervention: Theory and methodology* (7th ed.). St. Louis: Mosby.

American Academy of Orthopaedic Surgeons. (1987). *Emergency Care and Transportation of the Sick and Injured* (4th ed.). Park Ridge, IL: Author.

American College of Surgeons. (1993). *Advanced trauma life support student manual.* Chicago: The College.

Auerbach, P. (1995). *Wilderness medicine* (3rd ed.). St. Louis: Mosby.

Barkin, R. (Ed.). (1992). *Pediatric emergency medicine.* St. Louis: Mosby.

Billmire, M. E. & Myers, P. A. (1985). Serious head injury in infants: Accident or abuse? *Pediatrics, 75,* 340–342.

Bonica, J. (Ed.). (1980). *Obstetric analgesia and anesthesia* (2nd ed. rev.). Amsterdam: World Federation of Societies of Anesthesiologists.

Caldwell, E. (1978). The psychologic impact of trauma. *Nursing Clinic of North America, 13*(2), 247–54.

Campbell, J. (1988.). *Basic trauma life support: Advanced prehospital care* (2nd ed.). Englewood Cliffs, NJ: Prentice-Hall.

Campbell, J. E. (Ed.) (2000). *Basic trauma life support for paramedics and other advanced providers* (4th ed.). Upper Saddle River, NJ: Brady/Prentice Hall Health.

Centers for Disease Control: Division of Injury Control, Center for Environmental Health and Injury Control. (1990). Childhood injuries in the United States. *Am J Dis Child,* 144:627.

Chambers, E. & Belicki, K. (1998). Using sleep dysfunction to explore the nature of resilience in adult survivors of childhood abuse or trauma. In *Child Abuse Neglect.* Aug 22(8):753–8.

Chandra, N. C. & Hazinski, M. F. (Eds.). (1997). *Basic life support for healthcare providers.* Dallas: American Heart Association.

Childhelp USA. (2000). Major Forms of Child Abuse. Available online [http://www.childhelpusa.org/child/abuse.htm]. 800-4-A-CHILD 24-hour hotline, Scottsdale, AZ.

Collier, I., McCash, K. & Bartram, J. (1996). *Writing nursing diagnosis.* St. Louis: Mosby.

Colucciello, S. A. (1995). The treacherous and complex spectrum of maxillofacial trauma: Etiologies, evaluation, and emergency stabilization. *Emerg Med Rep, 16*(7), 59.

Coody, D., Brown, M., Montgomery, D., Flynn, A. & Yetman, R. (1994). Shaken baby syndrome: Identification and prevention for nurse practitioners. *Journal of Pediatric Health Care, 8*(2), 50–56.

Cooper, A. (1993). Critical management of chest, abdomen and extremity trauma. In P. R. Holbrook (Ed.), *Textbook of pediatric critical care.* Philadelphia: WB Saunders.

Creel, J. H., Jr. (1995). Mechanisms of injuries due to motion. In J. E. Campbell (Ed.), *Basic trauma life support.* Englewood Cliffs, NJ: Prentice Hall.

Cummins, R.O. (Ed.). (1997). *American Heart Association, fighting heart disease and stroke, advanced cardiac life support.* Dallas: American Heart Association.

Davis, H. (1991). Child abuse and neglect. In B. Zitelli & H. Davis (Eds.), *Atlas of pediatric physical diagnosis* (2nd ed.). St. Louis: Mosby.

Davis, R. J., Dean, M., Goldberg, A. L., Carson, B. S., Rosenbaum, A. E. & Rogers, M. C. (1987). Head and spinal cord injury. In M. Rogers (Ed.), *Textbook of pediatric intensive care.* Baltimore: Wilkins & Wilkins.

Dolan, M. (1992). Head trauma. In R. M. Barkin (Ed.), *Pediatric emergency medicine, concepts and clinical practice.* St. Louis: Mosby.

Edlich, R. F., Glassberg, H. H. & Tobiasen, J. A. (1994). Abbreviated burn severity index. *Current Concepts in Trauma Care, 7*(1), 20.

Ehrlich, F., Heldrich, F. & Tepas, J. (Eds.). (1987). *Pediatric emergency medicine.* Rockville, MD: Aspen.

Emergency Nurses Association. (1995). *Trauma nursing core course* (4th ed.). Chicago: The Association.

Esposito, T. J. (1994). Trauma during pregnancy. *Emer Med Clin North Amer, 12*(1), 167.

Esposito, T. J., Gens, D. R., Smith, L. G. & Scorpio, R. (1989). Evaluation of blunt abdominal trauma occurring during pregnancy. *Journal of Trauma, 29*(12), 1628–1632.

Feliciano, D. V., Moore, E. E. & Mattov, K. L. (Eds.). (1996). *Trauma* (3rd ed.). Stamford, CT: Appleton & Lange.

Fleming, A. (Ed.). (1993). *Facts, 1993.* Arlington, VA: Insurance Institutes for Highway Safety.

Goodman, M. H. (1990). The physical abuse of children: Then and now. *Nursing Practice Forum, 1,* 84–89.

Grant, H. D., Murray, R. H., Jr. & Bergeron, J. D. (Eds.). (1990). *Brady emergency care* (5th ed.). Englewood Cliffs, NJ: Prentice Hall.

Guerriero, W. G. & Devine, C. J., Jr. (1984). *Urologic injuries.* E. Norwalk, CT: Appleton-Century-Crofts.

Guyton, A. C. & Hall, J. E. (1996). *Textbook of medical physiology* (9th ed.). Philadelphia: WB Saunders.

Handysides, G. (1996). *Triage in emergency practice.* St. Louis: Mosby.

Henderson, V. J., Smith, R. S., Fry, W. R., Morabito, D., Peskin, G. W., Barkan, H. & Organ, C. H. (1994). Cardiac injuries: Analysis of an unselected series of 251 cases. *Journal of Trauma, 36*(3), 341–348.

Herman, J. L. (1992). *Trauma and Recovery.* New York: Basic Books.

Holleran, R. (1994). *Prehospital nursing: A collaborative approach.* St. Louis: Mosby.

Hollingsworth-Frielund, P., Andrews, J. & Hoyt, K. S. (1989). Preparing the hospital site review for trauma center designation: A survey of nurse evaluators. In: *J. Emergency Nursing,* 15(5): 405–409.

Hopkins, A. G. (1994). The trauma nurse's role with families in crisis. *Critical Care Nurse, 14*(2), 35–43.

Hyden, P. W. & Gallagher, T. A. (1992). Child abuse intervention in the emergency room. *Pediatric Clin North America, 39*(5), 1053–1081.

Jaworski, M. & Wirtz, K. (1995). Spinal trauma. In S. Kitt, J. Selfridge-Thomas, J. A. Proehl & J. Kaiser (Eds.), *Emergency nursing* (2nd ed.), pp. 357–376. Philadelphia: WB Saunders.

*Joint hearing of the House Commerce Committee, House of Representatives, and the Senate Labor and Human Resources Committee, Senate,* (1998).

Kelly, S. J. (1994). *Pediatric emergency nursing* (2nd ed.). Norwalk, CT: Appleton and Lange.

Kempe, C. H. (1962). The battered-child syndrome. *JAMA, 181,* 17–24.

Kidd, P. S. & Sturt, P. (1996). *Mosby's emergency nursing reference.* St. Louis: Mosby.

Kitt, S., Selfridge-Thomas, J., Proehl J. & Kaiser, J. (Eds.). (1995). *Emergency nursing: A physiologic and clinical perspective* (2nd ed.). Philadelphia: W. B. Saunders.

Kitt, S. & Kaiser, J. (1990). *Emergency nursing: A physiologic and clinical perspective.* Philadelphia: Saunders.

Kshettry, V. R. & Bolman, R. M. (1994). Chest trauma: Assessment, diagnosis and management. *Clinical Chest Medicine, 15*(1), 137–146.

Kubler-Ross, E. (1974). *On death and dying* (Rev. ed.). New York: MacMillan Publishing Company.

Laudicina, S. S. (1988). *Medicaid coverage and payment policies for organ transplants: Findings of a national survey.* Washington, DC: George Washington University, U. S. Department of Health and Human Services.

Lavery, J. P. & Staten-McCormick, M. (1995). Management of moderate to severe trauma in pregnancy. *Obstet Gynecol Clin North Am, 22*(1), 69.

Lewis, S. M., Collier, I. C. & Heitkemper, M. M. (1996). *Medical and surgical nursing: Assessment and management of clinical problems* (4th ed.). St. Louis: Mosby.

Maslow, A. H. (1954). *Motivation and personality.* New York: Harper and Row.

McSwain, N., Paturas, J. & Wertz, E. (Eds.). (1994). *Pre-hospital trauma life support.* St. Louis: Mosby.

Miller, R. (Ed.). (1981). *Anesthesia* (2nd ed., Vol. 2). New York: Churchill Livingstone.

Moore, A. D., Stambrook, M., Peters, L. C., Cardoso, E. R. & Kassum, D. A. (1990). Long-term multidimensional outcome following isolated traumatic brain injuries and traumatic brain injuries associated with multiple trauma. *Brain Injury, 4*(4), 379–389.

Morris, M.R. (1998). Elder abuse: What the law requires. *RN, 61*(8), 52–53.

National Center for Education in Maternal and Child Health. (1991). *Children's safety network: A data book of child and adolescent injury.* Washington, D.C.: Author.

National Center for Health Statistics. (1993). *Monthly vital statistics: Advance report of final mortality, 1993. 44*(7), 1996.

National Committee for Injury Prevention and Control. (1989). Injury prevention meeting the challenge. *American Journal of Preventive Medicine, 5*(3), 2.

National Safety Council. (1996). *Accident facts, 1996 ed.* [Brochure] Chicago.

Neff, J. & Kidd, P. (1993). *Trauma nursing: The art and science.* St. Louis: Mosby.

Nettina, S. & Gregonis, S. (1990). Assigning priorities. *Nursing, 20*(11), 86.

Neufeld, J. D. & Marx, J. A. (1992). Trauma in pregnancy. In P. Rosen, F. J. Baker, R. M. Barkin, G. R. Braen, R. H. Dailey, J. R. Hedges, R. S. Hockberger, R. C. Levy, J. A. Marx, & M. Smith (Eds.), *Emergency medicine: Concepts and clinical practice* (3rd ed.). St. Louis: Mosby.

Newberry, L. (Ed). (1998). *Sheehy's emergency nursing: Principles and practice* (4th ed.). St. Louis: Mosby.

Notice of Opportunity for Partnerships, 63 *Fed. Reg.* (1998, September 17).

O'Carroll, B. M. (1990 Mar/Apr). Eye Emergencies: Seeing Clear Solutions. *Rescue,* 17–29.

O'Carroll, B. M. (1991 Sept/Oct). Child neglect and abuse: Opening closed doors. *Rescue,* 48–66.

O'Carroll, B. M. (1992 Jan/Feb). Respiratory emergencies: A matter of life. *Rescue,* (Pt. 1), 26–38.

O'Carroll, B. M. (1992 Mar/Apr). Respiratory emergencies: A matter of life. *Rescue,* (Pt. 2), 19–37.

O'Keefe, M. F., Limmer, D., Grant, H. D., Murray, R. H. & Bergeron, J. D. (1998). *Brady Emergency Care* (8th ed.). Upper Saddle River, NJ: Brady/Prentice Hall.

Pate, J. W. (1989). Tracheobronchial and esophageal injuries. *Surg Clin North Am, 69*(1), 111–123.

Peitzman, A. B., Rhodes, M., Schwab, C. W. & Yealy, D. M. (Eds.). (1998). *The trauma manual.* Philadelphia: Lippincott-Raven.

Peterson, N. E. (1991). Current management of acute renal trauma. In S. W. Rous (Ed.), *Urology annual* (pp. 151–179). Norwalk, CT: Appleton & Lange.

President's Commission for the Study of Ethical Problems in Medicine and Biomedical Research. (1981). *Defining death: Medical, legal, and ethical issues in the determination of death.* Washington, D.C.

Ray, L. & Yuwiler, J. (1994). *Child and adolescent fatal injury databook.* San Diego: Children's Safety Network.

Reeder, S., Mastroianni, L., Martin, L. & Fitzpatrick, E. (1976). *Maternity nursing* (13th ed.). Philadelphia: Lippincott.

Sanders, M. J. (1995). *Mosby's paramedic textbook.* St. Louis: Mosby.

Sangstat: The Transplant Company. (1999). *Facts about transplantation.* [Online].

Schwartz, G. (Ed.). (1999). *Principles and Practice of Emergency Medicine* (4th ed.). Baltimore: Williams & Wilkins.

Sheehy, S. B. & Jimmerson, C. L. (1994). *Manual of clinical trauma care: The first hour.* St. Louis: Mosby Year Book.

Shoemaker, W. C. (1996). Resuscitation from severe hemorrhage. *Critical Care Medicine, 24,* 12–23.

Solomon, Z., Oppenheimer, B., Elizur, Y. & Waysman, M. (1990). Trauma deepens trauma: The consequences of recurrent combat stress reaction. *Israel Journal of Psychiatry and Related Sciences, 27*(4), 233–241.

Soud, T., Pieper, P. & Hazinski, M. F. (1992). Pediatric trauma. In M. F. Hazinski (Ed.), *Nursing care of the critically ill child* (2nd ed.). St. Louis: Mosby.

Soud, T. E. & Rogers, J. S. (1998). *Manual of pediatric emergency nursing.* St. Louis: Mosby.

Sparks, S. M. & Taylor, C. M. (1998). *Nursing diagnosis reference manual* (4th ed.). Springhouse, PA: Springhouse.

Stamatos, C. A., Sorensen, P. A. & Tefler, K. M. (1996). Meeting the challenge of the older trauma patient. *American Journal of Nursing, 96*(5), 40–48.

Teasdale, T. W., Christensen, A. L. & Pinner, E. M. (1993). Psychosocial rehabilitation of cranial trauma and stroke patients. *Brain Injury, 7*(6), 535–542.

*Think you know something about child abuse? (1993).* [Booklet]. Chicago: National Committee to Prevent Child Abuse.

Thomas, P. (1994, June 23). Study of rape in young girls. *Washington Post,* reprinted in *The Commercial Appeal,* pp. A1–A5.

Trunkey, D. D. & Lewis, F. R. (Eds.). (1986). *Current therapy of trauma.* Toronto: BC Decker.

United Network for Organ Sharing (UNOS). (1998, September). *U.S. organ donors by organ and donor type—1988 to 1997.*

United Network for Organ Sharing (UNOS). (1999, September). *UNOS president testifies in support of H.R. 2418: Legislation seeks to strengthen National Organ Transplant Act.* [News Release.]

U.S. Department of Health and Human Services. (1998). *Conference on increasing donation and transplantation: The challenge of evaluation.*

U.S. Department of Health and Human Services. HRSA Press Office. (1998). *Improving fairness and effectiveness in allocating organs for transplantation.*

Vachss, A. (1993). Rapists are single-minded. *Parade,* 4–6.

Walleck, C. (1994). Central nervous system II, spinal cord injury. In V. Cardona et al., (Eds.), *Trauma nursing* (2nd ed. pp. 435–465). Philadelphia: WB Saunders.

Walleck, C. & Mooney, K. (1994). In E. Barker (Ed.), *Neuroscience nursing.* St. Louis: Mosby.

Williams, R. A. (1991). Injuries in infants and small children resulting from witnessed and corroborated free falls. *Journal of Trauma, 31,* 1350–1352.

Wolfe, S. (1998). Look for signs of abuse. *RN, 61*(8), 48–51.

Wong, D. L. (1997). *Haley & Wong's essentials of pediatric nursing* (5th ed.). St. Louis: Mosby.

# INDEX

## A

ABC assessment, 13-14
abdominal cavity, 123-124
abdominal trauma
    assessment of, 16, 132-133, 224
    internal hemorrhage and, 46
    interventions for specific, 128-132
    mechanism of injury, 127-128
    nursing diagnoses related to, 135
    nursing strategies for, 134-135
    overview of, 123
    pediatric, 215-216
    signs of symptoms of, 133
    *See also* obstetric trauma
abducens (cranial nerve VI), 64
abruptio placentae, 161
acceleration-deceleration force, 215, 221
acceptance stage, 246
acid burns, 80-81, 198
acromioclavicular (ACL), 177
acute hospital care, 6-7
Acute Pulmonary Edema/Hypotension/Shock Algorithm, 37*f*
"Adam's apple," 24
adenoids, 25
adolescents
    anatomy/physical characteristics of, 210-213
    cardiovascular system of, 212
    depression/suicidal behavior in, 209
    gastrointestinal system of, 213
    musculoskeletal system of, 213
    neurologic system of, 212-213
    *See also* children; pediatric trauma
adult respiratory distress syndrome (ARDS), 110, 179, 195, 201, 202
advanced life support measures, 6
air bag injuries, 66, 80
airway anatomy/physiology
    assessment of pediatric, 222-223
    lower airways, 25
    pediatric, 25, 211
    upper airways, 24-25

airway management
    assessment, 13-14, 26-27
    burn injuries and, 202
    importance of, 23
    injury and obstruction, 26
    nursing strategies for, 30
airway stabilization
    manual techniques for, 27-29
    maxillofacial/neck trauma and, 70, 71
    mechanical methods for airway control, 29
    opening the airway, 27
alkali burns, 80-81, 198
all-terrain vehicles (ATVs), 209
American Association for the Surgery of Trauma, 145
American College of Surgeons, 7
American College of Surgeons Committee on Trauma, 12
*American Heart Association Advanced Cardiac Life Support Manual* (1997), 27
*American Journal of Nursing,* 229
American Nursing Association Standards, 12
amniotic fluid, 156
amniotic sac, 155-156
amputation of penile shaft, 148
anaphylactic shock, 40-41
anesthesia, 97
anger stage, 245-246
angiography, 145
angular joint movement, 172
angulation (fracture) of penis, 148
ankle fracture, 184
anterior cord syndrome, 96
anterior ligament rupture, 93*f*
anterior shoulder dislocation, 177
aorta
    basic anatomy of, 44-45
    effect of pregnant uterus on, 158*f*
aortic rupture, 46, 114
appendicular skeleton, 171-172
appendix, 126
aqueous humor, 76
ARDS (adult respiratory distress syndrome), 110, 179, 195, 201, 202
artery injury, 175

asphalt burns, 203
assessment. *See* trauma assessment
auscultation technique, 15
autonomic dysreflexia, 95-96
autonomic nervous system, 91
avulsion, 79, 148
axial loading, 93
axial skeleton, 171-172

**B**
Babinski's reflex, 214
back assessment, 224
bargaining stage, 246
basal metabolic rate, 234
basic life support measures, 6
battered child syndrome, 218-219
    *See also* child abuse
battle's sign, 69*f*
Bennett Amendment of 1972 (Social Security Act), 268
bite marks, 220
bladder injuries, 145-147, 216, 217
bladder rupture, 146*f*, 147*f*
blast injuries, 5
bleeding
    with escharotomy, 202
    fractures and estimated, 180*t*
    spinal cord injury and, 94
    treatment of ocular trauma, 79
blood pressure
    head injuries and, 58
    measurement of, 14-15
blood vessels
    cardiovascular system, 44-45
    musculoskeletal system and, 173
blood volumes, 45*t*
blunt trauma
    abdominal injury from, 127
    described, 5
    maxillofacial/neck trauma, 65-66
    musculoskeletal injuries due to, 173-174
    obstetric/gynecologic injuries due to, 161-162
    ocular injuries from, 77
bone fracture, 46
bone procurement, 266
bones, 171-172
bowel, 126
bowel injuries, 130
brain
    anatomy/physiology of, 53
    diffuse injuries of, 56-57, 214
    *See also* head injuries
brain death, 267-268

    *See also* death
breathing assessment
    burn injuries and, 202
    of children, 211, 223
    steps in, 14
    *See also* respiratory system
bronchial injury, 112
bronchial tree, 25
Brown-Séquard syndrome, 96
bruises, 220
burn depth, 195, 201
burn injuries
    assessment of, 200-202
    characterization and prognosis of, 197*f*
    chemical, 80-81, 198-199
    classified by depth, 193*f*
    as clinical findings of child abuse, 220
    elderly population and, 231
    electrical, 199-200
    epidemiology of, 191-192
    to eyes, 77, 80-81, 203
    mechanism of injury, 195
    nuclear radiation, 200
    nursing diagnoses related to, 204
    nursing strategies for, 202-204
    overview, 4, 191
    pathophysiology of, 193-195
    pediatric, 218
    temperature regulation and, 203
    thermal, 195-198
    wound care of, 203-204
    *See also* skin

**C**
capillary permeability, 193-194
Caplin, Arthur, 258
car seats, 208
carbon monoxide intoxication, 194, 199, 202
cardiac arrest, 46, 47
cardiac contusions/concussion, 113
cardiac muscle, 172
cardiac tamponade, 46, 116-117
cardiogenic (low output) shock, 34, 38-39
cardiotocography, 162
cardiovascular anatomy/physiology
    aging and changes to, 232
    blood, 45-46
    cardiac arrest, 46, 47
    of children and adolescents, 212
    circulation through heart, 44*f*
    heart, 43
    lungs, 45

pregnancy changes to, 157-158
resuscitation considerations, 46-47
thoracic trauma to, 108, 113-114
vessels, 44-45
Cardiovascular Triad, 35*t*
carotid arteries, 65
cartilage, 173
"cauliflower ear," 66
central cord syndrome, 96
central nervous system (CNS), 90
central venous pressure (CVP), 158
central zone of coagulation, 193
cerebrospinal fluid (CSF), 53, 55, 92
cervical injury, 96
Champion Sacco Trauma Score, 16, 17*f*-18*f*
chemical burns, 80-81, 198-199, 203
chemical injury, 194-195
chest
    anatomy and physiology of, 106-108
    assessment of, 16, 223-224
    cavity/related structures of, 107*f*
    injuries to back of, 109
    injury to wall of, 109-111
    *See also* thoracic trauma
child abuse
    definitions of, 219*t*
    failure to thrive, 222
    indications of, 221*f*
    Munchausen syndrome by proxy, 222
    significant clinical findings of, 220-221
child maltreatment
    assessment of, 222-224
    emotional abuse, 220
    neglect, 218
    nursing diagnoses related to, 225-226
    nursing strategies for, 224-225
    pediatric trauma due to, 3, 207-208
    physical abuse, 218-219
    sexual abuse, 219-220
    significant clinical findings of, 220-222
Child Protective Service, 208, 210
children
    airway anatomy of, 25
    anatomy/physical characteristics of, 210-213
    assessing burn injuries of, 201
    bladder of, 141
    breathing assessment of, 211, 223
    cardiovascular system of, 212
    elbow dislocation in, 177-178
    emotional abuse of, 220
    foreign bodies in vagina, urethra and bladder of, 149
    gastrointestinal system of, 213

head injuries in, 53
homicide of, 209-210
kidneys of, 140
musculoskeletal system of, 213
neurologic system of, 212-213
normal ranges of vital signs in, 212*t*
sexual abuse of, 219-220
spinal injury without radiographic abnormality in, 97
    *See also* adolescents; pediatric trauma
chin lift maneuver, 27
circulation
    assessing pediatric, 223
    assessment of, 14
    burn injuries and, 202-203
    spinal shock/sympathetic system, 100
circumduction joint movement, 172
Class I hypovolemic shock, 36
Class II hypovolemic shock, 36
Class III hypovolemic shock, 36
Class IV hypovolemic shock, 36, 38
clavicle fracture, 181
closed chest injury, 109
closed fracture, 180
closed/blunt abdominal injury, 127
cognition deterioration, 233
colon injuries, 130
comminuted fracture, 180
comorbid conditions, 234
compartment syndrome, 175-176
compound fracture, 180
compression injury
    abdominal trauma and, 127
    compartment syndrome due to, 175-176
    to spinal cord, 93, 95*f*
    to thorax, 109
computerized tomography (CT scan)
    for abdominal trauma, 132
    for genitourinary trauma, 145
concussion, 57
conjunctiva, 76
conjunctival laceration, 79
consent form, 263
contact burns, 198
contact lenses, 82-83
contrecoup, 54
contusion (head), 55
contusions (spinal injury), 97
"cool stage," 40
COPD (chronic obstructive pulmonary disease), 38
cornea, 76
cornea procurement, 266
corneal abrasion, 78

corneal laceration, 78-79
costovertebral angle (CVA), 140
coup, 54
Cowley, R. Adams, 7
cranial nerves, 53, 64
crepitus, 185-186
crisis intervention model, 246-247
critical burns, 196, 201
critical incident debriefing, 251
crush injuries, 176
CSF (cerebrospinal fluid), 53, 55

**D**
death
    conveying news to family of, 249*f*, 264
    determination of donor, 260, 262
    issues of brain, 267-268
Death/Organ/Tissue Donation checklist, 259, 260*f*
deceleration trauma, 127
deformity (spinal injury), 97
denial stage, 245
depression stage, 246
dermis, 192
diagnostic peritoneal lavage (DPL), 132, 162
diaphragm, 124
diaphragm injuries, 113, 128
diffuse axonal injury (DAI), 57
diffuse brain injuries, 56-57
direct fractures, 179
disability
    assessment of elder, 236
    assessment of pediatric, 223
    special needs patients with, 248
dislocated shoulder, 177*f*
dislocations, 176-177
distraction, 93
distributive (or vasogenic) shock, 34, 39-41
domestic violence, 3, 161
donors. *See* organ donors
drowning/near drowning injuries, 4

**E**
ecchymosis of tissue, 185
elbow dislocation, 177-178
elbow fracture, 181-182
elder abuse/neglect
    injuries due to, 3-4, 231-232
    nursing diagnoses related to, 238
    nursing strategies for, 238
    primary categories of, 234-235
    risk factors associated with, 325
    signs and symptoms of, 235
elder population, 232-234

elder trauma
    assessment of, 236-237
    burn injuries, 231
    epidemiology/mechanisms of injury, 230-232
    nursing diagnoses related to, 238
    nursing strategies for, 237-238
    overview of, 229-230
electric shock, 199
electrical burns, 203-204
electrolyte balance, 210-211
embryo, 156
emergency nursing specialty, 6
EMSS (emergency medical service systems), 6
    *See also* trauma centers
endocrine system (pregnancy), 159
endotracheal airway control, 29
endotracheal intubation, 24
EOA (esophageal obturator airway), 29
epidermis, 192
epidural hematoma, 55-56
epiglottis, 65
epiphyseal fracture, 180
erythrocytes, 45
escharotomy, 202
esophageal injury, 111
ET (endotracheal tube), 29
evisceration, 128
expiration, 108
exposed fragments, 186
exposure assessment, 223
extremities assessment, 16
eye procurement, 266
eye prostheses, 83
eyes
    anatomy/physiology of, 75-77
    assessment of pediatric, 223
    burn injuries to, 77, 80-81, 203
    *See also* ocular trauma
eyesight deterioration, 233

**F**
facial fractures, 67*f*, 68*f*
facial nerve (cranial nerve VII), 64
facial structures, 63-64
failure to thrive, 222
fallopian tubes, 144
falls, 3, 209, 230
false motion, 186
family
    conveying news of death to, 249*f*, 264
    donor evaluation prior to speaking with, 262
    obtaining consent from donor, 263-265

organ donation process and, 258-259

"required request" legislation and, 257-258

*See also* organ donors; patients

FARS (Fatal Accident Reporting System), 3

fascia, 192

*Federal Register,* 258

female genitalia, 149

female genitalia injuries, 216

*See also* genitourinary trauma

female reproductive system, 141, 143*f*, 144

femoral fracture, 183-184

fetus

described, 156

direct injury to, 162

primary assessment of mother and, 163

secondary assessment of mother and, 163-164

fibula fracture, 184

financial abuse/neglect, 235

finger dislocation, 178

fingertip injuries, 176

firearm injuries, 4, 210

first degree burns, 195

five stages of resolution, 245-246

flail chest (segment), 110, 112*f*

flame burns, 197

flash burns, 197

"flashbacks," 245

flexion-extension force, 215

flow (obstruction) shock, 41

fluid distribution, 210-211

fluid resuscitation, 203

foot fracture, 184

forearm fracture, 182

foreign bodies

abdominal trauma and, 132

in female genitalia, 149

injuries due to, 5

ocular injuries and, 77-78

foreskin, 149

fractures

classifications of, 179-180

as clinical finding of child abuse, 220-221

described, 179

estimated blood loss in, 180*t*

signs and symptoms of, 185-186

types of, 180-184

frontal bone (forehead), 64

**G**

gallbladder, 126

gastrointestinal system

children and adolescent, 213

pregnancy and, 159

genital injury, 148-150

genital/reproductive system, 141-144

genitourinary system

assessment of, 224

pregnancy and, 159

genitourinary trauma

assessment of, 150-151

interventions for specific, 144-150

mechanism of injury, 144

nursing diagnoses related to, 151

nursing strategies for, 151

overview of, 139

pediatric, 216-217

GES (General Estimates Systems), 3

gestation, 156

Glasgow Coma Scale (GCS), 57, 222, 236

gliding joint movement, 172

global rupture, 81-82

"golden hour" concept, 7

gravid, 156

Green, Nicholas, 255

greenstick fracture, 180

guarding behavior, 185

gynecologic trauma

nursing diagnoses related to, 166

nursing strategies for, 166

overview of, 165-166

*See also* obstetric trauma; rape

**H**

hand dislocation, 178

hand fracture, 182

*Harvard Criteria for Determination of Brain Death,* 257, 262

head

anatomy/physiology of, 52-53

assessment of, 15, 223

head injuries

assessment of, 57-58

child abuse and, 221

diffuse, 56-57

focal, 55-56

nursing strategies for, 58-59

pathophysiology of, 54

pediatric, 53, 213-214

shock and, 59

specific types of, 54

traumatic brain injury due to, 51

head tilt maneuver, 28

head tilt-chin lift maneuver, 28-29

hearing deterioration, 233

hearing impaired patients, 248
heart
  anatomy/physiology of, 43
  cardiac arrest and injury to, 46
  circulation through, 44*f*
heart valve procurement, 266
heart-lung transplants, 256
hematology system (pregnancy), 160
hematoma
  ear injuries, 66
  epidural, 55-56
  subdural, 56
hemithorax, 106
hemorrhagic shock, 46
hemothorax, 115-116
hip dislocation, 178
hip fracture, 183
hollow organs, 124, 125*f*
homicides, 209-210
  *See also* murder-suicides
hospital's internal reporting form, 263
humerus fracture, 181
hyoid bone, 24, 65
hyperemia zone of damage, 193-194
hyperextension, 93
hyperflexion, 93
hyphema, 79-80
hypotension
  acute pulmonary edema, shock, and, 37*f*
  neurogenic shock and, 39
  shock and, 36
hypothermia, 225
hypovolemic (low volume) shock, 34, 36, 38, 116

**I**

immunosupression, 256
impact trauma, 5
impalement injuries
  abdominal, 128
  orthopedic, 176
  spinal, 96-97
incomplete spinal cord injury, 96
increasing intracranial pressure (ICP), 54, 58
indirect fractures, 179
inferior vena cava, 158*f*
inferior vena cava syndrome, 157
inhalation chemical burns, 198-199
inspection technique, 15
inspiration, 107
intentional trauma, 3-4
intravenous pyelogram (IVP), 145
iris, 76

iris injury, 80

**J**

jaw thrust maneuver, 27-28, 99
joints, 172
jugular vein distention (JVD), 116
jugular veins, 65

**K**

kidney dialysis programs, 256, 268
kidney injuries, 144-145
kidney transplants, 256
kidneys, 140
kinetic energy mechanisms, 5
knee dislocation, 178-179
knee fracture, 184
knee injuries, 175

**L**

laboratory measurement, 15
lacerations
  conjunctival, 79
  corneal, 78-79
  of penile head, 149
  spinal injury, 97
large intestine, 126
laryngeal injury, 111
laryngopharynx, 24
larynx, 24, 25, 65, 111
lateral bend, 93
LeFort I, 68
LeFort II, 68
LeFort III, 68
lens, 76-77
lens injury, 80
leukocytes, 45
Level 1 urgency, 19
Level 2 urgency, 19
Level 3 urgency, 19
Level I trauma center, 7
Level II trauma center, 7
Level III trauma center, 7-8
ligaments, 173
light burns, 198
lightning burns, 200
light/radiation burns, 81
liver, 126
liver injuries, 130
long-term care/rehabilitation, 7
*Look, Listen, and Feel* assessment, 26-27, 28
loss of consciousness (LOC), 54, 55-56, 97
lower airway anatomy, 25
lower extremity fractures, 183-184

lumbar injury, 96
lungs, 45

**M**

magnetic resonance imaging (MRI), 145
male genitalia, 148
male genitalia injuries, 216
    *See also* genitourinary trauma
male reproductive system, 141, 142*f*
mandible, 64
mandibular fracture, 67-68
Mannitol, 203
maxilla, 64
maxillary fracture, 68
maxillofacial/neck trauma
    assessment of, 69-70
    described, 63
    fractures, 67*f*-68*f*
    major vessel and, 65
    major vessel injury, 67
    mechanism of injury, 65-66
    nursing diagnoses related to, 72
    nursing strategies for, 70-72
    soft-tissue, 66-67
    upper airway and, 64-65
Medawar, Sir Peter, 256
mediastinum, 106, 108
medical command, 6
Medicare, 268, 269
meninges, 52-53
mesentery, 124
metabolic shock, 34, 41-42
metabolism
    aging and changes to, 234
    pediatric, 210-211
minor burns, 196
moderate burns, 196
motor vehicle accidents, 2-3, 208-209, 230-231, 237
mouth, 64
Munchausen syndrome by proxy, 222
murder-suicides, 4
    *See also* homicides
muscle rupture, 175
musculoskeletal system
    aging and changes in, 233
    anatomy/physiology of, 171-173
    assessment of pediatric, 224
    of children and adolescents, 213
    impact of pregnancy on, 160
    mechanism of injury, 173-174
    pediatric trauma to, 217
    *See also* orthopedic trauma

myocardial contusion, 46

**N**

nasal fracture, 67
nasopharyngeal airway control, 29
nasopharynx, 24
National Center for Health Statistics, 2
National Clearinghouse on Child Abuse and Neglect, 3
National Organ Transplantation Act (1984), 258, 268, 269
neck assessment, 16, 223
    *See also* maxillofacial/neck trauma
neglect, 218
nerve root injuries, 96
nerves
    injury to peripheral, 175
    musculoskeletal system and, 173
    sensory, 192-193
nervous system
    aging and changes to, 233
    CNS and PNS of, 90-91
neurogenic shock, 39
neurologic assessment, 57-58
neurologic system
    of children/adolescents, 212-213
    pregnancy and, 159
next of kin identification, 265
    *See also* family
NHTSA (National Highway Traffic Safety Administration), 2
*The 1994 Uniform Crime Reports* (FBI), 4
non-English speaking patients, 248
nose, 64
nose assessment, 223
nuclear radiation exposure, 200
numbness (spinal injury), 98
"nursemaids' elbow," 178
nursing. *See* trauma nursing diagnoses; trauma nursing strategies

**O**

observation techniques, 15
obstetric trauma
    assessment of, 162-164
    interventions in specific, 161-162
    mechanism of injury, 160-161
    nursing diagnoses related to, 165
    nursing strategies for, 164-165
    overview of, 155
    *See also* abdominal trauma; gynecologic trauma
obstruction (flow) shock, 41
obstructive (or flow) obstruction, 34
ocular trauma

assessment of, 83
burn injuries and, 77, 80-81, 203
contusion, 78
interventions for specific, 77-83
mechanism of injury, 77
nursing diagnoses related to, 85
nursing strategies for, 84
overview of, 75
treatment of bleeding, 79
*See also* eye anatomy/physiology
oculomotor (cranial nerve III), 64
olfaction or smell technique, 15
Oklahoma Department of Health, 218
oliguria, 36
omentum, 124
Omnibus Budget Reconciliation Act (1986), 258
open chest injury, 109
open fracture, 180
open pneumothorax/sucking chest wound, 115
open/penetrating abdominal injury
described, 127-128
dressing an, 129*f*
OPOs (Organ Procurement Organizations), 258
orbital blowout fracture, 68-69
orbital complex, 64
orbital fracture, 82
organ donation
ethical considerations of, 267-268
financial considerations of, 268
future of, 268-269
historical background of, 256-257
hospital requirements regarding, 263
legislative background of, 257-258
nursing strategies for, 269
overview of, 255-256
process of, 258-265
procurement process, 265-267
organ donors
determination of death and, 260, 262
evaluation of, 262
medical examiner evaluation of, 263
recognition of, 259-260
types of U.S. (1988–1997), 259*t*
*See also* family; patients
Organ Injury Scaling Committee, 145
Organ Procurement and Transplantation Network
  (OPTN), 258
organs
  major body, 125*f*
  peritoneal space, 125, 126
oropharyngeal airway control, 29
oropharynx, 24, 25

orthopedic/neurovascular trauma
  amputations, 184-185
  assessment of, 185-186
  mechanism of injury, 173-174
  neurovascular problems associated with, 174-185
  nursing diagnoses related to, 187
  nursing strategies for, 186-187
  overview of, 171
  *See also* musculoskeletal system
ovaries, 14, 141
over rotation, 93
ovum, 156

**P**

pain
  genitourinary trauma, 150
  spinal injury, 98
palpation
  spinal cord assessment and, 99
  technique for, 15
pancreas, 127
pancreas injuries, 131
paradoxical movement, 110
paralysis, 97
parasympathetic autonomic system, 91
parietal peritoneum, 124
parietal pleura, 106
partner abuse, 3, 161
parturient, 156
passenger vehicle driver deaths (1998), 231*t*
  *See also* motor vehicle accidents
patella fracture, 184
patellar dislocation, 179
pathologic fracture, 180
patient history
  genitourinary trauma and, 150
  importance of, 14
  pediatric, 224
  spinal injury and, 98-99
patients
  assessment of spinal cord injury in, 98*f*
  burn injuries and status and age of, 201
  conveying to family death of, 249*f*
  immobilization of spinal cord injury, 100
  nursing care for shock in, 42-43
  nursing strategies for head injury, 58-59
  nursing strategies for special needs, 247-248
  *See also* assessment; family; organ donors
pedestrian injuries, 231
pediatric airway anatomy, 25
pediatric patient history, 224
pediatric trauma

abdominal injury, 215-216
    burn-related, 218
    due to head injuries, 53
    epidemiology and mechanisms of, 208-210
    genitourinary injury, 216-217
    head injury, 213-214
    musculoskeletal injury, 217
    nursing diagnoses related to, 225-226
    nursing strategies for, 224-225
    overview of, 207-208
    spinal cord injury, 214-215
    thoracic injury, 215
    *See also* child maltreatment
Pediatric Trauma Score (PTS), 222
pelvic fracture, 131, 162, 182-183
pelvis assessment, 224
penetrating injury
    bladder, 146
    described, 5
    eyes, 77
    kidneys, 144
    maxillofacial/neck trauma, 66
    musculoskeletal injuries due to, 173-174
    obstetric trauma due to, 160, 162
    spine, 96
    thorax, 109, 113
penile angulation, 148
penile tissue, 141
penile trauma, 148
percussion technique, 15
perforation of eye globe, 81-82
periorbital injury, 77
peripheral nerve injury, 175
peripheral nervous system (PNS), 90-91
peritoneal cavity, 124
peritoneal space, 124, 126-127
personal rights violations, 234
pharynx (throat), 24, 65
physical abuse, 218-219
    *See also* child maltreatment
placenta, 167
pneumothorax, 114
point tenderness, 185
posttraumatic stress disorder, 245
posterior dislocation of vertebrae, 93*f*
posterior hip dislocation, 178
posterior ligament rupture, 94*f*
posterior pharynx damage, 194
posterior shoulder dislocation, 177
PQRST (Provoking factors, Quality, Region/radiation
    factor, Severity and Time of onset), 14
pregnancy

additional system changes during, 159-160
    cardiovascular changes during, 157-158
    pulmonary changes during, 158-159
    terminology associated with, 155-156
    uterus changes during, 156-157
    *See also* obstetric trauma
prehospital care, 6
premature uterine contractions, 161
premature ventricular contractions (PVCs), 113
priapism, 98
primary assessment
    of child maltreatment, 222-223
    of maxillofacial/neck trauma, 69
    of obstetric/gynecology trauma, 163
    of trauma injuries, 13-14
    *See also* trauma assessment
problem-solving approach, 247
prostate gland, 141
prostheses (eye), 83
psychogenic shock, 34, 42
psychological abuse, 234
psychopathology theory, 232
psychosocial issues
    general perspective of, 243-244
    nursing diagnoses related to, 250
    nursing strategies for, 248-250
    special patients, 247-248
    stages of response to, 245-246
    stress due to trauma, 244-245
    suicide/suicide attempts, 247
pulmonary artery, 45
pulmonary circulation, 108
pulmonary contusion, 112-113
pulmonary system
    basic anatomy of, 106-108
    injuries to, 111-113, 194
    pregnancy changes to, 158-159
pulmonary veins, 45
pulse oximetry measurement, 14
pulse rate, 58
pupil, 76

**Q**

*Questions and Answers on Death and Dying* (Kubler-
    Ross), 245

**R**

raccoon eyes, 69*f*
radiation burns, 200
radiographic evaluation
    for abdominal trauma, 132
    for genitourinary trauma, 145
    for  obstetric trauma, 162

radionucleotide, 145

rape, 4, 149-150, 165-166

    *See also* gynecologic trauma; sexual abuse

rape-trauma syndrome, 166

rapid forward deceleration, 5

rapid vertical deceleration, 5

recreational activity injuries, 4

rectal injuries, 130

reflex, 91

rehabilitation care, 7

reimplantation of amputated part, 185

renal system

    aging and changes to, 234

    trauma to, 217

"required request" legislation, 257-258

respiratory patterns, 58

respiratory system

    aging and changes to, 232-233

    children/adolescent, 211

    difficulties of, 98

    measurement of, 14

    *See also* breathing assessment

resuscitation considerations, 46-47, 236

retina, 77

retinal detachment, 80

retroperitoneal space, 124, 127

Revised Trauma Score (RTS), 222

Rh-compatible blood, 158

rib fracture, 109-110

role theory, 231-232

rollerblading injuries, 209

rotation joint movement, 172

rule of nines, 196

rupture of eye globe, 81-82

## S

"sandwich generation," 235

SANE (sexual assault/abuse nurse examiners), 166

SART (sexual assault response teams), 166

scald burns, 196

scalp, 52

scapula fracture, 181

sclera, 76

seat belts, 160, 208-209

second degree burns, 195

secondary assessment

    of child maltreatment, 223-224

    of maxillofacial/neck trauma, 69-70

    of obstetric/gynecology trauma, 163-164

    of trauma injuries, 14-15

    *See also* primary assessment

Section 1138 (Social Security Act), 258

seminal vesicles, 141

sensory nerves, 192-193

septic shock, 40

sexual abuse, 219-220

sexual assault (rape), 4, 149-150, 165-166

shaken baby syndrome, 221

shock

    algorithm of acute pulmonary edema/hypotension and, 37*f*

    anaphylactic shock, 40-41

    cardiogenic (low output), 34, 38-39

    Cardiovascular Triad and, 35*t*

    causes of, 33-34

    distributive or vasogenic, 34, 39-41

    head injuries and, 59

    hemorrhagic, 46

    hypovolemic (low volume), 34, 36, 38, 116

    metabolic, 34, 41-42

    nursing diagnoses related to, 43

    nursing strategies for patient in, 42-43

    obstruction (flow), 41

    physiology of, 34

    pregnant women in, 157-158

    psychogenic, 34, 42

    recognizing, 34-36

    septic, 40

shock spinal, 95

shoulder dislocation, 177*f*

shoulder fracture, 181

sinus cavities, 64

skateboarding injuries, 209

skeletal (or voluntary muscle), 172

skin

    anatomy of, 192

    functions of, 192-193

    procurement of, 266

    *See also* burn injuries

skull, 52, 53*f*

skull fractures, 55

small bowel injuries, 130

small intestine, 126

smoke inhalation, 194-195

smooth muscle, 172

soft-tissue trauma

    maxillofacial and neck injury, 66-67

    orthopedic/neurovascular injury and, 174

solid organs, 124, 125*f*

somatic nervous system, 91

special needs patients, 247-248

spinal cord

    anatomy of, 92

    mechanism of injury to, 92-95

spinal column injury to, 95-97
*See also* trauma to the spine
spinal shock, 95
spleen, 126-127
spleen injuries, 130-131
sprain, 174-175
stabilization
airway, 27-29, 70, 71
manual head, 100*f*
of spinal cord and column injuries, 99-100
Standards of Emergency Nursing Practice, 12
stasis zone of damage, 193
state reporting form, 263
sternal fracture, 110-111
stomach, 125, 126
stomach injuries, 128, 130
straddle injury, 149
strain, 174
stressed caregiver theory, 232
subconjunctival hemorrhage, 79
subcutaneous emphysema, 114
subcutaneous tissue, 192
subdural hematoma, 56
subluxation, 179
sucking chest wound, 115
suicide/suicide attempts, 247
supine hypotensive syndrome, 157
surgical airway control, 29
Surgical Transplants Act (Sweden), 259
SVR (systemic vascular resistance), 34
sympathetic autonomic system, 91
synovial fluid, 172
synovial membrane, 172
systemic circulation, 108

**T**
tar burns, 203
TBSA (total body surface area), 196
teeth, 65
temperature
measurement of, 14
regulation of, 203
tenderness, 97
tendon rupture, 175
tendons, 173
tension pneumothorax, 114-115
testicles, 141
testicular trauma, 148
thermal burns, 81, 203
thermoregulation, 211, 234
third degree burns, 195-196
thoracic trauma

assessment of, 117-118*f*, 119*t*
cardiac/great vessel injuries due to, 113-114
cardiovascular system and, 108
categories of, 109
complications of, 114-117
conditions produced by, 111*f*
interventions for specific, 109-114
mechanism of injury, 108-109
negative pressure and, 107-108
nursing diagnoses related to, 120
nursing strategies for, 118-120
overview of, 105-106
pediatric, 215
pulmonary injury due to, 111-113
spinal cord injury and, 96
*See also* chest
tibia fracture, 184
tingling (spinal injury), 98
tissue ischemia, 175-176
tissue procurement, 265-266
tonsils, 25
topical chemical burns, 198
total body surface area (TBSA), 196
trachea (windpipe), 24-25, 65
tracheal injury, 111-112
*Traffic Safety Facts* (NHTSA), 2
transgenerational theory, 232
trauma
crisis intervention and, 246-247
defining, 1
epidemiology of, 2
injuries associated with, 2-4
means of impact, 5
psychosocial responses to, 245-246
stress due to, 244-245
suicide/suicide attempts in case of, 247
trauma assessment
ABC, 13-14
abdominal trauma, 16, 132-133, 224
airway, 13-14, 26-27
anaphylactic, 41
burn injuries, 200-202
cardiogenic (low output) shock, 39
Champion Sacco Trauma Score for, 16, 17*f*-18*f*
child maltreatment, 222-224
distributive (or vasogenic) shock, 39-40
elder trauma, 236-237
genitourinary trauma, 150-151
head injuries, 57-58
hypovolemic shock, 38
maxillofacial/neck trauma, 69-70
obstetric/gynecologic trauma, 162-164

ocular trauma, 83
orthopedic/neurovascular trauma, 185-186
principles of, 12-13
septic shock, 40
thoracic trauma, 117-118*f*, 119*t*
trauma to the spine, 14, 97-99
*See also* primary assessment; secondary assessment
trauma centers
acute hospital care at, 6-7
classification of, 7-8
long-term care/rehabilitation at, 7
origins of, 5-6
prehospital care and, 6
trauma nursing
importance of, 11
major body areas evaluation, 15-16
patient assessment, 12-15
process of, 12
triage, 16, 19
trauma nursing diagnoses
related to abdominal trauma, 135
related to burn injuries, 204
related to elder trauma/maltreatment, 238
related to genitourinary trauma, 151
related to gynecologic trauma, 166
related to head injury, 59
related to maxillofacial/neck injuries, 72
related to ocular trauma, 85
related to orthopedic/neurovascular trauma, 187
related to pediatric trauma/child maltreatment, 225-226
related to psychosocial issues, 250
related to shock, 43
related to spinal cord/column trauma, 101
related to thoracic trauma, 120
trauma nursing strategies
abdominal trauma, 134-135
airway management, 30
burn injuries, 202-204
conveying news of death to family, 249*f*, 264
crisis intervention, 246-247
critical incident debriefing, 251
elder trauma/abuse and neglect, 237-238
genitourinary trauma, 151
gynecologic trauma, 166
head injury patient, 58-59
maxillofacial/neck trauma, 70-72
obstetric trauma, 164-165
ocular trauma, 84
organ donation, 269
orthopedic/neurovascular trauma, 186-187
patient in shock, 42-43

pediatric trauma/child maltreatment, 224-225
psychosocial patient needs, 248-250
spinal cord and column injuries, 99-101
suicide/suicide attempt interventions, 247
thoracic injury, 118-120
trauma, 11-19
triage, 19
*Trauma and Recovery* (Herman), 245
Trauma Score (TS), 222
trauma to the spine
anterior ligament rupture, 93
assessment of, 14, 97-99
impalement, 96-97
injury without radiographic abnormality, 97
mechanism of injury, 92-95
nursing diagnoses related to, 101
nursing strategies for, 99-101
overview of, 89-90
pediatric, 214-215
penetrating injury, 96
pharmacological management of, 101
spinal cord anatomy, 92
spinal cord and, 95-97
traumatic amputations, 184-185
traumatic asphyxia, 116
traumatic brain injury (TBI), 51
triage nursing, 19
triage systems, 16, 19
trigeminal (cranial nerve V), 64
trochlear (cranial nerve IV), 64
Type I triage system (traffic director), 19
Type II triage system (spot checker), 19
Type III triage system (comprehensive), 19

**U**
ultrasound (US)
for abdominal injuries, 132
for genitourinary trauma, 145
for obstetric trauma, 162
umbilical cord, 156
unconsciousness, 54, 55-56, 97
Uniform Anatomical Gift Act (1968), 257, 269
UNOS (United Network of Organ Sharing), 255, 258
upper airway anatomy, 24-25
upper airway obstruction, 194
upper extremity fractures, 181-182
upper torso fractures, 180-181
ureters, 140-141
urethra, 141
urethra injuries, 147-148, 217
urgency categories assessment, 19
urinary bladder, 141

urinary system, 140*f*-141
U.S. Department of Health and Human Services (DHHS), 258
U.S. organ donors, 259*t*
uterine rupture, 161-162
uterus
 effects on IVC and aorta by pregnant, 158*f*
 pregnancy changes to, 156-157
 premature contractions during pregnancy, 161
 trauma to the, 144, 147

**V**
vagina, 144
vas deferens, 141
vascular organs, 124
vascular structure injuries, 131
vascular structures, 124
vasoconstriction, 36
Vasogenic (or distributive) shock, 34, 39-41
vena cavae, 45
vertebrae
 compression force causing injury to, 95*f*
 forward dislocation of the, 94*f*
 posterior dislocation of the, 93*f*
vessel injuries
 maxillofacial/neck trauma and, 67
 thoracic trauma and, 113-114

vessels (cardiovascular system), 44-45
violation of personal rights, 234
violence
 domestic, 3, 161
 trauma and, 3
 *See also* child abuse; elder abuse
visceral peritoneum, 124
visceral pleura, 106
vision impaired patients, 248
vital signs measurement, 14
vitreous humor, 77
vocal cords, 24, 25
voluntary (or skeletal muscle), 172
vomiting, 58

**W**
Worksheet for Organ and Tissue Donor Referral, 259, 261*f*
World Transplant Games, 269
wrist fracture, 182

**Z**
zones of burn damage, 193-194
zygoma, 64
zygoma fracture, 68

# PRETEST KEY

| | | |
|---|---|---|
| 1. | A | Introduction |
| 2. | B | Chapter 1 |
| 3. | C | Chapter 1 |
| 4. | D | Chapter 2 |
| 5. | B | Chapter 2 |
| 6. | C | Chapter 3 |
| 7. | B | Chapter 3 |
| 8. | D | Chapter 4 |
| 9. | A | Chapter 4 |
| 10. | C | Chapter 5 |
| 11. | B | Chapter 6 |
| 12. | D | Chapter 7 |
| 13. | A | Chapter 8 |
| 14. | B | Chapter 9 |
| 15. | C | Chapter 9 |
| 16. | B | Chapter 10 |
| 17. | D | Chapter 11 |
| 18. | A | Chapter 12 |
| 19. | C | Chapter 13 |
| 20. | B | Chapter 14 |
| 21. | C | Chapter 15 |
| 22. | B | Chapter 16 |
| 23. | B | Chapter 16 |
| 24. | A | Chapter 17 |
| 25. | A | Chapter 18 |